"I want every single woman, and every human who has loved (or even met) a woman, to read this essential book. This deeply personal memoir manages to encapsulate in its pages virtually every way society conspires to screw us over, from sexual assault to workplace harassment to the absurd and nearly fatal gender inequities in the healthcare system. And yet it is also warm and compassionate and, yes, hysterically funny. It is a page-turner that makes you scream in empathetic frustration and laugh so hard you have to put the book down. I'm honestly not sure whether I cried more because I was laughing or because I was so very sad."

  —AYELET WALDMAN, author of *A Really Good Day: How Microdosing Made a Mega Difference in My Mood, My Marriage, and My Life*

"*Ladyparts* is a beautifully written, boots-on-the-ground, first-person chronicle of everything that can go wrong with women's bodies and too often does. Deborah Copaken's book is an important addition to the field of women's health from the lens of a patient."

  —LISA MOSCONI, PHD, *New York Times* bestselling author of *The XX Brain*

"*Ladyparts* is an unmanicured middle finger to an archaic culture that shames women into suffering in silence. It is a bold love letter to 'women warriors,' championing self-reliance while tackling the societal obstacles unrelentingly thrown in that path. Deborah Copaken shines a light on her scars, bravely helping those who cover their own feel less alone."   —AJ MENDEZ, *New York Times* bestselling author of *Crazy Is My Superpower*

"*Ladyparts* is in equal measure raw, unshrinking, hilarious, and heartbreaking. Deborah Copaken has been both a war photographer in Afghanistan and a single working mother in America, but take a quick guess as to which experience has been more dangerous. Lucky for her, she lived through both to tell the tale. Lucky for us, she has transformed her unique traumas into wholly relatable gold. Few people write like Copaken: her ability to translate the workings of her dazzling mind into prose is without parallel."

—DONAL LOGUE, actor and co-author of
Trejo: My Life of Crime, Redemption, and Hollywood

"Deborah Copaken has written an amazing book. She uses her own body as a framing device. But through that lens, she's able to write movingly about everything you can imagine: love, divorce, war, parenting, cancer, gender inequality, dating apps, gourmet pie, you name it. I'm sorry that Copaken has had to battle so many Job-like challenges—but I'm delighted she is the heroine, not the victim, of her life. We need her to keep writing. We need this book, and many more, from her."   —A. J. JACOBS, *New York Times* bestselling
author of *The Year of Living Biblically* and *Thanks A Thousand*

"Filled with stories of what it's like to be a woman and a writer in America today, and heart-wrenching moments of injustice and redemption, this page-turner of a memoir is harrowing, hopeful, and urgent. If you are a woman, it will change the way you look at the parts that make you and the parts that you play. If you are a man, it will illuminate you. And if you are either, or neither, it will move you and transform you. This memoir is visceral and beautiful. Thank you, Deborah Copaken, for writing this brave and brilliant book. *Ladyparts* is an absolute mustread."   —ARIANA NEUMANN, author of *When Time Stopped*

"Utterly vital . . . *Ladyparts* enraged and amused me in equal measure. Deborah Copaken shows what it means to barely survive beyond the hallowed slice of privilege, where moving through the world in a woman's body can be dangerous, absurd, frustrating, beautiful, and sometimes all at once. . . . A wickedly smart, thoroughly investigated, and elegantly written takedown of the gender discrimination and institutional misogyny we have accepted for too long. This book howls for women in a world that too often only allows us a whisper."

—RACHEL LOUISE SNYDER, author of
No Visible Bruises and *What We've Lost Is Nothing*

"This book is a must-read for anyone who knows a woman, loves a woman, or is a woman. Copaken's sharp wit, heartfelt humor, and unabashed honesty turn what could be a tragic tale into a heroic journey of perseverance. Anyone who reads it will walk away feeling inspired."   —KATHERINE SCHWARZENEGGER,
New York Times bestselling author of The Gift of Forgiveness:
Inspiring Stories from Those Who Have Overcome the Unforgivable

"Every chapter of Deborah Copaken's memoir contains information about women's bodies that I couldn't believe no one had told me before. I was constantly outraged at what she had to endure to learn it all, but the book is so funny, smart, and entertaining that I'm grateful to have her as a guide. Ladyparts is essential reading for all women, and for the people who love them."

—MAILE MELOY, author of Do Not Become Alarmed

"Ladyparts is a memoir unlike any I've ever read—it's quite literally visceral, from the unforgettable first moment where Copaken crawls on the tile floor collecting what she takes to be her own bloody organs. With breathtaking candor, Copaken catalogs the calamities of her body, part by part, spinning out a raw, raucous, often hilarious account of herself—with so much insight and generosity that I finished the book feeling re-made."

—SEMI CHELLAS, award-wining writer/producer,
Mad Men and The Romanoffs

LADYPARTS

A MEMOIR

DEBORAH COPAKEN

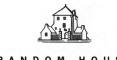

RANDOM HOUSE

NEW YORK

Published in the United States by Random House, an imprint and division
of Penguin Random House LLC, New York.

RANDOM HOUSE and the HOUSE colophon are registered trademarks of
Penguin Random House LLC.

Library of Congress Cataloging-in-Publication Data
Names: Copaken, Deborah, author.
Title: Ladyparts: a memoir / by Deborah Copaken.
Description: First edition. | New York: Random House, [2020]
Identifiers: LCCN 2020055455 (print) | LCCN 2020055456 (ebook) | ISBN 9781984855473
(hardcover) | ISBN 9781984855480 (ebook)
Subjects: LCSH: Copaken, Deborah. | Copaken, Deborah—Health. | Authors, American—21st
century—Biography. | Women authors—Biography. | Photojournalists—United States—
Biography. | Women photographers—United States—Biography. | Women—Health and hygiene.
Body image in women.
Classification: LCC PS3611.O3654 Z46 2020 (print) | LCC PS3611.O3654 (ebook) | DDC
818/.5403 [B]—dc23
LC record available at https://lccn.loc.gov/2020055455
LC ebook record available at https://lccn.loc.gov/2020055456

Printed in the United States of America on acid-free paper

randomhousebooks.com

2 4 6 8 9 7 5 3 1

First Edition

Book design by Jo Anne Metsch

For Sasha, again

&

in memory of Nora

"Above all, be the heroine of your life, not the victim."

—NORA EPHRON

"They were trying to save their souls—and who but a fool could fail to see that all that was the matter with their souls was that they had not been able to get a decent existence for their bodies?"

—UPTON SINCLAIR, *The Jungle*

Author's Note

The human brain is not a tape recorder. Which makes memoir-writing tricky. Have I transcribed every word of dialogue in these pages verbatim? No. Impossible. With the exception of emails, which leave an immutable record, and direct quotes from studies, all dialogue has been filtered through the distortion field of memory or, in some cases, trauma, leaving an ingrained if imperfect imprint. Have I nonetheless done my best to make sure all sentences placed between quotation marks, including my own, have been rendered as close to the essential truth of what was spoken? Yes. Absolutely.

Also, many names have been changed or in some cases completely omitted (e.g. "my ex," "my son," "my daughter," "the actor," "the PR firm"), and a few identifying characteristics have been deliberately left out for the sake of privacy, but both the people and the corporations inside here are real, not composites. Each scene in this book unfolds as it did in real life, without compression of events, flipping the timeline, or alteration of the narrative arc. But every scene, except where noted—for example, when I was unconscious—has been reconstructed solely from my perspective. I am the person on the gurney, not the one pushing it or watching it enter the operating room. That is to say: This is my blood-bath. My story. The stains on the floor are real, but their interpretations, as of any Rorschach blot, are mine alone.

Preface

The idea for this book came to me in the shower in the summer of 2018, a year after my near-death from vaginal cuff dehiscence.[*] Gazing down at my scar-covered torso, mentally dissecting each body part—the way a butcher approaches a cow or an advertiser a barely legal female—I realized that each excised or broken body part represented not only the chapter in time during which they failed me, they also, when strung together, served as a weirdly apt organizing principle around which to construct a narrative: organ by organ, nick by cut, each a useful metaphor for their parallel autobiographical upheavals.

To wit: My uterus was removed within hours of losing my mentor and surrogate mother to cancer as well as at the precise hour my daughter's body grabbed the reproductive baton. My breast grew a lump the same month I became a solo mother to my children and the den mother to a raucous commune of misfits in Harlem. My heart went on the fritz

---

[*] Should you choose to google this, which I do not recommend, I cannot be held responsible for the trauma of that image gallery. I looked it up the day after mine was repaired, and now I can't unsee those photos. Ever. You've been forewarned. I promise it will be described if not tastefully herein then with enough comic detachment to get us through it.

just as I was re-dipping a toe in love's lake. My cervix hung a closed-for-business sign on its door, right when new customers were finally showing up. My vagina tried to kill me as I was attempting a midlife act of rebirth. My brain had to escape halfway around the globe to learn how to turn down the volume after its scaffolding's near collapse. Finally lungs—which was not in my original book proposal—reminded us all that the right to a deep breath, particularly in America, is not a given.

The scars covering my female body, in other words, felt like the vague outline of a story begging to be fleshed out, body part by body part, like those connect-the-dots kindergarten worksheets that, when joined with a pencil in the correct numerical order, reveal an elephant, a snowman, a waggy-tailed puppy. Only this time it would be me, reconstructed. In fact, I realized, toweling off and getting dressed that morning, by objectifying my own body into its various parts—minus the misogyny—I could provide a useful microscope through which to contemplate the vastness of a whole life. Not only its nicks, cuts, and frequent slips on life's banana peels, but also its joys, triumphs, and belly laughs evoked not despite its seemingly unrelenting trips to the human body shop but *because of them*. Indeed, what had once felt like a constant ducking from turds in an endless shitstorm suddenly seemed not only like a cosmic gift from an overly generous muse—*Here, Deb, have another turd! And another! Whee!*—the mere act of reframing it thus suddenly gave me an umbrella. And the skeleton to describe it.

This same flash of insight had occurred once prior, in a now-defunct coffee shop called Xando on Broadway and West 76th Street in New York. It was May of 1998, around 7:30 A.M. I was clutching a double-wide stroller with my then one- and two-year-olds in it when I suddenly understood exactly how to organize the trauma and chaos of my early years as a war photographer into something resembling order. Each memory frame of that visual tale, I realized, depicted not only a specific war in a specific setting—Afghanistan, Israel, Romania, Zimbabwe, the USSR, etc.—it also contained a male figure lurking just off-screen: an abuser, a casual fling, a good Samaritan, a troubled lover, a husband, my firstborn son. I fished a pen from my purse. Found a napkin. *I will flip Mulvey's male gaze,* I thought, scribbling the names of these men onto that coffee shop napkin, *by ironically naming each chapter of my life as an independent woman out in the world, at war, after the man (or, in one case, little boy) standing outside the frame.* I, the female, would be the seer. They, the males, would be the objects, whether of my affection, scorn, lust, gratitude, or love. *The female gaze,* I wrote underneath the names, underlining it twice: a daily reminder to myself of how to frame the story.

Ladyparts is both an obvious bookend to that format as well as a continuation of the female gaze, only this time I'm objectifying my own body. Not to erase my personhood, as a man would, but to reclaim it.

That being said, yes: Over the past twenty years since *Shutterbabe*'s[*] publication, both my body and I have driven over what some might consider an unusual number of narrative potholes: medical, marital, financial, professional, personal, emotional, and holy shit, who could have seen that one coming? There's the FBI knocking at my door. I've also frequently and sometimes at great personal cost felt compelled to use my mouth and firmly planted feet to fight back, while simultaneously managing four free falls at once: the media industry, a marriage, my health, and the American middle class.

Does my voice, from all that shouting, have an edge to it? Fuck yes. I know I speak for many women in America when I say we are tired of this. We are tired of being the default caretakers. We are tired of corporate malfeasance and government indifference to the needs of working families. We are tired of modulating our "tone" when that word gets used as a weapon against us. We are tired of being paid less than men, interrupted when we speak, fired at will, and tossed aside the minute we hit our perimenopausal stride. We are tired of doing all the work and getting none of the credit. We are tired of being told to lean in while being forced out. We are tired of required NDAs; of rapists in robes; of data gaps, healthcare traps, and scientific neglect.

We are tired of headlines such as this one, from the first week following that annus horribilis, 2020, when the massive holes in the fabric of our country's safety net were finally revealed by the black light of a novel virus: "The US economy lost 140,000 jobs in December. All of them

---

[*] I wanted *Shuttergirl* or *Develop Stop Fix*, but I was told the decision was not mine to make. Sad, since the book was about subverting the male gaze not capitulating to it, but hey: Here I am, back at my old home, Random House. Twenty years, seven books, three publishers, and one #MeToo movement later. New people are in charge now. It's all water under sexism's bridge.

were held by women." And we're tired of how all of this has affected not only our psyches, our professional choices, our quality of life, and our bottom lines, but also our bodies.

Because yes, my body is covered by an unusual number of surgical scars. No doubt. But aside from the pace and extent of their etchings, are my dings unusual? Do they make me distinctive? No. In fact, what they make me is everywoman, born with female organs into a gutting world that, by dint of those organs, refuses to see her or hear her or pay her or study her or support her or treat her as equal.

So. Welcome to my body! Come on inside. I'll give you the nickel tour.

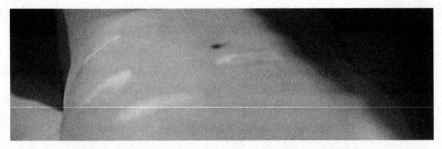

Bandages, post-trachelectomy, June 2017, © Deborah Copaken

Contents

PART I

VAGINA

2017

Fireworks

JULY 2, 2017

I'm crawling around on the bathroom floor, picking up pieces of myself. These pieces are not metaphor. They are actual pieces. Plumsized, beet-colored, with the consistency and sheen of chicken liver, three of them have shot out of me like shells from a cannon.

I am bleeding out. But my brain, starved of blood and in shock at the sight of so much of it, cannot process this information. Instead, I've become convinced that the ordnance sliding around my bathroom floor are my internal organs, which I must rescue so someone can put them back inside me.

I head to the kitchen to hunt for Tupperware. Not just any Tupperware. The glass kind. Heaven forbid my liver and kidney should come into contact with BPAs. It does not occur to me, in my befuddled state, that had my internal organs actually fallen from my body, I would not have the pulse with which to rummage in my kitchen cabinet in search of a container to store them.

It is Saturday night—no, now Sunday morning, just after midnight—of the July Fourth weekend, 2017. Pads and underwear have become useless against these pyrotechnics, so it's just me and my bathrobe, hemorrhaging. Outside, bootleg fireworks are erupting into the sky. Inside, gravity has forced another palm-sized chunk to plunge—splat!—onto the kitchen floor. And the rocket's red glare, indeed: Happy Independence Day to me! (Added bonus, I'm mid-divorce.) I scoop up the large mass and put it in the glass container with the others.

With the blobs now safely stored in carcinogen-free glass on the top shelf of my fridge—I've seen enough medical procedurals to know about the importance, when transporting human organs, of picnic coolers—I call the answering service for my surgeon, who three weeks earlier had removed my cervix. This post-op emergency, which I'm not yet prepared to call an emergency, is unusual. In fact, of all trachelectomies—that's the clinical name for cervix removal—performed in the U.S., only a small percentage result in "vaginal cuff dehiscence": the clinical name for uh-oh, the stitches where they sewed up the top of your vaginal canal have come undone, and now you're a blood clot howitzer.

I am twelve hours, without medical intervention, from my own death. Possibly less.

At this point, however, I know none of this. Neither the number of hours I have left nor the technical name for what's happening. I just know I'm exhausted and bleeding profusely. That I'm still deep in the weeds of recovering from major surgery. That I'd already gone to the emergency room near family court six days after surgery, after nearly passing out from pain while representing myself at a custody hearing, but the hospital had sent me home, saying everything looked fine.

I am loath to cry wolf again. But my apartment looks like a crime scene. So I'm crying medium-sized dog, possibly rabid. Alas, no one from the hospital is calling me back, so I'm crying into the void anyway. I call the answering service again. I text them a photo of one of the masses in the palm of my hand for size context. Nada.

I feel like medicine's needy girlfriend, ghosted by the hospital.

It has now magically jumped from midnight to 1:30 in the morning. Like a Truffaut film. *Qu'est-ce que c'est, degueulasse?* What is disgusting? I mean, for starters, the bathroom floor.

Part of me can't help but wonder if all of these bloody missiles are, in fact, metaphor: the expulsion of decades of marital sludge. But while I am grateful for my escape from a toxic, lonely marriage, I've recently been as alone as I've ever been, as lonely as I've ever felt. My eldest has been living with his girlfriend in Bangkok, where he's teaching English.

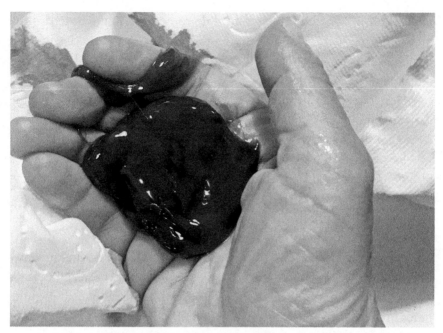

New York, NY, July 2, 2017, © Deborah Copaken

My youngest is away at summer camp. My middle one has been in the Middle East, so I've been walking the dog and doing the dishes and taking out the trash and lugging laundry back and forth from the communal laundry room in the basement on my own.

None of these tasks are on the list of acceptable activities on the hospital handout they give you when they kick you out the morning after surgery and tell you to rest. But having been recently downsized, I can't afford the added cost of a home health aide. Or, frankly, food or shelter. Aside from the few freelance gigs I've been able to cobble together from bed, I now have zero income combined with an extra $2,314.20 a month in COBRA* fees, which has always struck me as one of the more insulting cosmic ironies of losing a job in America: *Bye! Have a nice life! Here's zero months of severance plus an extra rent's worth of healthcare costs.*

The rest of the night becomes fuzzy, as I slip in and out of conscious-

---

* COBRA, I was surprised to learn, stands for the Consolidated Omnibus Budget Reconciliation Act, not Crap Option Bewilderment of Ruinous Assholery. For the non-Americans reading this, COBRA is a limited number of government-mandated months of insurance continuation for American workers who lose or leave a job, and it's always heart-stoppingly expensive.

ness, so I'll just mention the scenes I do remember in the order I think they occurred. This is not me trying to sound postmodern. It's just the jump-cut way in which I recall them, devoid of the normal transitions that streamline a narrative.

"Hey, sweetie, sorry to wake you . . ." I finally wake my sleeping daughter, feeling guilty about so doing. She's just arrived home from Tel Aviv, after many layovers and no sleep. Birthright* wasn't around when I was her age, so my first trip to Israel was also my first assignment as a photojournalist, to cover the first *intifada*. Rocks and CNN trucks. The boys would always wait around for the trucks to show up before throwing their rocks. McLuhan was right. The medium is always the message. What are these blobs trying to transmit to me?

"I think my kidney fell out," I say to my daughter, clutching my mystery masses, "so I might have to go to the hospital. But you stay here with Lucas and walk him in the morning." Lucas is our dog. Like all dogs, he hates fireworks. To self-soothe, he's been sitting on my face.

My daughter's bleary eyes widen. She is staring at the contents of my Tupperware container.

The crack of fireworks. Technicolor bursts outside the window. The dog barks. The world spins.

"Mom! Oh my god! That's not your kidney. If it were your kidney, you'd be dead." She examines the blobs, unsqueamish. She's premed, studying neuroscience. "I think they're giant blood clots," she says. "We have to get you to the hospital. Now."

"I'm tired. And no one's calling me back. Maybe we should wait until tomorrow."

She gets up and notes the pools of blood on the bathroom floor. In my bed. Down the hallway. In the kitchen near the refrigerator. I did my best to clean up the mess until I ran out of paper towels. "Are you kidding? Let's go. I'm calling 911."

"No! Absolutely not. We can't afford it." I'm currently living off the remains of my meager 401K, facing a huge tax penalty for its early withdrawal. After months of illness followed by major surgery with co-pays

---

* A somewhat controversial Zionist organization that funds fifty thousand free educational trips to Israel for young Jewish adults each year. "Enjoy the country. Ignore the dogma," I'd told her before she left, to which she'd said, "Duh, of course." We both knew I'd be unable to afford to send her there on my own.

and monthly COBRA fees, I have just under $3,000 in cash reserves left and zero credit cards. I've read too many cautionary tales of surprise bills as high as $8,000 for ambulance transport. I'm hemorrhaging enough already.

"Fine," she says, "call an Uber."

I remain firm. "No. I'll take the subway. And you're not coming with me. You have to stay here with the dog."

She doesn't listen. I am being pulled outside by the arm.

Streetlamps. Darkness. I smell pot.

"No one says pot anymore," says my daughter. "It's weed. Call an Uber. Now!" The numbers 1:43 A.M. atop the smiles of my three sun-kissed children on the face of my phone. I search for the white U inside the little black square, remembering that 143, according to Mr. Rogers, equals *I love you*. Funny how that stuff stays. I=1; love=4; you=3. It took me awhile to figure out the code.

"I love you," I tell my daughter. UberPool is half the price of UberX, so I choose that. Your driver will be Faraj. How many other passengers could Faraj possibly have at 1:43 in the morning? None, as it will turn out. If I live, I can use the money I'll save to replenish our supply of paper towels.

My daughter squeezes my hand. "I love you, too."

More fireworks. It feels like we're in a movie. I'd rather be in bed.

My daughter to the driver: "Yes, it's an emergency!"

Warm blood. Lots of it. Under me. On the seat of the Uber, down my legs, pooling in my shoes. An uber pool in an UberPool. I feel awful for the mess my body has unleashed. An apology to Faraj.

"Don't worry," he says. "Just go. God bless." Two decades earlier, when my water had broken all over the floor of a taxi, the driver had spoken those exact words. *Don't worry. Just go. God bless.*

I empty my wallet of bills and try to hand them to Faraj. He won't accept them. I try and fail again.

He brings his hand to his heart.

"*Salaam alaikum*," I say. Words learned in Ramallah, while living for a week with a Palestinian family under lockdown. That was the real tragedy of the *intifada*: not the David/Goliath scenes manufactured for CNN, but the hidden indignities of second-class citizenship, poverty, and home confinement.

A woman's body is the same. All of the bad stuff happens inside, off-screen. So when you go to the emergency room and say, "It hurts," as I did two weeks earlier, they nod as if they're listening, leave you on a gurney in the hallway for hours, hand you two aspirin, and send you home. It's almost a relief to be bleeding so profusely. To have tangible proof of the pain inside. Doctors and CNN trucks pay attention to pyrotechnics.

No one ever bought my photos of the Palestinian family stuck inside their home. Guns and rocks were my bread and butter.

"*Alaikum salaam*," he says.

The twenty-foot distance between car and emergency room seems as unbridgeable as it had after my water broke. My daughter offers me her shoulder to lean on as we exit. I am both grateful and ashamed. How, in the twenty years between soiled taxis, have our roles reversed?

I have absolutely no memory of entering the hospital, but a trail of blood says I did.

Emergency room receptionist, asking my daughter for my name. All of the words are outside me now. Other voices have taken over the task of speaking them. My name? It's unretrievable.

My name! A brief snap back from the post-verbal abyss. My name: something that should be simple but isn't. Because my divorce is taking longer than expected—nearly four years at this point, for lack of funds to pay lawyers—I've petitioned the court on my own to revert to my birth name pre-divorce, only to be told by a desk clerk that I need my ex's signed and notarized permission to do so.

"Permission?" I'd said. "That's sexist."

"No," said the clerk, "men have to do it, too."

"You must be flooded with such cases."

"Give them Daddy's last name!" I say to my daughter, one last gasp of cogency before everything goes dark. It has been over a month since I'd handed my ex the name change permission paperwork, on a bench between our two apartments. The exchange had felt tawdry, like a dime-bag drug deal. He has yet to get the papers notarized. I wonder if they'll insist on using my married name on my death certificate, should it come to that. If nothing else, I must stay alive to avoid that.

The world tilts. My body falls, seemingly in slow motion. This is a thing, backed by science: a perception of time expanding and slowing down during a moment of trauma. Upon contact with the hospital floor, my rib breaks.

The glass Tupperware container flies out of my hand, splattering onto the ground, drenching the sleeve of my daughter's flannel shirt with her mother's blood and covering the hospital floor with shards of broken glass. I have no memory of this. I am told it was quickly mopped up.

"It hurts to breathe!" I shout. Is anyone listening?

Overhead lights. Green, fluorescent glow. Voices yelling. What's happening?

"We have to move her to another stretcher. There's too much blood." How long have I been here?

Hands under me. A sleepover levitation: light as a feather, stiff as a board. Air underneath, then, boom, solid stretcher below. The antiseptic stench of the prior one being hosed down with bleach. I peek. Bad idea. A voice: "Get her into a room! Now!"

Darkness.

Irrational anger as the nurse uses scissors to cut off my green yoga pants, now soaked red. "No, please! They're my favorites!" Too late. They're in the trash. Relief at having a tangible object outside of myself onto which to misdirect my feelings.

Beeping.

The constant gush of liquid underneath me. Imagine a gallon of milk, turned on its side. Glug, glug, glug. How much blood does a body hold? Tiny droplets of sweat on my upper lip. I am salt. On its return to the sea. I can actually feel my body dying. My brain is less scared of this than I'd always assumed it would be. I feel more like an observer of my disintegration rather than a participant. I take comfort in this, in case I have a future in which that information might be useful.

Darkness. Beeping.

More enormous clots flying out. No. Not a thousand, my daughter corrects me. She's been counting. We're up to sixteen. Her voice: "Oh god, oh my god . . ." Then, into the hallway: "Someone please get in here! Now!" She's five foot zero. Her voice sounds much taller.

The eighteenth giant clot emerges. My daughter's face, the one she puts on when she's trying too hard to seem okay. I see your fake composure, young lady, and I raise you fake levity. "A *chai!*" I say. *Chai* is the Hebrew word for eighteen. But also for life. It's one of the first things they teach you in Hebrew school. My daughter laughs.

Religious Jews don't believe in cremation. They bury the body the next day. I'm not a religious Jew. I'm more of a bagel Jew. I want to remind my daughter to cremate my body and sprinkle the ashes into the Seine if I die, but now's not the right time. Plus we've talked about this already. She knows my wishes. And I'll be dead so what do I care if she actually carries them out? It was just a plan, to have one. Seems silly, now that it's real. *Find the nearest tree*, I want to tell her, *and call it a day*, but I've lost the ability to turn thought into speech.

Darkness. Beeping.

A nurse shoves fist-sized hunks of gauze up me: "This is not going to stop it, but we have no other solution until the surgeon gets here."

Pressure. So much mounting pressure from the gauze plugging up the hole where my viscera are trying to escape. Ow! Ow! Eject!

I leap off the bed to relieve the pressure. Voices are yelling at me to lie back down, but I can't. My need for gravity overrides their desire for obedience. The cork is already halfway out of the bottle. "It's coming out! It's coming out!" I yell. The blood-soaked gauze shoots out of me and lands with a splash in a bedpan held out by a nurse like a catcher's mitt. For a too-silent moment, all of us are in shock. Did that just happen? Was that . . . *thing* actually inside me? The clot-covered gauze ball looks monstrous, more like a prop from a horror film than a real object. "Score!" I say. My daughter laughs. Score, indeed. Levity is all we have.

Darkness. Beeping.

My child's voice, finally breaking, as she leaves the room and whispers into her phone. "Jen? Jen? Oh my god, Jen! It's awful. When can you get here?" Jen is my sister, a choreographer who lives in the Bay Area. She is in New York this holiday weekend, unusually, for some R & R with her family but also to research footage from the original *Fiddler on the Roof* in the Lincoln Center archives.

A *Fiddler* earworm: Is this the little girl I carried? Horror, once again, at the thought of putting my twenty-year-old daughter through this ordeal. Simultaneous gratitude for her poise and ferocity. I gave birth to my own savior out of the canal trying to kill me. My brain bends in on itself, pondering this.

One time, when she was thirteen, she said she was going to hang out with a friend. In truth, she met two friends who'd shared an entire bottle of vodka and had called her in a panic. She got there just in time. Contacted both of their parents and an ambulance. Spoke to the paramedics. Saved two lives.

The girls' parents were furious. At their daughters' poor choices, yes, but more, I had the impression, at the cost of the ambulance.

The surgeon's flip-flops. Tiny grains of sand. I've interrupted her beach vacation. "I'm so sorry," I say.

"Don't be," she says. "It's my job." She's faceless. My only memory is of her legs, moving around the stretcher, and of her voice, after she does the pelvic exam and gasps: "We need to get her into the OR now. I don't care. Bump someone if you have to. Yes, now!"

We are still waiting.

Lisa, my friend and literary agent, is now in the room. Cool. How did that happen? My daughter texted her, after having searched for allies in my phone. Lisa's my rock. She hosted a fiftieth birthday lunch for me the previous year, against my protestations. Lots of talk about what to do with the dog. There's an app on the phone. "Wag!"? No, I don't have it. Another problem I can't solve.

Darkness. Beeping.

My sister has arrived. After Lisa, I think, but I'm not sure? The soothing chatter of three women at my feet. Beautiful women, all of whom look as if they come from the same shtetl. Even Lisa, who's not related to us. I half expect them to break out into "Matchmaker." I have a team! I've been alone all my life, in ways large and small. In marriage, most of all. Their laughter masks worry. I hear its undertones. What time is it? What are we waiting for?

Hallway lights rush by, a tracking shot. As does my life. Jump cuts within jump cuts, in no particular order: preschool apple juice, pumpkin patch, red Schwinn, blue eyes: Dad's. Gone too soon.

"I wish Dad were here," I say. Out loud? Later, I'll ask my sister: Did I cry out for Dad?

"No, just your yoga pants."

My shtetl, halted by a double door. Team Deb is not allowed to go through. "You're going to be fine," they say, unconvincingly, growing smaller.

Liars. They have to say that. Where's the surgeon?

There she is. Masked. Now I'll never know what she looks like. She'll be forever entombed in my memory as sandy toes.

An operating room. Frigid air. Overhead lights. Blinding circle above. Legs spread below. I was just here. Three weeks ago. Five incisions, as yet unhealed. Things become disambiguated now, like on my first acid trip, when money became work, and cops became human aggression, and doorknobs stood for the problem of egress. The circle above becomes life. As do my spread legs below, which thrice produced life, but now expose viscera trying to escape into the birth canal and kill me.

I'm watching this all from above, a bleeding body on a slab, arms spread, wrists bound. Jew, Muslim, Buddhist, Hindu, atheist, it doesn't matter: We are all Christ under the knife. The speculum goes in. *L'chaim!* Dear Science: I will not die for your sins. That cervix should have been removed years ago, when you took out my uterus. Back then you claimed it played a role in sexual pleasure. In the passive voice: *It is believed to play a role in sexual pleasure.* You told me to keep it in, when I could have told you—any woman could have—that the clitoris is the only game in that town. That a cervix, unmoored, has no role in a body other than wreaking havoc. This havoc. These masks. This clattering of metal scalpels.

Gas. A voice. "Count backward from ten." Ten. Nine. Eight . . .

Fade to black.

Six years earlier . . .

PART II

UTERUS

2011–2012
(with two quick detours back to 2001)

Lunch with Nora, Freds

MAY 2011

The only thing a uterus is good for after a certain point is causing pain and killing you. Why are we even talking about this?" Nora jams a fork into her chopped chicken salad, the one she insisted I order as well. "If your doctor says it needs to come out, yank it out." A quarter century my senior, draped in black and bescarved, Nora speaks her mind the way others breathe: an involuntary reflex, not a choice.

"But the uterus . . ." I say, spearing a slice of egg. "It's so . . ."

"Symbolic?"

"Yes. Don't roll your eyes."

"I'm not rolling my eyes." She leans in. "I'm trying to get you to face a, well, it's not even a hard truth. It's an easy one. Promise me the minute you leave this lunch you'll pick up the phone and schedule the hysterectomy today. Not tomorrow. *Today*."

"Why the rush?"

"Why the hesitation?" Nora has leukemia. She knows this. I do not. "Wait. Don't tell me you're planning on having more babies."

"Ha!" I laugh. I'm forty-five. "No. Of course not. I couldn't get pregnant at this point if I tried."

She cocks her head. Raises an eyebrow.

"What?"

"You get pregnant when you don't try."

I've been pregnant five times. Two of those pregnancies were planned, three were not, and I've had no miscarriages. If my uterus were a math problem, it would look like this: 5 pregnancies — 3 live births = 2 abortions. The first was at seventeen. I'd taken all necessary precautions, but the diaphragm Planned Parenthood had given me had not done the one job we'd carefully planned for it to do: keep me from parenthood.

The second was in 2000, after the births of my first two children. The entire staff of the ultrasound office were called in to bear witness to the tiny blastula next to my IUD. "Oh, wow, look at that! So unusual!" they said, as thrilled by the rare sighting inside my womb as I was shook. I was thirty-four years old, in weekly couples therapy that wasn't working, and I'd been taking an oral medication for a toenail fungus that was contra-indicated for pregnancy.

Once again, I went in for a D&C, this time at a hospital instead of an abortion clinic, so I didn't have to deal with screaming protestors outside or with the hour of patronizing questions inside, asking me if I was sure that I was sure that I was sure. "Yes, I'm sure that I'm sure!" I'd said at seventeen, exasperated, for what felt like the twentieth time. Why would I be sitting there naked under my hospital gown, missing a day of school, with my parents waiting for me in the other room, if I weren't?

My fifth pregnancy, at thirty-nine, was also unplanned, but I made a deliberate, hopeful choice to keep the child, my younger son, born in 2006, just after I turned forty. The marriage was turning around, or so I thought. His father promised, this time, to help.

To be born with a uterus is to be constantly aware of it. Not just when it's suddenly colonized by a fertilized egg, or when it's actively growing a fetus, or every month, when it produces an ovum or bleeds, but every day from the moment you learn what it does, how it does it, and that at some unknowable moment in the future, it will leave the first of many impossible-to-remove stains.

Who am I without my uterus?

"Please," says Nora. "You don't need it anymore. It served you well, but that part of your life is over. The sooner you accept this the better. How great is this chicken salad?"

"Delicious."

We are seated at her preferred table at Freds, a restaurant on the ninth floor of Barneys, between a large column and a wall of windows. The column provides some privacy from her gawkers, as does the one near our usual table at E.A.T., which is the other place we sometimes go to have what have now become, over the course of a decade, our regular lunches. At E.A.T. we get the three-salad plate: cucumber and dill, always, plus two wildcards. At Freds, it's the chopped chicken salad. I once tried branching off and ordering the daily special, but no. I quickly understood that Nora's strong opinions derived from nearly always being right: Freds's chicken salad actually *is* the best item on the menu. Why order anything else?

To many of these lunches, Nora often arrives bearing gifts, along with careful verbal instructions for their use: Dr. Hauschka's lemon oil ("Dump at least half a bottle in the bath water. Don't skimp. If you like it, I'll get you more . . ."); a black button-down cardigan from Zara ("I bought five of them, they were so cheap. You can wear it on your book tour. Look, the buttons look just like a Chanel . . ."); a bracelet with multifaceted stones ("I'm too old to wear this, you're not . . ."); a mirrored picture frame ("I'm sure you have a beautiful black-and-white photo that would look nice in this, but make sure it's black-and-white. Color won't work").

"I don't know," I say. "Won't I feel like less of a woman without a uterus?"

"Oh, please." Nora rolls her eyes again. "Would you rather not have a uterus or be dead? That's the question you should be asking yourself. You'll still be every inch a woman after it's gone, you just won't bleed anymore, and trust me, if only for that, get it done tomorrow. They go in with robots now. You'll barely have a scar. So what is this adeno . . . how do you pronounce the thing you have?"

"Adenomyosis," I say, quickly googling it on my phone to make sure I get the definition right. I read from my screen: "A chronic condition of the uterus in which its inner lining breaks through the myometrium, causing extensive bleeding, anemia, heavy cramping, and severe bloating."

"Sounds delightful. I see now why you'd want to keep it."

I laugh. Then I sigh. I'd put up with this disease most of my adult life because, like most women who get adenomyosis, I had no idea I had it.

"How are your periods?" my gynecologist would ask every year, and every year I would answer, "Heavy," but with a tone that implied I had everything down there under control. I was bleeding ten to fifteen days out of every month, I couldn't make it through one of those days without downing at least sixteen ibuprofen, the maximum daily dosage, and I had given up on even super tampons, as they were useless against the flow, but so what? That's what being a woman entailed, right?

To manage the situation and give less of my income to Procter & Gamble, I'd started using a DivaCup, a breast-shaped silicone vessel you shove up the vagina like a cervical cap, just under the cervix,[*] to catch the flow. The DivaCup holds one ounce of blood. I was emptying it every thirty minutes to keep it from overflowing. To put this in perspective, the average period lasts between four to six days and produces, in total, approximately one DivaCup full of blood. I was producing one ounce of blood *every half hour*. For an average of twelve days straight. At night, unable to change the cup while I slept, I soaked through maxi pads the size of airline pillows, ruining hundreds of dollars' worth of bed sheets until I realized I could just sleep atop those waterproof pads they give you postpartum, the kind they also give to incontinent old people and dogs.

"How heavy?" my doctor would ask, raising her eyebrows.

"Oh, you know, normal heavy. Annoying but no big deal."

We women are taught, from an early age, to minimize. I don't mean we're actually taught this in school. I mean society teaches us to minimize our woes and to internalize its skeptical view of our pain so as not to be labeled crybabies or "hysterical": a meaningless, sexist diagnosis of unspecified female malaise, which, in the nineteenth and twentieth centuries, could sometimes mean you'd walk out of your doctor's office minus a clitoris. Why didn't I tell my doctor I had viselike cramps, slept on a doggy wee-wee pad half the month, and produced over 576 times the normal amount of blood each period? Because what's an extra 575 ounces of blood every month? A rounding error.

Every woman in a paper robe, facing her doctor, knows she is silently being judged. This is not paranoia or exaggeration. It is proven fact,

---

[*] My male editor thought I should add this description for my male readers. Women, I know you know.

based on numerous studies. I started collecting these studies, like charms on a bracelet. Women in an emergency room will wait an average of sixty-five minutes to be given pain medication, while men wait only forty-nine. Women who receive coronary bypass surgery are only half as likely to be given pain medication as men who've undergone the same surgery. If a woman claims her pain is a 7 on a scale of 10, her doctor will assume 5, while men's self-reported pain is taken at face value: A 7 is a 7 or maybe even an 8. This is neither the doctor's fault nor the patient's. It stems from a history, since the dawn of medicine, of treating women, though we outlive men, as the weaker, more sickly sex, plagued by "hysteria" of the female psyche (*hysteria*, of course, means "of the womb").

Dysmenorrhea (period pain), which one British professor of reproductive health described as "almost as bad as a heart attack," is so severely understudied and underfunded, most doctors have little to offer aside from NSAIDs and a shrug. At the same time, a recent double-blind, randomized, controlled trial of sildenafil citrate—that's Viagra, to you and me—found "total pain relief [of period cramps] over 4 consecutive hours" with "no observed adverse effects."

Wait. Hold the fuck up, I thought, when I first read that in a book. Viagra was found to provide *total pain relief* of period cramps *over four consecutive hours* with *no adverse side effects*? You mean the holy frigging grail of monthly ladyparts pain for which every woman I know has been searching her whole life actually . . . exists? And no one told us?

If you're a woman reading this, and you hadn't already heard the news, go ahead and take a minute or two to compose yourself after screaming. Go on. Close your eyes. Breathe deep. Smash a dish.

I'll wait.

So why isn't Viagra immediately prescribed these days to women suffering from severe dysmenorrhea? Simple. Lack of follow-up studies. Once researchers had clinically proven Viagra's lucrative use on flaccid penises, funding for our uteri—which could be equally if not more lucrative, considering 90 percent of them bleed and cramp every month—was cut off before a larger sample size study could be undertaken. In fact, Dr. Richard Legro, the lead scientist, had his grant application for further studies of the effects of Viagra on dysmenorrhea not only rejected—twice—by the NIH, no one ever reviewed it. "The reviewers did not see dysmenorrhea as a priority public health issue," he said.

Why? Because "men don't care about or understand dysmenorrhea." And men, of course, still hold the research purse strings.

I'd had dysmenorrhea my entire post-adolescent life, but it grew exponentially worse in 1995, after the birth of my first child. It wasn't until *sixteen years* later, however, just after my annual checkup in 2011, that my general practitioner became visibly alarmed. "A *seven*? This can't be right," said Dr. Bertie Bregman, seeing my finger-prick hemoglobin level and asking the nurse to run the test again. The results came back, once again, as 7 grams per deciliter. Anemia, in a woman, begins at any number less than 12 grams per deciliter. "How are you even standing?"

I was sitting. "I've been a little tired." (*I'm exhausted! All the time!*)

"How are your periods?"

(*Have you seen Niagara Falls?*) "Heavy."

"What about your energy level? Are you able to work and take care of the kids?"

"I do my best." (*I mean, who the fuck else is going to do it?*)

This time, however, sensing that I was being heard by a caring diagnostician, I elaborated. The fifteen-day periods. The emptying of the one-ounce DivaCup every half hour. The grape-sized clots. The nightly blood bath. Concomitant bowel issues. Intractable pain.

Luckily, Dr. Bregman was unnerved enough by my grocery list of vampire delicacies that he ordered further studies, which came back with the diagnosis of adenomyosis: a disease that had most likely been going on, judging by the size of my uterus, for decades. My uterus had grown so large, in fact, that it was impinging on the abilities of its backdoor neighbor, my rectum, to function properly. No wonder pooping during periods had grown so painful and difficult, I'd have to brace myself and mentally prepare each time.

"Look," said my doctor at our follow-up, after I got a second opinion from my gynecologist, who confirmed the diagnosis and urged the same uterus-yanking solution. "We can either hospitalize you every month for anemia or you can go ahead and get a hysterectomy. It's your choice but not really? I don't think getting transfusions every month is a sustainable life choice."

"Whatever it's called," says Nora, "I want you to promise me you'll get that hysterectomy *this year*. Also, I don't like the new cover they sent you for *The Red Book*."

"The one with the woman lying on a park bench, with the book in her hand?"

"Yes. Is it too late to change it?"

"I don't think so."

"Good. She looks dead. Like the book was so boring *it killed her*."

Ten years earlier, Nora had cold-called my home, annoyed that she'd had to get my number through a mutual friend. Throughout her life, if you dialed 411 and asked for her home number, you'd get it. "Why would you ever *not* be listed?" she'd said. "What if someone needs to get in touch with you?" But first she said, "Hi, Deb, this is Nora Ephron. I loved your memoir, and I'd like to take you out to lunch."

"Yeah, right," I said. "And I'm Joan of Arc. Meg, is this you?" Meg, my friend, is an excellent mimic. Nora had adapted Meg's novel *This Is My Life*, and the two had remained close. Meg knew Nora was my hero. Screenwriter, director, novelist, humorist, essayist, journalist: Nora did all the things I'd ever wanted to do but better, faster, stronger, and able if not to leap tall buildings in a single bound then at least to memorialize them on screen in such a way that the Empire State Building in *Sleepless in Seattle* will always be my Empire State Building. I saw *Heartburn* three times when it first came out; *When Harry Met Sally* too many times to count.

Nora's essays in *Esquire*, masterworks of the form, set the bar for all of us who came after. In fact, I draw a direct line from reading Nora's "A Few Words About Breasts" in *Esquire* to my first fumbling efforts as a teenager in the pages of *Seventeen* to my first memoir, *Shutterbabe*, which would eventually conjure Nora, genielike, into my life.

What Nora did in those essays, before and better than anyone else, was to subvert the inward-looking me-me-me of male gonzo journalism and rework it with a self-mocking dash of Dorothy Parker to serve the higher purpose of a collective *we*: the personal as a poignant and sometimes hilarious path to the universal. She'd choose the most humiliating parts of herself—her frizzy hair, the sag of her neck, the fact of being the only intern in the JFK White House at whom the president did not make a pass—and feature them front and center not as self-abasement but as her superpower. "When you slip on a banana peel, people laugh at you," she wrote. "But when you tell people you slipped on a banana peel, it's your laugh."

"No, Deb. This is Nora. And I'd like to invite you to lunch." The voice alternated between female tenor and male soprano with an undertone of school principal.

I froze. It *was* her. Nora ephing Ephron. On the other end of my phone. So what does one say to the woman whose work you've admired your entire life? For starters, not this: "Ummmm . . ."

"Are you still there?" said Nora.

"Yes, sorry. Lunch?"

A long, uncomfortable pause. "Is that a yes?" she said.

"Sorry. Yes!"

"Great. How about this Wednesday at E.A.T., 1 P.M.?"

"The one on Madison?"

"Is there another E.A.T. I don't know about?"

Some moments in life are so pivotal, some relationships so crucial, you remember exactly where you were and what you were clutching—bubble wrap, in this instance—when your world altered. I'd been standing in the foyer of my old apartment on the Upper West Side when Nora first called, staring at a wall of family photos that needed to come down. The dark, airless 1.5-bedroom on the ground floor of 70 Riverside Drive was located over a parking garage that would overheat every summer, rendering the kitchen tiles too hot for bare feet. Our windows framed the last stop of the M79 bus route. Buses idled there 24/7, blasting a constant, toxic cloud of apt metaphor into the master bedroom.

Moving boxes were everywhere. My husband and I were eight years into our marriage, seven years into breathing bus fumes, six years into parenthood, and five days away from seeing whether more light, air, and space could keep our marriage from collapsing. Our then two children had outgrown their half bedroom. Our upper respiratory systems, compromised by carbon monoxide, had succumbed to every cough, flu, and cold in the Tri-State area. I craved the slant of sunlight through the slats of a window, even if only for a New York minute.

Our new living room, bright and fume-free, had an oblique southern view of the World Trade Center. Until four months later, when it didn't.

That Clear Blue Morning

SEPTEMBER 11, 2001

That clear blue morning, deflecting questions from my then four-year-old, her still-baby thighs gripping my hip as we watched, from the roof, solid mass disintegrate into twin plumes — "Are they going to fly a plane into our building next?" (*No, I promise, that's not going to happen . . .*); "Where's Daddy?" (*I'm sure he's on his way back home right now . . .*); "What's going to happen to the kids?" (*Which kids?*); "The kids of the people in the fire?" — I felt fresh tremors of my own family's implosion. As much as I was horrified at the thought of my children's father not making it home from his office across the street from that pyre of steel and charred flesh, a small, shame-filled part of me wondered what a passive reprieve from our conflict and pain would feel like.

Phones were jammed. Transportation had shut down. So for those first chaotic hours after the planes hit, I had no word from him. Emails, on the other hand, were landing in my inbox faster than I could respond, many of them too painful to process. Ted Hennessy, a friend from college, was a passenger on one of the planes. Carlton Valvo, father of Dante, a second grader in my son's school, was trapped in the tower. Mike Pescherine, uncle of Max, my son's best friend, was trapped there as well. Yes, I replied to Tom and Maria, Max's parents. I'd come by with the kids and food later that night to hold vigil. Maybe Mike would make it out of the rubble, who knew? That was the magical thinking we still had in those first hours. That a person might survive a fire followed by a hundred-floor plunge. We'd all had dinner together just a few weeks earlier. Between the main course and dessert, Mike had proudly announced that his wife Lyn was pregnant with their first child.

I slammed shut my computer. It was too much. The smoke had now wafted uptown, into our apartment. It smelled acrid, toxic. I closed the windows before strapping my daughter into a baby seat on the back of my bike to hand-deliver the film I'd shot of the burning towers to my photo agent, who'd put out an SOS for whatever images any of us in New York might have snapped that morning.

Riding downtown on the Hudson River bike path, against an amoeba flow of the vacant-faced heading uptown on foot, felt like being back at war, so familiar was the march and scope of human trauma moving step-by-step together, away from the violence, backlit against smoke. I wanted to stop and shoot off a few frames of this, but my daughter had fallen asleep in the baby seat, clutching my camera bag, and the bike would have toppled over had I left her alone to climb a tree to get the shot. Instead, the image would lodge itself in my memory such that I have not

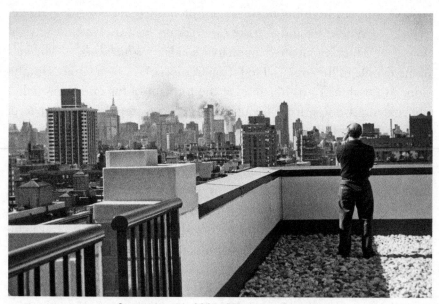

September 11, 2001, © Deborah Copaken

been able to ride down the Hudson River bike path since without seeing those dust-covered ghosts.

"Oh, gosh. I'm sorry. I forgot you have a toddler," whispered my agent, Jeffrey, when I pushed the bike and napping child out of the elevator and asked him to hold it upright as I fumbled in the bag for the film. I apologized for not being able to head farther downtown into the heart of the chaos. I still had to fetch my son. His first grade teacher had suggested we not pick them up until the end of the day, to give them some semblance of normalcy, but now I was having second thoughts.

I hopped on the bike and pedaled as fast as I could back uptown, away from what would turn out to be lethal air. But what to do with the four-year-old, still asleep in her baby seat? My son's school was too far from our home for her to walk; I'd given away her stroller; our usual babysitter was trapped across the river in Brooklyn; the city was on lockdown, with all subway, taxi, car, and bus travel forbidden; and I could fit only one child on the bike at a time. It felt like one of those brain teasers in which the farmer has a fox, a chicken, and a bag of grain but can take only one item across the river at a time.

"Where is he?" I said out loud, pedaling past the Intrepid, one of my husband's favorite museums, tears falling hard as the reverberations of overhead fighter jets rattled my rib cage. What I meant was *Where is my husband at this exact moment in time? Is he dead? Is he alive?* but also *Where is he always?*

In the spring of 1995, two weeks before our first child's due date, he'd insisted we visit the *Intrepid*, a former World War II aircraft carrier docked in the Hudson River. The ship had survived five kamikaze attacks and one torpedo strike. I, on the other hand, could barely survive its steep, narrow staircase. Halfway up, bent over in pain and winded from the pressure of womb upon lungs, I stopped. "I can't make it," I said. "I'm so sorry. Go on without me. I'll wait for you on a bench downstairs."

"No!" said my husband, visibly upset. "You promised!" He loved war museums. I'd found this endearing, at first, his love of history, armaments, and though I would not necessarily choose to visit a war museum during my downtime, I went along with it in every city we visited because that's what marriage is about, I thought. Compromise.

Trapped between Memorial Day weekend tourists, not wanting to make a scene, I kept climbing up the stairs until I reached the top, where I was promptly left sitting on the floor. (There were no benches, or at least none I could immediately locate.) I thought about heading back down the stairs to sit by the water, on an actual bench, on a beautiful Sunday in May, but I figured my husband would take a quick look around and then come back to find me. Instead, he toured the ship on his own for what felt like forever while I sat on the floor waiting. And waiting. And waiting. *Where is he?* I wondered. Portable cellphones were still three years away. The Braxton-Hicks contractions grew more and more intense with each passing minute. Or were those real contractions? (They were real.)

"Where were you?" I said, choking back tears, when he finally returned.

"What? I was visiting the museum," he said.

Two hours later, in Rockefeller Park, a downtown landfill in the shadow of the Twin Towers, my water broke.

Now, six years later, back home from the photo agency, I unstrapped my sleeping daughter from the bike, put her down for a nap, and tried to reach someone to watch her while I fetched my son. But the phone lines were still jammed. And while the many parenting books on my shelves had excellent tips on sleep training, hiding vegetables in sauces, and dealing with toddler tantrums, none of them had any advice on dealing with school pickup during a terrorist attack.

Then, a reprieve: A neighborhood father showed up, in person, asking if I needed any help. I thanked him, left him in my apartment with my sleeping toddler, and immediately jumped on my husband's bike, which was equipped with a tagalong for an older child. I pedaled east across Manhattan with R.E.M.'s "It's the End of the World" ricocheting through my head, an unending earworm. New York City, absent its cars and people, unfurled in ominous silence between sirens, sparkling beneath cerulean skies. I felt guilty for noticing and appreciating this.

"You're late," said my son, his bottom lip quivering, when I finally fell to my knees and hugged him. It was just after lunch, but he was nevertheless one of the last first graders to be picked up. I guess all the other parents decided not to wait until the end of the school day either.

"I'm sorry, sweetie," I said, choking back my own tears. "I got here as fast as I could."

"Max's uncle is in the building. And Dante's daddy."

"I know. I heard. It's terrible." I held him as he crumbled.

"Is Daddy okay?" He'd just visited his father's office at 5 World Trade Center the previous week. They'd gone all the way up to the Windows on the World to check out the view.

"Daddy's fine," I said, leaving out the part about not having heard from him for several hours. Cellphone towers had been jammed since the attack, so it was understandable, but why hadn't he called our landline from his office or from a payphone*, just to let us know he was okay? Men and women dying in buildings, in harrowing voicemails made public, had figured out ways to call their spouses and kids to say, "I love you." It had now been five hours since he left for work.

No. No. Stop catastrophizing, I chastised myself. *He's fine. He's just being him.*

A year into our relationship, in a busy train station in Milan, I'd left my husband—then boyfriend—alone for five minutes while I fetched us two bottles of water. When I returned to the spot where I'd left him, he was gone. He stayed gone—this was also in the pre-cellphone era—for over an hour, not understanding my tears and fury when I finally found him. "Where have you been?" I'd said. "I've been looking for you everywhere!"

"Exploring," he said, hurt and confused by my anger.

So much of what I loved about this man was his guilelessness: his intense curiosity, his childlike awe and innocence, which could sometimes manifest as a kind of accidental ignorance. Ignorance, however, need not be willful for it to be destructive.

My son and I exited his school as yet another rumble of fighter jets zoomed above. We looked up. What was happening in the sky? Were more planes trying to crash into more buildings? "How do you know Daddy's fine?" said my son.

"I just do," I said, fairly confident of my statement at the time, but then, upon our return home, a new question had hit my inbox, from multiple correspondents: Did I know whether or not my husband had gone to the breakfast at the Windows on the World?

What breakfast at the Windows on the World? I looked it up. My heart sank.

---

* Only later would I find out that payphones, too, had been rendered useless.

The ill-fated breakfast had been organized by the eerily named Risk Waters Group for delegates in the financial sector working in tech. My husband, at the time, was in the financial sector, working in tech. Had he been invited to that breakfast? We hardly ever discussed our day-to-day professional minutiae. Or really anything for that matter. I did my writing, he did whatever he spent his day doing, maybe we'd speak for five minutes at the end of the day, after I'd fed, bathed, and read to the kids, loaded the dishwasher, folded the laundry, signed the permission slips, and sorted plastic figurines from Lego bricks from wayward spirals of pasta before sitting down to sneak in another hour or two of writing. I'd given up asking where he was or begging him to come home in time for dinner. By that point, it seemed easier to go to bed at 10 P.M. than to stay up late for his arrival and ignite yet another argument about the imbalance in our domestic duties, the strain it was putting on my career, or how lonely I felt in our marriage.

All this to say, I had every reason to believe he was there at that breakfast at the Windows on the World and every reason to believe he was not. And also every reason to believe he could have been somewhere else entirely. Exploring.

Should I make a missing person sign? The next day, the city would be choked with them, as if everyone in New York had had the exact same thought at the exact same moment, printing photos of their loved ones under "Missing!" and "Have you seen my daddy?" and "Last seen at 7 A.M., please call Juanita with any information."

No, I thought. Stop panicking. He's just being him. A month into our courtship, back in Paris in 1990, I'd arrived at the appointed time to the brasserie he'd picked for our date. Fifteen minutes dripped by. Then twenty. Then forty-five. I asked the maître d', several times, if anyone had called for me. "*Non,*" I was told, with increasing pity and annoyance.

So much for that relationship, I thought, stomping home, too angry to cry. But then I walked in, and my phone rang. "Please," he begged, full of remorse. Please try to understand: His French wasn't good enough to explain that he'd been held up at work. Plus he didn't have the number of the restaurant.

"You didn't have . . . the number? Why didn't you look it up on the Minitel?" The Minitel was France's internet before the internet, a little box of magic France Télécom provided with your phone service. You could talk to strangers on it. Sext before sexting was even a verb. Find any phone number in France.

"I was stuck in a meeting," he said. He offered to cook me dinner the next night in recompense. At first I said no. Then, believing everyone deserves a second chance, I changed my mind.

Years later, I would read that Maya Angelou quote—"When someone shows you who they are, believe them the first time."—and think back to that choice. But I'd said yes to his home-cooked penance, which was delicious, and then the next morning, when he left for work, he accidentally locked me inside his apartment. He apologized profusely for that, too—I'd had to cancel an important meeting with the photo editor of Géo—and now here we were: him, AWOL once again, but presumably making his way home from a terrorist attack; me, hunkering down with our children, pretending everything was okay.

When he finally walked in the door, several hours after the attack, I wept. As despairing as I was about the state of our marital dyad, no part of me would have wanted my young children, now smothering him with kisses, to have been deprived of their father. In fact, it was at that moment that I doubled down on my commitment to fix whatever was broken.

The next day, September 12, 2001, was our eighth wedding anniversary. But between the thousands of missing faces staring out from those hand-lettered flyers; the armed National Guards on every corner; the deaths of friends and community members; the implosion, with the towers, of my husband's job; and the fact that our dinner reservation was now located across from a still-smoldering mass grave, it didn't seem right to start sifting through our marital dirt in search of the salvageable.

I had no name for our particular dysfunction. Or, rather, I was not yet ready to name it. For to name it would have been to end it. And if I was good at coping under less-than-ideal circumstances, I was even better at denial. We're just going through a rough patch, I'd tell myself. Close friends. A married sister. Nora. We're not getting along.

But it wasn't just that we were not getting along. We couldn't agree on anything. Not on where to live: I wanted to cut our housing expenses and move to Brooklyn; he wanted to keep white-knuckling it in Manhattan. Not on how to divide domestic responsibilities: "You're the mother, it's your job," he'd say to every one of my requests for help, as if Betty Friedan had never howled into the void. Not on how to balance our various work responsibilities: He believed his took precedence over mine, even during that long stretch of years when I was the primary wage earner. Not on how to save money or speak civilly or stop hurting our children's psyches with our sniping. And not, most saliently, on how to love.

Ten years passed.

Lunch with Nora, East Hampton

JULY 2011

can't do this anymore," I finally admit to Nora. I call her early, too distraught to elaborate, after a particularly disturbing interaction with my husband the previous night. The final edit of my new novel is due on my editor's desk in a week. I am supposed to be spending the morning communing with my red pen. But the words on the manuscript pages look scrambled. My brain is frozen, unable to move past the incident.

"I'm reserving you a jitney ticket right now," says Nora, sending me the link while we are still on the phone. She's in her home in East Hampton, writing *Lucky Guy*, the play about a tabloid journalist dying from cancer that will turn out to be her final work. "I'll meet you at the bus stop. Don't eat. I'm making lunch." Five years earlier, when I'd called to say I couldn't attend the baby shower she was throwing for me, because I'd been confined to bed rest for the remainder of my pregnancy, she showed up at my apartment with a dozen lobsters, two home-made lemon meringue pies, our mutual friends, and her sleeves rolled up to do the dishes when the party was over.

Until today, I've told no one but my shrink about the darker corners of my marriage. There's the shame of speaking the words out loud, but also the shame, self-blame, and dissonance of believing myself to be a strong and capable woman who is simultaneously too weak to leave a dysfunctional marriage. Or even to admit it is dysfunctional. (*We're just going through a rough patch. We're not getting along.*) I also don't want to speak ill of the father of my children to anyone, let alone to my mentor and superhero. But that afternoon, in Nora's light-filled kitchen, feeling both safe in her maternal presence and confident of her discretion, I unearth all of it. Every last bone.

Later, after the exorcism, Nora's husband Nick joins us for lunch, placing his hands gently on his wife's shoulders before kissing the top of her head. "Is this for real?" I say dubiously, air-circling their conjoined heads with my finger. "Is this as good as it seems?" It's almost cloying, the way the light haloes their happy coupledom: Harry and Sally, in their golden years. My jealousy of their bond burns almost as brightly as my admiration.

"No," says Nick. "It's better."

"Deb!" Nora laughs, standing up and walking to the kitchen counter. "He's my third husband. If you can't get it right by your third marriage, well . . . come. Help me carry the salad to the table." She slices thick slabs of peasant bread. "Are you staying over tonight?"

"I can't," I say. "I have to pick up my son from the camp bus stop at 5:30."

Nora purses her lips and tilts her head down, leaving only her eyebrows in place. "Might his father be able to do that?"

"I'll ask," I say, knowing before dialing his number what the answer will be.

To this day, I'm still angry at myself for not saying to him, "I don't care. Figure it out. I'm not coming home. I'm too angry and hurt right now. I'm sleeping at Nora's." But I hated discord more than I minded picking up the kids or the slack.

After lunch, Nora drives me back to the jitney and scribbles the name and number of her friend Joyce, a Jungian therapist whose specialty is treating couples at an impasse. My husband and I had stopped seeing our previous couples shrink several years earlier, when she showed up for lice check on the first day of our older son's kindergarten, and the three of us stood there, speechless, suddenly realizing that our kids were in the same school. "You know I'm here for you," Nora says, "if you decide to pull the plug, but please: Try to fix the marriage before taking any drastic measures."

"I think we're too far gone," I say. "I think it's too late."

"You know I always say this, but I'll say it again: Marriages come and go, but divorce is forever. He loves you. I've seen it with my own eyes. Even if he is an excellent liar." Nora and I would often take turns cooking for and hosting twenty-person dinner parties that would end in hours-long, knock-down, drag-out mafia games, during which one of my husband's lies once rattled all of us.

Lies, of course, were part of the game if you drew one of the three mafia cards: You had to lie and say you were a villager, to fool the other villagers into believing you weren't in the mafia, while simultaneously urging them to kill off their innocent neighbors.

On the night of his infamous lie, my husband was in the mafia, I was not. Meaning, he knew who else still left in the game was on his team. I was a villager and therefore playing blind. It was down to the wire, with only a few players left. If we villagers killed one of our own, the mafia would win. If we killed a mafioso, the village would win. My husband looked me straight in the eye, in front of eighteen of our mutual friends, and said, "Deb, look at me. I love you. You're my wife. You know I would never lie to you. I promise. I *swear* to you. I'm not in the mafia. If you kill me instead of Adam, the mafia will win." This was an unusual, last-ditch tactic. Laying the trust in one's marriage on the line, and publicly at that, was a move of desperation. I'd seen it used only a few times before, but always for the good of the village. Trusting him, thinking maybe he was even the commandant, falling on his own sword to save the village, I voted with him to kill off our friend Adam, the last villager standing. And with that one kill, the mafia won.

Everyone laughed about it afterward. Especially me. But the more I thought about it in the months that followed, the more I was unnerved by a simple truth his lie had unveiled. It wasn't that I felt humiliated. Or that I was shocked by or angry about the lie. It's that it had felt too familiar, our not being on the same team. And now that private and troubling part of us, on which, I realized, I was expending far too much energy keeping hidden, was out there, public, for all our friends to see.

"Yeah, that mafia lie was definitely odd, but whatever," I say to Nora. "It's not about his lies or his love." My husband told me he loved me often. I didn't doubt the truth of his feelings. "It's about empathy. Or rather his lack of it. And how that absence is slowly killing me."

"Joyce is a genius," she says. "Call her."

Empathy

JULY 2011

Joyce's bright, white, and welcoming office is on West 67th Street, just off Central Park West, and she makes you take your shoes off at the front door: a disarming trick every shrink should copy, as it immediately removes the artifice of decorum and sets patients at ease. Exposing one's feet, I now firmly believe, is the gateway to exposing the psyche. It's also an apt reminder, when you leave weekly couples therapy, that each person in a marriage stands in their own shoes, and that the work of marriage is to try to understand how those other shoes might fit, were you to stand in them. "Why are you here?" Joyce asks.

"Because she made me," jokes my husband.

I laugh. His sense of humor is another one of the reasons I fell in love with him. Then I immediately feel the pinprick of tears. "Empathy," I say, and the deluge begins.

Alas empathy, we will soon find out—a key ingredient in mature love if not *the* key ingredient—is beyond the capabilities of the man I chose to marry. As in literally, neurologically beyond them. For years I did not understand this. I thought he was deliberately not trying to stand in my shoes, which only furthered my frustration and anger. It takes Joyce, twenty-one years into our relationship, to suggest a lack of empathy might simply be my husband's set point. And that the daily harm caused by this might be wholly unintentional.

Watching us interact in her office, week after week, she notes that the man who once vowed to love, honor, and cherish the woman sitting next to him never once places his hand on her thigh or shoulder when she cries. He simply stays on his side of the couch, watching my tears fall. This leads to a consultation with an autism expert, who gives us each an emotional intelligence (EQ) test. The test assesses empathy, scored from 0 to 80, with 0 being the least empathic, 80 being the most. I score a 68. My husband gets an 8: one of the lowest the doctor has ever measured.

The approximate cutoff is 30 for what was then called Asperger's syndrome (AS) but what is now called falling within the high-functioning range of autism spectrum disorder (ASD). "Mind blindness," it can also be called. Meaning, neurologically, he could neither intuit what was going on in my mind nor react appropriately when I told him how I was feeling. In the nature/nurture divide, I'd always assumed my husband's emotional shortcomings were due to his upbringing and therefore not insurmountable, given the right dollop of love, intention, and therapy. That his biography was to blame for our marital woes, not his neurology.

I was wrong.

To be fair, it was an honest mistake. He'd recounted the tale of his upbringing on our first date: the deadbeat father; emigrating from Brezhnev's Russia to the U.S. with his single mother and identical twin brother when he was nine; being orphaned at fifteen when his mother died; the struggle to fit in, both with the Orthodox kids in his yeshiva, after having been raised by an a-religious mother, and with the modern Orthodox family who took him in after she died. We were twenty-four years old at the time, sitting on the banks of the Seine in Paris, where we both then lived. His story hooked me. Made me cry. Made me forgive all of the little quirks and idiosyncrasies I saw early on. I pictured his émigré mother, the brilliant art historian, working as a diamond sorter to make ends meet. Sacrificing herself in a foreign land so that her sons might have a better life, only to die, soon thereafter, of heart disease.

In retrospect, I probably fell in love with her that first night more than with him: with her moxie, her bravery, her willingness to sacrifice herself for the sake of her sons' futures. And part of him, whether consciously or not, understood this. "Women always leave me," said my future husband that same night, his first gauntlet of many: *I dare you to be the woman who stays.* The next gauntlet was the houseplant he left in my apartment as a homecoming surprise when I was off covering postcoup Romania. "Take care of me," said the note affixed to its leaves. "I need lots of water, sunlight, and, most of all, love."

Two weeks before I'd walked into my home to see that plant aglow in afternoon light, I'd witnessed a dead Romanian orphan being disemboweled with a rusty saw on a slab of wood after he'd hit his head, too many times, against a piss-stained wall. This was in Vulturești, in 1990, at the now infamous Hospital for the Irrecoverables, where Romanian children with disabilities were left to suffer in conditions so shocking, they still haunt me: bedframes with no mattresses; tattered, filthy clothes; a toddler's ankle tied to his bed; Dickensian gruel slurped ravenously and spoonless into, well, I wouldn't necessarily call them bellies. More like skin stretched drum-tight over bone.

The disembowelment of the dead boy, I was told, was Romanian law. Every organ of every Romanian corpse had to be removed then placed back inside, but you only had to show proof of their removal to be in compliance of the ridiculous law: a long scar down the middle of the

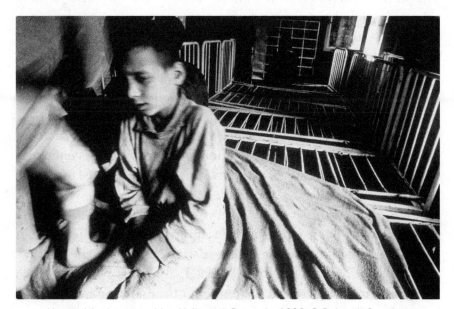

Hospital for Irrecoverables, Vulturești, Romania, 1990, © Deborah Copaken

body, another across the forehead, which was peeled down to expose the brain, the sight of which caused me to retch.

"Now what?" I'd asked the woman with the rusty saw, through a translator, as she stood in front of the boy's emptied corpse, now surrounded by his lifeless organs. She was not trained as a doctor, a coroner, or even a nurse. She was a poor village woman, whose job it was to care for too many abandoned and disabled kids with zero resources with which to care for them. Would she write up a report of her findings? Did she have the proper tools to measure his heart, his lungs, his brain? Would any of this data provide any insight into his suffering or death?

"Now we put the pieces back inside," she'd said with a shrug. As if this were a game of Operation. I had to leave the room once more to throw up.

Two weeks later, when I walked into my apartment in Paris, and I saw that backlit houseplant my future husband had left as a surprise, with its note asking for love, care, sunlight, and water, did some part of my subconscious decide: *Here's an orphan I can save?* Yes. Absolutely.

And here was a nurturer, his subconscious must have decided, he could claim. Most marriages in which one partner has Asperger's and the other does not are forged precisely on this dynamic. We'd fallen straight into a trap so typical for a neuroatypical/neurotypical relationship, it was mundane.

After his diagnosis—a relief to both of us, as it explained everything we'd been up against as a couple—I read every book I could on the subject of Asperger's and intimate relationships, discovering passage after passage describing our dynamic in textbook detail. "There can be a strong maternal compassion for the person's limited social abilities," wrote Tony Attwood in *The Complete Guide to Asperger's Syndrome*, "with a belief that his social confusion and lack of social confidence were due to his circumstances as a child, and can be repaired over time. Love will change everything."

I was, it suddenly dawned on me, reading these books, 100 percent complicit in my own unmet needs from the start. Therefore at least 50 percent responsible for the broken marriage that followed. Nowhere in that note left on the houseplant or later, in our marital vows, which we each wrote privately, did my future husband ever promise or even mention reciprocal care. I had simply convinced myself, without any concrete evidence to the contrary, that if I nourished the parched soil of this once-broken child, he would grow into the kind of man who'd produce the emotional oxygen I, too, needed to survive. Instead, over the course of the next two decades, I struggled to breathe. "You have no empathy!" I would scream, over and over again.

"I don't even know what that means!" he'd shout back, visibly shaken and hurt. I thought he was being deliberately dense.

"No," says our Asperger's therapist, Dr. Richard Perry, decades after the steps of this dance were firmly entrenched. "He's not being deliberately dense. He literally does not know what you mean."

How did this dynamic play out in day-to-day life? In ways, I told our therapist, both large and small. If I stepped on a shard of glass or cut my finger in lieu of an onion and said, "Ow!" this did not elicit an "Are you okay?" but rather either a kind of stunned silence or rebuke for not wearing shoes or being clumsy. My tears over the death of a beloved professor evoked an "Eh, death," with a blasé flick of his hand. He once stepped outside a restaurant to take a non-emergency call from his twin brother at the beginning of our fifth wedding anniversary dinner, before the appetizers had arrived, and didn't return to the table until after the main course had grown cold. When our boiler broke one particularly cold week in February and left us with no heat or hot water, and I emerged blue-lipped from a cold shower and asked him to please bring me a dry towel, as he'd taken mine, his response was a terse, "No."

One of the clearest signs of a person with Asperger's, Dr. Perry tells us, is that what often seems to be an intentional infliction of pain is actually completely unintentional. This rings painfully true. My husband isn't cruel, I say, but his actions—or in many cases his lack of actions— are. Not only to me, although I bear the brunt of it, but sometimes with our kids and friends, too.

When our four-year-old was admitted to the hospital with what would turn out to be Kawasaki disease—the leading cause of heart attacks in children under the age of five—and I pleaded with him to come to the hospital to help me, he went out for drinks for his boss's birthday instead. Fifteen years earlier, when our eldest, then eight months old, produced several diapers full of gelatinous blood, the pediatrician on call correctly suspected intussusception and urged us to meet her at the hospital immediately. "Deb, it's ten o'clock!" said the father of our critically bleeding child. "Couldn't you have waited until morning?" Intussusception, the doctor had told me on the phone—though common in infant boys between the ages of five and nine months—is an intestinal blockage which, if left untreated, is uniformly fatal.

That's not to say he was a bad father. Unlike his own absent father, he wasn't. In fact, in so many important ways, he was better than most, particularly after the kids turned five. ("Call me when they're five," he'd often say. It took me a while to realize he wasn't joking.) He could sit for hours with them in front of a bowl of fruit, teaching them how to draw. During summer vacations, he had the energy, enthusiasm, and creativity of a camp counselor. He loved exploring foreign cities and experiencing art and music and nature with them, often planning hikes and trips and excursions weeks in advance.

But these carefully wrought plans could also be extremely rigid. If he'd planned to take our children to a museum, but they wanted to go bowling instead, the resulting dissonance could ruin the weekend. Meanwhile, his sudden impulse or desire to do a new activity, once something else was already in full swing, resulted in moments such as the time we were hosting our friends Rebecca and Matt for dinner, and he stood up, just as the four of us were all sitting down to eat, announced he was going to the gym, and walked out the door.

It wasn't until two decades into our marriage, while speaking with Dr. Perry, that I would learn that hosting meals—a task my husband seemed unusually adept at both planning and enjoying—was so stressful to him that he would have to periodically get up and leave the table, go into our bedroom, and lie down on the floor to stare up at the ceiling and regenerate, a habit I'd always chalked up to frequent bathroom breaks. This was doubly confusing to learn as he was, more often than not, the initiator and executor of these meals, such as the all-day cassoulet feast he personally planned, cooked, and organized every winter for years.

Preparing that meal, which our children once mistook for a national holiday ("What do other families do on Cassoulet Day?"), took three full days of painstaking, bean-by-bean, sausage-by-duck steps, which he would then carefully notate in a growing multipage file on his computer. I finally read that mad scientist document, for the first time, after we were asked to co-write an essay in a food anthology, which would take its title from our essay, "The Cassoulet Saved Our Marriage." Our contribution was written in the form of emails back and forth between us: his heartbreakingly hopeful and minimizing; mine burdened with the deep ambivalence and sadness that would augur our end. I begged the editor to please consider changing the title of the book—she couldn't—as it was being published at the precise moment that our marriage was in free fall.

But the real revelation of co-writing that essay with him for me was this: Until I saw his multipage, minute-by-minute, step-by-step cassoulet document, with its yearly honing of precise methods and temperatures and times, I hadn't realized that the three-day preparation of the dish was not the challenge he had to get through every year before enjoying the meal with friends but rather the point of the exercise entirely. Serving it to our guests, including Nora, Nick, and others, was the challenge.

There were other oddities I mistook for lovable eccentricities, prediagnosis, that I would later come to understand were obvious signposts of high-functioning autism as well. His encyclopedic knowledge of armaments was so precise that when I spotted tanks rolling down Gorky Street on the first morning of the Soviet coup, and I yelled, "Oh my god! Tanks! Run!" his immediate response was to stand still in Red Square and correct my inaccuracy. "No, they're not tanks. They're APCs. BTR-60s, to be exact. Why would you call them tanks?" When peak oil was suddenly in the news, he became so obsessed with reading and talking about it, I would have to make excuses to the friends upon whom he'd meticulously unload his doomsday scenarios as they tried to change the subject.

All of these personality quirks and empathy-challenged moments I would have been able to accept in the name of keeping our marriage together, I tell our autism therapist, had our marital bed, which should have been our raft, not, instead, become our Titanic.

Other women married to Aspie men speak of similar daily struggles, in which their partners view intimacy through a utilitarian lens or their needs become misaligned. "Whenever I tell him that I am too tired for an encounter," one said, "he tries to convince me that I don't need to do anything. He says, 'You can even go to sleep,' as if that would make it easier. Usually, I'm too tired to explain to him why this reasoning makes me sick to my stomach."

Trying to keep the peace and keep my marriage intact, I would periodically give in to my husband's needs in lieu of my own: the worst re-sponse, in retrospect—albeit textbook as well—as it created both frustration on his part and porous boundaries on mine. These porous boundaries, which I fully own and regret, only fueled his insistence on continuing to cross them, creating a vicious circle of despair instead of connection.

In most marriages that fail, including mine, the off-course grooves marking these circles become so deep and entrenched that the turntable keeps skipping, ruining the song. At that point in the discord, when only dissonance and repetition remain, both partners are to blame for keep-ing it going. Chicken, egg, it doesn't matter who started it. The sound of that skipping record is now untenable to both, the needle stuck forever in the same spot. The unkind actions of one keep leading to the angry and defensive reactions of the other, creating an infinite negative feed-back loop, which in our case looked something like this: His lack of empathy, absence from the home and its responsibilities, and constant attempts to assert control led to my tears and tantrums; my tears and tantrums made him less likely to come home and more likely to want to assert control. Rinse, repeat. Ad infinitum.

Lost in this maelstrom was love.

Because I could not come up with an exit strategy that did not in-volve the dissolution of our marriage; because ending our marriage, I knew, would inflict pain on our children; because marital vows, to me, were still sacrosanct; because no one in my family had ever divorced except Great-Aunt Ruth, one week after her wedding, and that was only because her husband had brought his mother along on the honeymoon; because until that fateful lunch at Nora's, when I finally spoke the words out loud, I'd been too ashamed to open up about the more troubling matters of intimacy to friends and family; because making ends meet as a married couple in America was already a challenge with one partner on the spectrum, the other with all of her professional eggs in media's shrinking basket, and a middle class dissolving faster than you could say "subprime mortgage crisis"; because our health insurance was tied to my husband's job, not mine; because single motherhood, I rightly assumed, would be financially and emotionally challenging; because homeless-ness and bankruptcy were not the irrational fears of a doomsday catastro-phist but rather both real and imminent; because my bed had become a place of fear and sadness instead of one of safety and love; because of all of these things, I kept embarking on mini escapes from the marriage. Many of which I hid, even from myself, in the guise of professional pursuits.

"Why didn't you just leave?" people will often ask today, as if that thought hadn't occurred to me several times each day or multiple times in a single hour. But like most women in similar relationships, where it takes seven attempts, on average, to finally pack it up and leave, my first forays into flight took the form of these temporary departures.

Escape

2001–2003

A few weeks after 9/11, I convinced O, *The Oprah Magazine* to send my then six-year-old son and me back to my early stomping grounds, Peshawar, Pakistan, to deliver aid to Afghan refugee children at the start of the U.S. ground war. I'd traded war photography for TV news, followed by book publishing and magazine journalism, wanting to minimize my children's exposure to a dead mother. But in those anthrax-filled weeks following 9/11, when staying in New York felt as risky as covering a war, parents in my son's first grade class had suddenly begun questioning why our children's teacher had launched a class humanitarian project of selling the students' handmade bookmarks to raise money for Afghan refugees. "Why are we raising money for Afghan refugees, isn't that like raising money for the enemy?" I heard one of them ask, which is when something inside me snapped.

I'd covered the end of the war in Afghanistan in 1989, the one to which the U.S. had sent Stinger missiles in the name of containing Soviet communism, when I was a twenty-two-year-old cub reporter on her second big assignment. I knew the damage we'd left in our wake, the moral corruption of our aid, how all of it eventually came back to haunt us via the attack my daughter and I had witnessed from our roof. "We'll get the money there ourselves," I rashly promised my son's teacher, explaining that we could do so in relative safety if we stuck to the camps in Peshawar, miles away from the ground war in Afghanistan.

Over the course of ten days, this was what we did, adding toys, fruit leathers, school supplies, and whatever sports equipment we could carry, while also going from school to school and refugee camp to refugee camp with a missionary zeal, hoping to convince a bunch of war-traumatized kids that not all of us in the U.S. wanted them dead.

One day, in the lobby of the Pearl Continental Hotel, I befriended *Wall Street Journal* correspondent Daniel Pearl, one of the only other journalists who stayed behind in Peshawar after the start of the conflict. My son had been in the men's bathroom off the lobby for too long, so I asked Danny to please check in on him. "He's fine!" said Danny, returning with a smile. "He's doing his thing and singing show tunes." As we waited for my son to emerge, I asked Danny why he hadn't run off across the border like everyone else. The hotel, once overbooked and teeming with journalists, was now nearly empty. "My wife's pregnant with our first child," he said. He didn't want to put himself in undue danger. He was covering a different side of the story, he said. A relatively safer side.

"Same," I said, telling him of our exploits.

Three months later, Danny was beheaded by al-Qaeda kingpin Khalid Sheikh Mohammed, who would later claim personal responsibility for wielding the knife. I was on my paperback book tour when I read the news. In some hotel somewhere, bawling.

Some of my friends and family members had expressed concern and, in a few cases, horror over my bringing a six-year-old to Peshawar. I obviously understood their finger-wagging, but I do not regret our trip. In fact, my now adult son still remembers our daily visits to refugee camps, if vaguely, as a seminal moment in his own understanding of the world and his place in it. He'd brought his own Legos to give the children, but instead of playing together, each tried to hoard and hide pieces in hands, pockets, and mouths. "No!" he'd said. "Don't do that. We have to build something together. Look, like this . . ." The kids immediately understood and started cooperating on a single structure.

On the night after our return, when his little sister whined about being deprived of a second cupcake after dinner, he stood up on his chair, pointed his finger at her, and said, "There are places in the world *where there are no cupcakes!*"

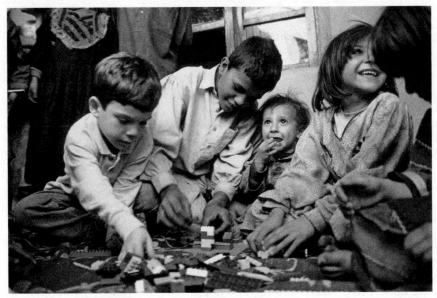

Kachagari Refugee Camp. Peshawar, Pakistan, November 2001, © Deborah Copaken

Viewing our trip now, however, through unfogged goggles, it's clear that providing aid to refugees and showing my child his obligations as a human toward other humans were not my only motivations. Much less romantically, we needed the money. My husband had lost both his physical office building and his job in the wake of 9/11, and O, The Oprah Magazine, for whom I was both writing and shooting the accompanying photos, paid well on both fronts. One of my primary motivations, however, was a ten-day reprieve from my marriage. Which begs the obvious question: How unhappy at home must a woman be to bring her young son to the borderlands of a war?

Soon after arriving home from Peshawar, suffering from clinical depression and seeking further escape, I rented the cheapest office I could find, in a former fabric factory on lower Broadway that had not yet been sold to developers, where I would retreat every day to write my second book, the novel *Suicide Wood* (later retitled by my publisher to *Between Here and April*[*]). That this unheated, filthy room, for which I was paying $179 a month, was dark, drafty, and in disrepair, with a view of an air

---

[*] I wanted to keep *Suicide Wood* but was told, once again, I had no say in the matter. My publisher felt a Dante reference in the title might harm sales. The novel is an allegory of *The Inferno*.

shaft through a blackened window, felt apt for the task at hand: mining the blackest coals within me.

I based the novel on the true story of my best friend from first grade, Connie Hummel, whose mother had killed her, herself, and Connie's two siblings in 1972 by attaching a vacuum hose to the tailpipe of the family car. I then forced my stand-in protagonist, the book's narrator, Lizzie, to live through many of the pains and miseries at the heart of my own marriage, only tempered: In the margins next to one particular scene, later excised, my agent had written, "Too much. Too horrific. Strains the bounds of credulity." I left that scene in the novel when I turned it in, only to be chastised again in red ink by my editor's hand. "No," she said, when I called her on the phone and asked her to keep it. "I'm sorry. But I don't buy it. No woman would ever put up with that kind of abuse in a marriage. Not even a weak one, and Lizzie's not weak." I wasn't capable yet of telling either of them — or anyone — that I knew an allegedly strong woman who had and would: me.

Though I'm less ashamed to admit this today than I would have been back then, there were many days, during the decades-long, drawn-out death spiral of my marriage, when I, like my protagonist, craved the escape of nothingness. My kids, at particularly low points, were the only anchors keeping me from taking out a shovel and digging my own grave.

"The overwhelming majority of non-Asperger's syndrome partners stated that their mental health had significantly deteriorated due to the relationship," writes Tony Attwood, a clinical psychologist who specializes in the field. Moreover, many reported a deterioration in physical health as well.

Fearing that I might harm myself, I sought treatment under the care of a psychiatrist, in whose office, week after week, the continual pattern of pain and escape, action and reaction, suddenly became clear, stretching all the way back through childhood. Volatility? Be the straight-A student beyond reproach. Assault, rape? Run off to war and enmesh yourself with abusive lovers. Pain? Escape it. By any means necessary.

I even escaped, periodically, back into cigarettes, after having quit in my late twenties, sneaking one every so often between the kids' bedtime and mine, blowing smoke through the security bars on my kitchen window like an inmate in solitary. I escaped, too, into every piece of literature of marital discord I could get my hands on: Roth and Updike,

Tolstoy and Flaubert, Woolf, Plath, and yes, Ephron, whose *Heartburn*, upon rereading, made my heart ache with recognition. I also escaped in the late '90s—I'm ashamed to admit this as well—into an inappropriately close relationship with a neighborhood father, who was dealing with his own downward marital trajectory: a freemasonry of fellow sufferers, as Dickens might have called it.

My therapist called it an emotional affair.

At the time, I justified our constant email and phone contact, in the twisted synapses of my mind, as a necessary corrective. For both of us. Here was a man, I told myself, equally unhappy in his own marriage, who actually heard and saw me as I heard and saw him; whose empathy and attentions were not only dependable but sometimes too much so. The more I examine those months and words from the distance of years and language, however, the more I see the mirage of us for what it was (two drowning people pulling each other under) and what it was not (love).

The neighborhood dad and I cut ties when he separated from his wife and started bringing up a different marriage: ours. I wanted to fix what was broken in the marriage I had, I told him, not jump into another catastrophe. He needed to leave me alone—stop emailing, stop calling, stop making me mix CDs and inviting me out dancing, stop showing up at my office, uninvited—so I could do the necessary work of repair, unburdened by extraneous complications. His constant attentions were becoming both millstone and liability. So when he called on the morning of 9/11, a few months after I'd asked him to please respect my wishes and leave me alone, the conversation went something like this:

HIM: "Turn on your TV."
ME: "I told you to stop calling me."
HIM: "I know, but . . . a plane flew into the World Trade Center."

I pictured a small aircraft, a wayward gust of wind. "That's no reason to contact me. Please, leave me alone."

"Jesus Christ, just turn on your TV!"

I turned on my TV just in time to watch the second plane fly into the towers. You know the rest, except what I left out, in my earlier telling, was that the neighborhood dad who showed up at my apartment and offered to watch my daughter while I fetched my son across town was him. Part of me was enraged that he'd used the excuse of a terrorist attack to reconnect. The other part was both grateful and on stone-cold autopilot: My six-year-old was far away and frightened during an unfurling tragedy, and I needed to bring him home. Now, every time anyone mentions where they were on 9/11, or how they found out—meaning often, particularly for those of us who live in New York—I am forced to reconcile not only with the national pain of that day and grief over lost friends, but also with my moral shortcomings.

It would take another twelve years, a third child, the death of my father, and two more moving vans for me to finally admit, first to Nora, then to myself, that there was not enough bubble wrap in the world to protect our family.

Lunch with Nora, E.A.T.

DECEMBER 2011

ou're not eating," says Nora. We are sitting at our usual table at
E.A.T., a restaurant around the corner from Nora's apartment, but
today not even the cucumber and dill is doing it for me. Stress has eaten
my appetite. Anemia from my worsening adenomyosis has eaten my red
blood cells. *The Red Book*, my new baby, is coming out in April, with all
of the pre-publication responsibilities this entails: a book trailer, essays,
a new website, social media promotion—anything and everything to get
the news of its birth out there, now that local newspapers are dead. My
human babies are sixteen, fourteen, and five, with all of the responsibilities that they entail. My father's death has left an empathy hole in my
life where once he stood.

"I had a big breakfast," I say. "I'm not hungry."

"No. Sorry," says Nora. "You are not allowed to add anorexia onto
adeno . . . whatever it's called. Did you schedule that surgery yet?"

"Adenomyosis. And no. I have not scheduled the hysterectomy yet. I
can't have a major operation right now. It's not a good time. I'll do it after
my novel comes out. Where can I get a yahrzeit candle around here?"

Nora laughs. "On the Upper East Side?" She gestures out the window to Madison Avenue, bustling with holiday shoppers. "I'm sure even
the dry cleaners have them."

Jews light commemorative candles—yahrzeit candles—every year on the eve of the anniversary of a parent's death. *Yahrzeit* is a Yiddish word that means simply "time of year." It is early December, 2011, that time of year, which is to say one day shy of three years since my father's death.

I laugh. "True." Then my bottom lip starts to quiver.

Nora, unusually, takes her hand and places it atop mine. Though I've come to rely on her these days more as surrogate mother than mentor, she's not the touchy-feely kind. Her maternal love takes the form of unsentimental, direct truths, spoken plainly but with humor, encouragement, and a brush-yourself-off-and-keep-going practicality. But not today. Today she's fine wallowing along with me. "I know," she says, seeming to tear up as well. "He was a special guy."

At the book party for my novel in 2008, Nora and my father, Richard Copaken—a lawyer, weekend artist, and self-proclaimed movie buff who, in his final years had started a company that used algorithms to predict the future success of films—had spent most of the night together huddled in the corner, chatting. They were the same age, sixty-seven, born a month apart. They were both dealing with cancer diagnoses, although only my father had gone public with his—pancreatic, stage 4, prognosis: imminent death. At that point, Nora hadn't even told her sons about hers.

Which is weird, as she was the self-proclaimed Queen of Indiscretion. Years before it was public knowledge, she told me and anyone else who would listen that Deep Throat was Mark Felt. At one of my dinner parties, when my good friend and downstairs neighbor Marco, a journalist for Italian *Vanity Fair,* asked Nora if she was working on a new movie, she said yes, but it was a secret, and she was sorry, but she wasn't allowed to talk about it. Then she proceeded to tell him every last detail about *Julie and Julia,* including the fact that she'd just spoken to Meryl Streep that afternoon about coming on as its lead.

I sometimes wonder if she shared the secret of her illness with my dad that night at my book party, so intense was their conversation. He was the kind of person in whom you would confide such a thing. Particularly if you saw, from the way his suit jacket hung from his shoulders like an air mattress after deflation, that his time here was limited: a few weeks, as it turned out. But by the time I found out Nora was sick, it was too late to ask her.

"He's amazing," Nora would later say, having met him for the first time that night. Everyone who met my father said the same, from taxi drivers to teachers, homeless men to heads of state. The writer Malcolm Gladwell wrote a profile of him for *The New Yorker* after meeting him, describing his guileless glee, his giant Charlie Brown head, the way he was not afraid to cry in public when describing film scenes that moved him. His existence, in many ways, had allowed me to stay in my marriage far beyond its expiration date: He was the one who showed up to wheel me out of the hospital after an emergency appendectomy; who answered my calls with open ears and soothing words; who slept on my children's bedroom floor—speaking of air mattresses—for six weeks to be the on-set guardian for my eldest, who had been tapped to play a role in a film, when I was on bed rest during my pregnancy with my youngest. "I couldn't believe how completely at ease he was with his diagnosis," Nora continued. "Cracking jokes about the born-again plumber who came over to fix the toilet but ended up telling him to take Jesus into his heart."

Dad loved Harold, his plumber. He helped his son get into college. They spent hours gabbing in the kitchen together, after whichever clog Harold had come to fix was unclogged. When born-again Harold found out Dad was dying, he was distraught. He sat him down and spoke his mind. My Jewish father just nodded and promised Harold he would do whatever it took to stay alive, including accepting Jesus into his heart, if that would make Harold feel better. "I have to say," Dad later wrote on happydickissick.com, the blog I helped him create to keep friends and family apprised of his health, "whether it was Christ's will or just Harold's plumbing skills, the toilet now flushes beautifully."

"Look," says Nora, switching back to her no-nonsense self. "In terms of the hysterectomy, what exactly are you worried about when you imagine going under the knife? Aside from the whole 'not feeling like a woman anymore' because really, stop."

"I'm not worried about going under the knife," I say, moving the pieces of cucumber around on my plate like pawns on a chessboard. "I'm worried about the aftermath. About being helpless with a man who's not shown himself to be helpful when I'm incapacitated. Remember what happened after my appendectomy?"

"Yes," says Nora. "That was less than ideal."

Fun fact no one tells you when you get pregnant, or at least no one ever told me: The risk of acute appendicitis in postpartum women over the age of thirty-five—otherwise known as a "geriatric pregnancy" or "advanced maternal age"—is 84 percent greater than the risk to the general public. And so four months after giving birth to my youngest in 2006, when I was forty years old, I found myself writhing in pain on the emergency room floor, frantically trying to finish an edit of one of my essays with Dan Jones, the editor of *The New York Times* Modern Love column, before being admitted for an appendectomy. But the emergency room was crowded, the hospital guard kept yelling at me to get up off the floor and sit on a chair, and I kept telling him that sitting, right now, was not an option for my body. Then I had to explain to Dan what all of the yelling and commotion was about. "Wait, what?" said Dan, when he found out where I was and why and that I'd called him to finish the edit before calling my spouse to come join me. He insisted I hang up the phone and call my husband before we finish the edit, so someone could be my advocate in the hospital and get me admitted. How to explain to Dan that my husband's presence during times of need could be a kind of absence? Couldn't he divine that from the essay?

"Maybe he'll surprise you," says Nora. "Plus you can't get from point A—my uterus is diseased and needs to come out—to point B—it's out—if you don't take that first step. You look completely wan. Anemic. What are you, forty-four?"

"Forty-five."

"Your skin should not be that shade of gray at my age, let alone yours. So no more excuses. Get it done." Nora's tone is unusually urgent: a demand this time, not a suggestion. In seven months, she will be dead. She's in full-on mother-hen, affairs-in-order mode. "Or at least just promise me you'll make the appointment to get a hysterectomy as soon as possible. I'll come visit. I promise."

"Okay, okay, I'll schedule the surgery for after my book comes out." I fiddle with my wedding band: a new tic.

Nora notices. She notices everything. "How are things going with Joyce?"

I laugh. "Joyce is great. Really great at her job. Thank you for the recommendation."

"And the marriage?

I sigh. Not wanting to disappoint Nora, but unable to find hopeful words.

My desperation for love—to be seen and heard and understood and mirrored—has become pathological. I feel lonely all the time. I'd had lunch earlier that year with an old boyfriend who lived across the country and was in town for work, and we'd struck up a lengthy email correspondence afterward. We'd met and fallen in love in Jamaica in our early twenties, spent a week together in London when he was studying there, and then our budding relationship abruptly ended not because we'd broken up or fallen out of love, but because when he'd flown to Paris to spend the weekend with me at my place, he'd lost the scrap of paper with my address and phone number on it and wound up spending two nights alone in a youth hostel instead.

For twenty years, I thought he'd stood me up.

"It was nuts," he finally explained to me, of the missed connection nearly impossible to fathom in the age of the internet. I was unlisted. He'd wandered around Paris the whole weekend, trying to come up with any clues: the name of my photo agency, my neighborhood, an address, anything. Two years after that thwarted weekend, a friend of his had come back to the U.S. from a vacation in Paris with a stack of photos, and there I was, apparently, in the background of several of his snapshots of Père Lachaise, the Parisian cemetery in which Jim Morrison is buried. I'd had an assignment from *Libération* that day, to shoot the anniversary of Morrison's death. "That's my old girlfriend!" my once-boyfriend said to his friend. "Did you talk to her? Did you get her number?"

The friend hadn't. But even if he had, it wouldn't have mattered. By the time he saw those photos, I was already living with my future husband. When Google came along, the lost boyfriend googled my name. A photo appeared of my older kids and me in an article about my first book. Until then, he said, he'd still held out some vague hope we might find each other. He then married and started a family with the next woman who came along. And so life goes.

With this man, because he was not part of my social circle and never would be; because our relationship had ended the way it had, and we had a lot of catching up to do; because he'd known a past me that had not yet been beaten down by my present self; and because I had the shield of physical distance and a blinking cursor on a screen, I felt comfortable being brutally honest about the day-to-day exigencies of living with a spouse on the spectrum. His responses floored me with their perception and empathy. How was it that this person with whom I'd spent only a few weeks in my early twenties and who lived three thousand miles away saw me more clearly than my spouse of two decades? That was the kind of love I wanted: To be known. To be seen. To be heard and understood. No, not by the lost boyfriend—he was married, with three kids, to a wonderful woman—but by someone like him or, in the absence of an empathic substitute, by no one: The loneliness of single parenthood, I finally decided, would be preferable to feeling alone in my marriage.

And with this too-obvious epiphany—an epiphany I should have had years before—I finally spoke the words out loud in couples therapy: "I want a divorce." My husband, shocked, asked for one more chance to get things right. With our therapist's blessing, after a discussion of specific changes to be made as conditions for staying in the marriage, I agreed.

That week, the man I married put tangible effort into being a loving partner and a good father. He communicated clearly. He came home in time for dinner. He helped with the dishes. He listened. He tried. He turned down NPR when the kids asked him to and apologized when he messed up. He was kind and thoughtful in our intimate spaces. He paid careful attention to the needs of others. He brought home flowers. He did not complain or induce guilt when I went out to my monthly Torah class, whose topic that week was, ironically, empathy. Specifically the moment in Exodus when Moses asks God why he, of all humans, should be the one to lead the Jews out of Egypt. To which God says, "I will be with you." Not, "Buck up, kid, you've got this!" or "Because I'm too busy," or "So what, what's the big deal?" but a simple expression of empathy for the difficult journey ahead and a promise to be present throughout it: "I will be with you." Which is all I'd ever wanted out of my marriage.

Through tears of gratitude at couples therapy at the end of that week, I said that if that's the kind of spouse he could be from now on, I was absolutely willing to give our marriage another shot: to forget all his injuries and oddities and move forward into a clean-slate future.

It was a Friday night. I cooked us dinner: roast chicken, potatoes, spinach, a challah. We lit candles. He cleared the table. I swept the floor. The kids scurried off to their rooms, leaving us knee to knee on the couch, holding hands like moony teenagers and listening to The National's "Slow Show": my then favorite song, his less-than-favorite, but this time he didn't skip to the next song with an "Ugh, I hate this, it's so whiny." He simply let it play, knowing its notes brought me joy.

Finally, I thought, tearing up from the simple delights of a conflict-free Friday night: a real marriage. We can do this. I thanked him for his efforts. Said I noticed them and was grateful. Told him that if we could keep going forward like this, we'd make it. But then his BlackBerry buzzed, notifying him of new emails, and he fished it out of his back pocket to read them. There, on the face of his phone, a dozen or so emails from Jdate—a dating app for Jews seeking to date other Jews— suddenly went scrolling by, one atop the other, a waterfall of wishful Wendys and randy Rebeccas. He immediately tried to turn the screen away from me, but it was too late. I'd already drowned.

"Why are you getting emails from Jdate?" I said, feeling suddenly sick, on the verge of regurgitating challah and chicken all over the living room rug.

"It's just spam," he said.

"Please don't lie to me," I said. "The cover-up is always worse than the crime. I get it. I said I wanted a divorce last week, so you signed up for Jdate to see what else is out there, and now—"

He cut me off. Looked me straight in the eye, just like he did during our mafia game at Nora's. "I swear to god, Deb. Look at me. I did not sign up for Jdate. It's just spam."

"Stop lying!" I said. "Companies don't send spam fifteen emails at a time! And why would they target you anyway? You're middle-aged and married! Just admit it, please, and let's deal with this new wrinkle next Friday with Joyce and move on honestly from there."

"I'm not lying!" He doubled down. "I swear to god! I swear on our children's lives!"

The gaslighting went on for five days, back and forth, back and forth—"Stop lying!" "I'm not!" "Stop lying!" "I'm not!"—until finally, on the fifth morning, after the kids had left for school and were out of earshot, I lost it. I screamed. I cursed. I strained my vocal cords until they broke—unfortunate, as I was scheduled to perform live storytelling at the 92nd Street Y that same night. I called him a fucking gaslighter and an asshole and a dick and a liar and everything horrific and ugly and insulting in between. "Stop lying to me! Stop lying to me! Stop lying to me!" I wailed, unable to control myself. Snot poured out of my nose. I was part trapped animal, part monster on the verge of ripping off his head with my giant monster teeth. If he was telling the story of our marriage, he could point to that morning and say, "My wife was totally unhinged." Because in that moment, like Ingrid Bergman in *Gaslight*, I was. After about an hour or so of this ugliness, he finally admitted the truth. "Okay, fine, I signed up for Jdate! So what? What's the big deal?"

I shook my head and walked out. If he couldn't understand why this was a big deal to me—or, rather, why his five days of lying about it were—we were done.

"How's my marriage?" I say to Nora. "About as healthy as my uterus."

"Are you still corresponding with that old boyfriend?"

"No. It was palliative but stupid."

"Thank god," says Nora. "That would have gone nowhere good."

Nora grabs for the bill when it comes as usual.

"No," I say. "This time I want to pay. Please. I insist."

"Okay, okay," she says, after several rounds of this, finally releasing her hold on the server book. "But, I need to say something, and I don't want you to get upset." She pauses, weighing her words. "He doesn't have Asperger's, you know. I'm sure of it."

"What? No, stop." This is the only argument we will ever have in our eleven-year friendship, the only time her well-earned confidence about always being right gets in the way of the truth. It's partially my fault. For years I have shielded her, my trusted confidante, from my marriage's uglier moments the same way I've shielded my various doctors from what was really going on inside my body. Why? A combination of shame and not wanting to complain. "You're wrong," I say.

In many ways, Nora's and my backstories are similar: both the eldest of four girls; both writers of personal essays; both authors of memoirs and novels; both mothers of firstborn sons with the same first name. But we've become so enamored of our similarities, I haven't wanted to point out our one major difference: When her second husband, Watergate wunderkind Carl Bernstein, did something unforgivable—he cheated on her when she was pregnant with her second child—she walked out the door and never looked back. When my husband did something unforgivable, I pushed it aside, telling no one, and stayed. And stayed. And stayed. And stayed. Repressing the memory until it lodged in my body like a neglected splinter: a vague ache, somewhere there under the skin, but when you touch it, fire.

Asperger's, no Asperger's, in the end, what did labels matter? Bruises need not be visible to be calamitous, and I stayed in a sometimes abusive and empathyless marriage for decades instead of leaving it. That's on me and solely on me, and I regret not leaving years earlier. It's not that I couldn't leave, as much as I told myself otherwise. It's that I chose, every day, to stay. I was the peacekeeper as a child as well. It's a learned behavior, this avoidance and suppression. Always saying sorry first and solo, even if it's not your fault. Presenting a false front to the world for the sake of family loyalty: the ultimate self-annihilating omertà. But once you've learned this behavior, like a drunk party guest it lingers, permanently occupying the sleeper sofa of your psyche. Even now, after years of therapy, knowing everything I do about my own propensity for peacekeeping and minimizing, I'll still catch myself saying a cheerful "No worries!" to someone who's hurt me. When what I want to say is "Fuck you."

"I'm not wrong about the Asperger's," says Nora. "But we're going to drop this conversation right now, because I see that I've upset you."

"You are wrong, and we're not going to drop it," I say. With rare people, I'm sometimes able to suppress the suppression, to go to war with the peacekeeping. Nora, at the end of her life, was one of them. My husband's diagnosis, I tell her, in so many words, is not the daily special instead of the chicken salad at Freds or the beets instead of the cucumbers with dill at E.A.T. You can't just choose no Asperger's over Asperger's on the menu because you have a hunch the doctor is wrong. "He was diagnosed," I remind her, "by one of the foremost experts in autism spectrum disorders in New York City. He scored 8 out of a possible 80 points on the EQ test. He has all the hallmarks of the disorder and then some, whatever you want to call it, Asperger's or garden variety lack of empathy." Nora knows all of this. We've gone over it countless times. Plus no one knows what goes on in a marriage except the couple in it, and even they are living two different realities of the same relationship.

"But he's so at ease at our dinner parties. And he truly seems to love you. It doesn't make sense. I know people who are far more dysfunctional than he is. I've seen Asperger's up close, and I'm telling you: He doesn't have it."

"It's a ruse, his ease," I say. "He mimics it. He was a child actor, remember?" When his mother lost her job after applying for asylum under Brezhnev and became a refusenik, he and his twin brother made up the difference in lost income by acting in Russian films. "He's a chameleon. It's a survival skill. When he's with his friend Joe, he starts talking with Joe's Reno drawl and Hollywood swagger. When he's with his Orthodox family, he might as well be a Hasid. When he's with you and Nick, he becomes the urban sophisticate. He knows how to watch and listen carefully and learn behaviors. He watched rom-coms, for example, to figure out how to woo me."

"Seriously?" says Nora, rom-com auteur.

"Yes, seriously." At the end of our first heady weekend together in Paris, he'd insisted we each walk around the Pompidou on different sides of it, so we could feel the pain and loneliness of being apart again, after forty-eight straight hours of uninterrupted time together. I hadn't wanted to do this—why masochistically impose an artificial rom-com trope of separating the new lovers before bringing them back together when you didn't have to—but I went along with it.

Our subsequent reunion hug, in front of a line of moviegoers, was, indeed, cinematic and indelible, but not in the way he might have planned. It took years, in fact, of reliving that moment in my head, over and over again, to understand that the story of us was not the story of a couple who happily reunited with a public hug in front of a queue of moviegoers after an artificial separation. It was the story of a woman who agreed, against her better judgment and desires, to engage in an unnecessary moment of imposed pain for the sake of another's pleasure.

Nora is shaking her head, confused. "You mean he studied what men did in rom-coms and then . . . copied it?"

"More or less, yes," I say, "but here's the thing: Rom-coms always end with a wedding, right? Or just before it. Or just after, with maybe a montage of the happy couple a year later with their brand-new baby, like at the end of *Four Weddings and a Funeral*. But without a road map for the after part of happily ever after, he's had to learn on the job. Deprived of a model for fatherhood, he's had to create his own. Yes, he loves his children, and unlike his own father, he stuck around, and he 'loves me'" — I make air quotes — "in his own way, sure, okay. Because I take care of him. Ease his way. Deal with the kids and our home and earn money and help him translate the world through my neurotypical eyes. But he has no idea how to reciprocate care, and aside from that one week before the Jdate fiasco, he hasn't seemed particularly interested in learning how to fake it, as so many people with Asperger's learn to do. He himself was *relieved* at the diagnosis: It made him understand the giant disconnect between who he thinks he is and how others see him."

I give her one more example, the one that always comes to mind, simultaneously breaking my heart and making me laugh in equal measure: I'm sitting with our two older kids on an Amtrak train on the Sunday night after Thanksgiving, waiting for him to show up. He's wandered off again to explore. My daughter is eight months old, her older brother just turned two. They are appropriately squirmy, apoplectic, and exhausted after the long weekend at my parents'. From the stench of it, each needs a diaper change. "Yes, this seat is taken," I say, for the hundredth time, as frustrated and angry passengers on the standing-room-only train glare at me. The train doors shut. We start to move. *Oh, well,* I think. *He didn't make it.* I give away the empty seat to a kind older woman, who engages my toddler with her compact mirror while I feed the baby. A few minutes later, my husband appears at the far end of the aisle, beaming his guileless smile — a smile I will always love, despite everything — and carrying a large cylindrical duffel bag on his shoulder, perpendicular to the aisle. As he walks toward us, overjoyed at having finally spotted his family on the crowded train, he bonks every single aisle passenger on the head with his bag, one by one. Each passenger cries out, "Ow!" or "Hey!" or "What the fuck, man?" to no avail. My husband doesn't hear them. Doesn't see them. Doesn't notice the destruction in his wake. He has one goal, us, and he keeps walking toward it with that million-watt smile, oblivious.

"Okay, fine. I'll stop," says Nora. She gives me the dreaded Nora Stare™: a raised eyebrow, chin down, crooked mouth rebuke. "But that doesn't mean I think you're right."

I laugh. "I wouldn't want you any other way." I look across the table at this daughterless woman who has all but adopted me, my friend Meg, and several other women as well: Rebecca Traister, Lena Dunham, Meghan Daum, Natasha Lyonne. Who never judges my actions but rather tries to understand and, if necessary, redirect. Who listens to what I have to say and adjusts her response accordingly. Who champions my work, even when it's not going well, and loves my children as if they were her own. "Saw that adorable son of yours on the street," she'd recently written in an email, "or rather, he spotted us. He is divine. We had a big hello and a conversation about your new apt and then he crossed the street and was embraced by another group of people entirely. How's the apt?" I'm suddenly overcome with teary gratitude for her continuing presence in my life; for her constant reaching out with kind words and gifts; for her sense of humor and joie de vivre; for her love of food and entertaining; for her fierce intelligence and strong opinions; and yes, even for her pushbacks. I say, "I love you, you know. Even though you don't believe my husband has Asperger's."

"I know," she says, rolling her eyes. Raw sentimentality unnerves her. "And I love you right back. But whether he has Asperger's or not is immaterial. He is who he is, and you married him for whatever that was, so I'm asking you please: Give him one more shot. For me, okay? Not for you. That Jdate thing was, well, it was just *idiotic*. But it's not reason enough to get divorced."

"Fine," I say, picturing at least a hundred other reasons. "I promise. I'll give him one more shot."

And for the first and last time, Nora lets me pay for lunch. "Oh! You know who has yahrzeit candles?" she says, as we walk out. "Eli's. Go there. In the back. You can't miss them."

"Perfect," I say. To get to Eli's, I have to drive right past Nora's apartment. "Wanna ride?" I say, gesturing to my Vespa. I'm joking, of course. She would never. Plus she lives one short block and two long blocks away: a five-minute walk, if that.

"I hate that you ride that thing," she says, not for the first time. But in an expensive city, where I don't own a car, and taxis are unaffordable, and the crosstown bus is slow, and I have three kids who need to be shuttled east and west across a city with north and south subways, it has been a lifesaver. Plus, I got it for free, in exchange for shooting six years of Christmas card portraits of a wealthy acquaintance who'd bought it as a fortieth birthday present for her soon-to-be ex-husband. Nora knows this, so she usually doesn't push it, but today she does. "You know, one wrong turn, and boom. No more Deb," she says, shaking her head.

"I promise," I say. "I'm really careful when I ride it."

"It's not you I'm worried about." She flags down a taxi. On cue, it nearly crashes into two other cars while screeching over two lanes without signaling. She holds out her hands. "I rest my case."

I laugh and hug her goodbye. "Wait, where are you going?" I say. She always walks back home after lunch at E.A.T.

"Home," she says, getting into the taxi.

"Are you feeling okay?" This is so unlike her.

"I'm *fine*," she says. She shuts the door and rolls down the window. "Schedule that surgery, already, please! And be nice to your husband. One more shot, okay? For my sake."

"Okay, okay," I say. I watch the blur of yellow that is Nora disappear up Madison. Then I put on my helmet and zoom off to buy a memorial candle for my dead father.

Where's the Husband?

JUNE 2012

I schedule the hysterectomy for the last week in June 2012, after my book tour is done. My surgeon asks me what kind of hysterectomy I want: full, partial, or supracervical? I have no idea what those things mean, I tell her, so she takes me through the options like a waiter presenting the daily specials. With a full hysterectomy, which includes the removal of the ovaries, I'd lose hormonal benefits. Since my mother didn't go through menopause until she was much older than I am, and there's no history of ovarian cancer in my family, we decide the benefits of keeping the ovaries and their regulating hormones outweigh the potential risks. As for the cervix, I am told, "It is believed to play a role in sexual pleasure." Huh? I am wary of passive voice conjecture. Particularly with regard to the mechanics and proper functioning of my body. *It is believed?* Who believes this? Is there proof? A study? Hello? Anything? I get a second opinion, and the second doctor tells me the same thing: "We don't know," she tells me, "but there are theories that the cervix is somehow related to female orgasm."

"We don't *know?*" I say. "We've landed men on the moon, but we don't know the basic physiological roots of female pleasure? How is that even possible?"

She sighs. "I know," she says. "It seems nuts. But most studies of human anatomy and disease have been done on men. For example, if you get a hip or knee replaced, you're getting a hip or knee designed for a man."

"Great," I say. "I'll keep that in mind if my five-foot-two female body ever needs a new hip built for a six-foot-tall man."

It will take another four years—until 2016!—for an accurate 3D model of the clitoris to be created and for any lingering theories of cervical participation in orgasm to be debunked. Following the 2012 advice of these two doctors, however, and not wanting to give up my one surefire shot of pleasure in a life so often short on it, I choose the supracervical item on the hysterectomy menu: the removal of just the uterus, leaving the cervix and ovaries intact.

"I'm dying to see you," I write Nora, the morning after my surgery, at the precise moment when she, unbeknownst to me or to any of her other surrogate daughters, is the one doing the hard work of dying.

The last time I'd seen her—an unusually long interval because of book tour responsibilities—was at my forty-sixth birthday dinner in March. The next morning, over email, she'd sent me a photo she'd taken from her vantage point as the cake emerged candlelit behind her. The photo was in color and shot with her iPhone in extremely low light. She was unhappy with how dark it was, so I'd lobbed it back to her, brightened and transformed into black-and-white. "Look what I did with it," I wrote. "Love it. I even have cleavage in it. Which makes you a magician."

Two hours later, seeing how I was able to pump light into the darkened image, she sent me one more: "Bruce at the Apollo," she wrote, just before midnight. "What can you do with this?" Indeed it was Bruce Springsteen, up close, his face darkened by shadow, in the aisle of the famous Harlem theater two nights prior. I lightened the dark side of his face as best I could with Lightroom and sent her back the image once again in black-and-white.

"Amazing shot, Nora," I wrote. "So Christ-like. Brava." The images were nothing alike and yet somehow, side by side, they were exactly alike: two humans, caught on the right side of a well-composed frame in an act of joy. Nora always derided her photography skills, but she was wrong. Just because she was shooting in low light didn't mean she hadn't captured perfect luminance or herself. Every artist, in whatever me-

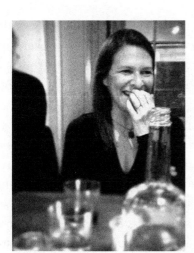

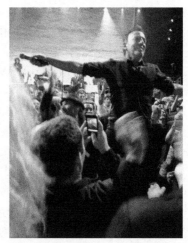

March 11, 2012, © Nora Ephron

Bruce Springsteen at the Apollo, March 9, 2012, © Nora Ephron

dium, is always communicating the same message, over and over again: This is how I see the world.

I loved how Nora saw the world.

The last time we'd spoken on the phone was the day in mid-April when *The Red Book* had hit *The New York Times* bestseller list, and she'd called me on my book tour stop in D.C. to congratulate me. "See! I told you," she said. "We'll celebrate when you're back."

The last time we'd corresponded over email had been a few weeks prior, when I'd sent her an article I'd published on Erich Segal's *The Class* in *The New York Times Book Review,* in which I'd quoted an old essay of hers from *Esquire.* She'd written back, "Terrific. It came out great. Xxx." Of course it had. She'd helped edit it. From her sick bed, as it turns out, though I did not know this then.

I continue typing from my own bed: "Just back from my hysterectomy, which is now complicated by a surgery-induced hernia that may have to be repaired ASAP. Meaning, god knows when I'll be on my feet again, but wanted to see what your summer looks like so we can plan something in, I dunno, late July? Silly, I know, but I miss you. xx, D."

Unusually, she does not write back. Or even call. I'm unnerved by this, particularly since she's been badgering me to get the surgery now for over a year, and she always responds to my emails within an hour or two, max. I shut my computer, take a painkiller, and fall asleep.

The hysterectomy—which, just as Nora had predicted, was done with robot arms—had lasted a little over eight hours. I'd woken up in recovery to the sounds of the nurses whispering: "Where's the husband? Has anyone seen the husband? We can't reach him. Is there another number?"

"What?" I said, suddenly cogent if groggy and in pain.

"We can't find your husband," said the unfamiliar faces now hovering over my head. "Is there anyone else we can call at this time?"

"Ahhhhhhhhhh!!!!!" I screamed, feeling the hernia pop out. "Ahhhh-hhhhhhhhhhhhhhhh!!!!!!"

I started thrashing along with my screaming, trying to pull out various IVs and tubes, until suddenly I was being strapped down to the gurney with restraints. "Lorazepam!" said a voice off to the left of my head. Post-operative delirium, they would later call it. A common side effect of anesthesia, particularly in elderly patients. But I was not elderly. I was forty-six years old and, aside from the bum uterus that had brought me there, in otherwise excellent shape. Perhaps the anesthesia had exacerbated my agitated postoperative state, but if delirium is defined by mental incoherence, then I was most certainly not delirious. I was 100 percent fucking coherent. And out of my coherent fucking mind. "Where is he?" I cried out. "Where is he where is he where IS HE? Ahhhhhhhhhhhh!!!!!!!!!"

Then tears, leaking out fast and strong. Of course he wasn't there. He never was. "I miss my dad . . . I miss my dad . . . I miss my dad . . . I miss my dad . . ." I said, gulping air between words.

"Do you want us to call your father?" said the nurse.

"No!" I said. "He's dead. Call Nora, please."

"Who's Nora?" said the nurse.

"Nora Ephron. She's listed. Call 411. That's E-p-h-r- . . ."

"Nora Ephron . . . the filmmaker? The one who did *When Harry Met Sally?*"

"Yes! She promised she'd come help me if my husband flaked. Please call her."

"She's delirious," I heard the nurses whisper. Then, out loud, to me, "Are you in pain?"

"Yes," I said. "A lot." If you only knew how much.

She explained how the morphine button worked. "Press right here, but only when you need it," she said. Define "need," I thought. A sudden godly warmth gushed through my blood. No wonder people get addicted to heroin. Am I allowed to take this button home with me?

When I awoke from the morphine haze, my husband magically appeared, clutching a bouquet of flowers. In the eighth hour after my planned eight hours of surgery, he'd gone out in search of blooms and food. I started weeping anew. It was like a bad O. Henry plot: an act of love, those flowers, when the only present I actually needed, then or ever, was his presence.

"You don't like them?" he said, looking hurt.

"No, they're beautiful," I said. "Thank you. It's just . . . no one knew where you were. I was all alone."

"No you weren't," he said. "You had the nurses."

"But I wanted . . . my husband in the room when I came to. They couldn't find you. You weren't answering your cellphone."

"I didn't hear it. Plus, I'm here now," he said. "What's the difference?"

The difference, I wanted to tell him, was too vast to explain if I had to explain it.

Back home the next morning, I awake in my bed after a long nap. I check my inbox once again for an email from Nora. Nothing. Weird. It's been hours since I sent her my missive from my hospital bed. She's normally so prompt with her replies. My stomach grumbles. I'd had to fast the night before surgery, and the first solid food they'd tried to serve me this morning, the day after surgery, was so unappetizing, I'd asked the nurse to please take away the tray before throwing up. In other words, I have not eaten any food in three days. "Hey, sweetie, could you please bring me some food?" I say. My husband is rocking back and forth in the nursing chair we still keep around, even though our youngest is now six. He likes to rock in it while he talks on the phone—"stimming," this is called, short for self-stimulation, which we all do to some extent. I'm a hair-twirler, for example. You might be a nail-biter or a pencil-tapper. Frequent rocking, however, is, more often than not, a symptom of ASD.

He holds up his finger: Hold on. He's on a work call. He's found work again, after another hiatus, and I'm glad for this, so I wait patiently for another hour or so until he hangs up. When he does, I ask, once again, for food. "I have to make one more call," he says, and proceeds to dial the phone.

"Please!" I beg. "I'm really hungry. Can you bring me a sandwich first? Or anything. I don't care."

"No," he says. "It's a conference call."

"So be on the call while you get the food. Wear headphones. Put yourself on mute. They'll understand! Your wife just got out of surgery." Multitasking, I know, is not his strong suit, but I am now so hungry I'm not thinking straight.

"Shhh!" he snaps, trying to listen in on the conference call and respond. "No. No, we can't do that . . ." he says. "That would require . . ." In a few weeks, I will understand his stress. This company, too, will go belly up, and he will lose yet another job through no fault of his own.

I lift the bottom of my shirt, exposing a bloated, sliced up belly with several pieces of medical tape covering various stitches. They had to pump air around the uterus in order to remove it, I was told. It will be a while until I deflate. I don't have the mental capacity yet to mourn what's missing. The pain where the organ that used to define me as female once lived has become untenable, so I pop another Percocet and wait for my husband to get off the phone. Another hour passes. Maybe two. I pass out. I wake up. I pass out and wake up again. At this point I'm so delirious with pain and hunger, I'm losing the thread of time. "Food!" I scream. "Please! I need food!" He's answering email now. Or I don't know what he's doing, but he's not getting up to bring me food. I call Nora's cellphone. No answer. Where is she? Why isn't she answering her phone? "Please!" I shout from my bed. "Please, I need food!"

"Just give me one more minute!" he says. "Jesus Christ."

"No stairs, no heavy lifting," the surgeon had warned us. A flight of stairs separates me from sustenance. We live in Harlem now, in the top two and a half floors of a narrow brownstone we rented after our third child was born, and the rent on our Upper West Side home was hiked up beyond what we could afford.

On the third floor of the brownstone, which is where our apartment begins, sits the master bedroom: Getting up here, after arriving home from the hospital the day after surgery, had required my husband to push the small of my back as I ascended at an angle, as if I were a dining room table: a climb so painful I can still, typing these words, feel the agony of it. On the fourth floor is the kitchen and dining area. Mounting that flight of stairs alone seems impossible, post-op, without a hand at my back, but I have no other option. The kids are in school. None of the restaurants I know and like will deliver above 96th Street. Hamilton Heights, my area of Harlem, has few options in terms of restaurants in the spring of 2012, and none, that I know, will deliver. All of my friends live too far away to make it here in the next five minutes, which is all I can take before I will lose it.

I climb out of bed, hunched over in pain.

"Stop being so dramatic. I'll get you some food in a minute. Get back in bed!" my husband shouts, but he does not try to stop me or step in to help, and I don't have time to wait. I need food. Now.

I crawl up the steps, one at a time, on hands and knees. The pain is shocking in its breadth and scope, not just inside my now empty pelvic cavity but all over my abdominal area, including externally on each point of entry as well. At the halfway point up the stairs, I pause. Unsure I'll be able to make it. I look down at my white T-shirt, now dotted with drops of blood from the still-raw incisions that have begun to bleed from the strain of climbing. Eight more steps. Then three. Now one. I stand up, leaning on the banister to ease the pain as I make my way into the kitchen, but it hurts too much to stand. I'm crawling on hands and knees again, reduced to pre-toddlerhood.

I'm desperate to talk to Nora. I want to tell her I'm sorry: I'm sorry we disagree about my husband's Asperger's; I'm sorry I can't put up with it anymore, whatever "it" is called. I'm also sorry I listened to her and gave him one more shot. His last straws have been so numerous at this point, the burden of this pain now lies solely on my shoulders: my inaction, my lack of agency, my staying when I should have left years ago. I was less than honest with you, Nora. Even this morning, in my email, I wrote to say the hernia was surgery-induced when in fact it popped out when I started screaming after hearing they couldn't find my husband. I've told you some of the disturbing things I've experienced in this marriage but not all of them because, also, who has time? Our lunches were only an hour to two tops, with a lot of ground to cover each meal, and I didn't want to spend the entirety of those hours complaining about something that was fully within my control to end. She will understand. She has to. If she could walk out on her husband for cheating on her while her uterus was filled with child, surely I can walk out on mine for negligence after its dissection and removal. In fact, if I'm to adhere to the rule she herself wrote and lived by—"Above all, be the heroine of your life, not the victim"—then my only options right now are to find food and get divorced. In that order.

I reach the refrigerator door, but, hard as I try, I cannot open it. My Ginsued stomach muscles hurt too much when I try to pull on the handle. Who knew pulling a fridge door requires so much core strength? I slump to the floor defeated, my back against the refrigerator. An ugly cry geysers out of my throat, blubbery and full-snottled.

Then suddenly, there on the kitchen counter, I spot my salvation: three yellow bananas, within easy reach. I pull myself up, nearly screaming in pain now, and grab them, slinking back onto the floor to peel and swallow each one with all the grace of Goodall's chimps. That is to say indecorously and as fast as primately possible.

Later that day, back in bed, I'm awoken to a series of urgent texts from a friend, asking if I've heard the news: Apparently Nora is in the hospital, gravely ill. What????!!!!! I quickly scan Google for any hint of this. Nothing. I call Nora's cellphone again. She doesn't pick up. "These rumors better be untrue," I frantically write in the subject header of my next email, weeping. "I can't imagine life without you. Please please please. I love you. I love you. I love you."

That night, after midnight, my husband's cellphone rings on his desk across the bedroom. I scan the darkened room to look for him. He's not there. I let it keep ringing until it stops. Whoever it is can leave a message. A few seconds later, the phone starts ringing again. The third time it rings, I yell my husband's name. "Your phone! Are you there?" Nothing. I pull myself up out of bed, gasping with pain, to retrieve the phone from the desk, on which our son's name appears. It's the beginning of his summer vacation. He's between his junior and senior year of high school. He'd left for a friend's party hours earlier. "What's going on?" I say, picking up. "Are you okay?"

"Oh, Mom!" he says. "I'm so sorry. I deliberately didn't call your phone. I didn't want to wake you up. Are you okay? Are you in pain?"

"I'm fine," I lie. "What's going on?"

"Ugh, I'm so sorry. I'm stuck downstairs in a taxi without enough money to pay the driver. I just need three more dollars. I'll pay you back, I promise. Can you ask Dad to bring them? The guy won't let me leave the cab until I pay."

"Of course," I say. "No problem."

My deal with my teenagers has always been thus: I take the subway, so you take the subway. If you're going to stay out late enough at a party that it would feel too risky to take the subway home, please take a taxi, but it's your responsibility to pay for it. That way, the burden of getting home at a decent hour lies on their shoulders, not mine.

I walk to the bedroom door, propping myself up with my hand on the jamb, and shout upstairs to my husband, calling his name once again.

"What?" he shouts back. I can hear the low hum of the TV two flights up.

"Please come down," I say.

"Why?" I hear.

"Our son is stuck in a cab downstairs!" I can feel the hernia popping out with every word. "Please, come down. It hurts to shout. He needs three dollars."

"I'm watching a movie. Can you bring it to him?"

"Jesus Christ, no!" It's been one day since my uterus was removed. Yes, in any normal first world society, I would still be in the hospital, recovering under the care of nurses. In the UK, the NHS would allow me to stay in the hospital for up to five days. In France or Canada, I'd get up to four. But this is America. Hospitals have to turn a profit. I'm much more valuable to them undergoing the removal of my uterus than I am lying in bed recovering from it. So I went in for surgery one morning and was back home within twenty-four hours.

"Okay, okay, tell him I'll be down in a second."

"Mom! Just hand the phone to Dad," says my son. "You shouldn't have to deal with this."

"I can't," I say. "I'm in my room, and Dad's upstairs watching TV. Don't worry. He says he'll be down in a minute."

"Thanks, Mom. I love you. I'm so sorry I woke you up."

"Don't worry about it. I love you, too."

Ten minutes later, my husband's phone rings again. This time I've put it on my bedside table, so I don't have to get up out of bed to fetch it. It's my son again. "Mom! Why are you answering Dad's phone again? Where's Dad?" he says.

"He didn't bring you the money?"

"No! Not yet! And the meter keeps running. I now need, um, eight dollars I think? Plus tip. And the driver's getting pissed. What's going on?"

"I'll get him," I say.

I hang up the phone to shield my son from my primal scream. This scream goes on. And on. And on and on and on, seemingly forever. I've arranged for our other two children to be at sleepovers, thank god, because the guttural noises coming out of my throat are frightening even to me. I'm spouting a combination of profanities and demonic howls. The hernia is now sticking out of my inflated pelvis as large and visible as, well, a baby's hand if I had to name it. I need to stop screaming to keep it from pushing out farther, but I can no longer control myself.

"What is wrong with you?" says my husband, finally descending the stairs. "You're going to wake up the neighbors!"

"I'm going to wake up the neighbors?" I say. "That's what you're worried about? WAKING UP THE FUCKING NEIGHBORS? I just had my uterus removed *yesterday*! How about worrying about me? How about worrying about your son, who's been stuck in a cab downstairs with an angry cabbie for fifteen minutes?"

"Stop being so dramatic!" he says: his go-to retort anytime I get upset.

"Look at this!" I lift my shirt and point to the hernia, which is now sticking out of one of the larger incisions and oozing. I am literally turned inside out with rage.

"Eyew," he says. "What's that?"

"Fury!!!!!" I say, weeping harder. "That's it. I want a divorce. No more second chances. No more thirty-fifth chances. We'll figure this out in the morning, but please sleep upstairs tonight. I can't even look at you, I'm so angry."

"No," he says. "I'll sleep wherever I want."

I cry myself to sleep, next to him.

Nora's death is officially announced the next day. I have to shut off the TV and radio to keep from weeping every time her face or voice is broadcast. Her husband, Nick, invites us all to the apartment the following night to eat the chicken salad sandwiches Nora herself, ever the den mother, has picked out and ordered for the occasion from William Poll. I'm still in a lot of post-op pain, and I can't stand for more than a few minutes at a time, but I make it down the stairs and take a cab to Nora and Nick's—No, I think, *it's now just Nick's*—crying anew.

I hug Nick. He recounts the story of Nora's jellyfish sting, after which her cancer had suddenly and mysteriously gone into remission for several years. Exhausted from the effort of standing, I sink into the fluffy cushions of Nora's white couch, feeling suddenly enveloped by her. "All couches should be white," she once told me. "That way you can bleach the slipcovers when you wash them, and it always looks brand-new. Plus white is bright and fresh and always looks good in a room. There's no reason to have a couch in any other color."

I'm in shock. All of us in that room are, since most of us hadn't known she was sick. There's Meg Ryan, on the other end of the white couch, weeping. There's Rosie O'Donnell, chatting with one of Nora's sisters, wearing a thousand-yard stare. There's J.J. Sacha, Nora's assistant, trying to make everything better as usual, but this is one wrinkle he cannot smooth. There's Barbara Walters, shaking her head with tears in her eyes. There's Diane Sokolow, one of Nora's best friends and my favorite running charades partner, coming toward me with open arms. "Why didn't she tell us?" I say. It's the question on nearly everyone's lips. At her memorial service two weeks later, Meryl Streep will accurately express the pain of this not knowing, transforming her hands, during her eulogy, into Nora's: upturned like the queen's and slowly twisting outward, then inward, her thumb meeting the tips of her fingers. Tom Hanks and his wife, Rita Wilson, will perform as Nick and Nora, on a typical night at home. The whiplash between laughter and tears will be fierce, as in any of Nora's films. A year later, during a different tribute, Hanks will talk about her accessibility as a maternal figure, despite the fact that being a mother, he'll say, was the least instinctive of Nora's abilities.

No, I'll think. Being a mother was what she was at her core. Not just to me. To everyone she loved.

Back home, I'm stopped by my teenage daughter as I head into the bathroom.

"Mom," she says, shutting the door behind us. "I need to tell you something really personal, but I've been worried about telling you while you're recovering. I didn't want to bother you. The coincidence is just too . . . weird."

"Hit me," I say.

"Okay, so," she says, "while you were in the hospital? Like, literally during the exact hours when they were removing your uterus?"

"Yes?" I say.

"I got my period."

"What?!!! No!!! That's so crazy! Congratulations!" I hug her. I kiss her. I am filled with sudden ecstasy. The torch has been passed. Life goes on. What comes out of me next can only be described as craughing: that particular combination of crying and laughter during which neither emotion quite wins. They simply exist, side by side, in perfect balance. "Wait. Do you have everything you need? Oh my god, I'm so sorry I wasn't here for that. Do you even know how to use a —"

"Mom! Oh my god, stop. Yes. I'm the last one of my friends to get it. They taught me everything."

"Okay, okay, but promise me one thing," I say, channeling Nora.

"Sure," she says, "what?"

"Promise me you'll never be afraid to talk to me about anything."

"Oh my god, Mom. Chill. It's just my period."

"No, no!" I laugh. "I'm not talking about periods. I mean, like . . . anything."

"Duh, of course," she says, shutting the door behind her, and suddenly it strikes me: Of *course* Nora told no one about her illness. The transmission of woes is a one-way street, from child to mother. A good mother never burdens her child with her woes. She waits until they become so heavy, they either break her or kill her, whichever comes first.

"What happened?" says my surgeon, palpating the hernia still protruding from one of the incisions, when I go back to the hospital the next morning to see her. She'd felt it before I left the hospital, back when it was still tiny, and had simply said to take it easy: It would probably retreat on its own once the incisions had healed.

What happened? I don't even know where to begin. "I got upset with my husband and started shouting," I say. Sure. That works. Keep it vague, as usual. When you actually try to explain, people look at you as if you're crazy.

The literature of autism spectrum disorders refers to this as Cassandra syndrome. Cassandra, in Greek myths, was the Princess of Troy who was consigned to uttering true prophecies no one ever believed. Similarly, with Cassandra syndrome, it's nearly impossible to explain to outsiders—let alone to yourself—the true scope of what's going on inside your home: the chronic, repetitive, psychological trauma that can occur behind the curtain of an intimate relationship with someone on the spectrum.

"Why were you shouting at him?" says the surgeon.

"All the normal reasons," I say. You know, like when you're home from the hospital, and he won't bring you food. Or when your son's stuck in a taxi without any money, and he keeps watching TV.

My doctor lowers her eyebrows, concerned. "Do you have enough help at home? You shouldn't be doing any chores of any kind."

"I'm fine," I say.

She orders a CT scan. I swallow the contrast dye prior, not knowing that I am allergic to contrast dye. I bring home fiery, itchy hives covering the entire surface of my body, because of course this happens. After a week of itching and scratching my skin until it bleeds, the hives fade. Soon thereafter, the hernia retreats into the pelvic cavity behind the muscle wall on its own.

I ask my husband, once again, for a divorce. Once again he refuses to accept that we are over. This, again, according to the literature, is typical in a marriage to someone on the spectrum. So I decide simply to act as if I'm separated and getting divorced, even though we're still living under the same roof. As it turns out, he will continue to stay in both our apartment and our marital bed for the next year and three months, even going so far as to book a family vacation we cannot afford in the hopes of salvaging our relationship.

Two months after my hysterectomy, feeling somewhat better, I escape once again, this time to Sun Valley, Idaho, to present two lectures at the Sun Valley Writers' Conference. There, I meet and fall into bed with the author of a novel that had hit it out of the ballpark that year. I show him my still-fresh scars. They do not make him flinch. In fact, just the opposite: He asks questions, shows empathy for the ordeal. His calm and shy presence are healing. His dry sense of humor makes me laugh. When "Livin' on a Prayer" pops up on the speaker, he suddenly pumps his fist above the bed, without missing a beat, and starts to sing: "Whoa, we're halfway there, whoa, livin' on a prayer . . ." I laugh. Once I start, I can't stop, and this laughter transports me to a new place: joy. So this is what I've been missing, I think, giggling, staring out at the mountain I'd just scaled, with only some residual post-op pain. This is the magic possible, even between strangers.

I suddenly have the distinct feeling that Nora is in the room with me, shaking her head. Giving me her Nora Stare™. This will continue happening throughout the rest of my life, whenever I'm doing something she would neither have done herself nor approved of in others. "Him?" she says. "Seriously, *him*? Mr. It-boy novelist?"

"No, no!" I respond in my head. "It's not what you think." He's nine years younger, still capable of starting a family. I'm forty-six with three kids and no uterus. As it turns out, the novelist and I will never set eyes on each other again. We will barely even text, after we each return to our homes in distant cities, and only then for a day or two to say "Thank you" and "Did you get back okay?," "Yes," but still: carpe fucking diem. "Don't worry, Nora. He's just the catalyst. I have the rest of my life to figure out what comes next."

PART III

BREAST

2013–2014

NINE

Landslide

SEPTEMBER 2013

The first time I feel the lump, I'm driving my eldest to his first year of college on the day my marriage ends. I would have preferred to spread out these plot points, were I in charge, but you get what you get, and you don't get upset. Which is a kind of shitty thing we say to our kids, now that I think about it. Better would be: "You get what you get, and if you do get upset—which is totally normal, because sometimes what you get blows—you'll have to learn to sit with those feelings and breathe through them. Preferably in sweatpants."

Less catchy, but much healthier in terms of acknowledging the corrosive effects of cortisol, the stress hormone that gets triggered whenever we experience adversity and have to swallow our feelings. Or as Lorenzo Cohen, director of the Integrative Medicine Program at MD Anderson Cancer Center, put it more bluntly, "Stress makes your body more hospitable to cancer." Chronic stress, in fact—such as the kind that might be experienced day after day in an emotionally challenging long-term marriage—inhibits a natural process called anoikis, which destroys diseased cells and prevents them from spreading. Indeed, a number of different studies have shown a causal effect between chronic stress and the production of certain growth factors that can actually speed the development of cancer.

The lump, when I palpate it, is hard. Noticeable. Located on the outside curve of my left breast. Before I reach over and feel it with my right hand, I first feel it as a nagging presence: not painful, like the mastitis I contracted breastfeeding each child, but extant, demanding attention, like a toddler's hand on a shirttail. Of course, I think, confirming its existence. Just when my health insurance has run out.

I'd previously been covered under my TV producer jobs at ABC and NBC News, where I wrote and produced long-form news stories between 1992 and 1998, first at *Day One*, then at *Dateline NBC*. Prior to that, when I was based in Paris for four years, I didn't need health insurance: I just went to a doctor whenever I needed one and never paid a centime, and the monthly cost of my birth control pills was negligible. When I sold *Shutterbabe* in 1998, for twice my *Dateline* salary, I switched to my husband's plan, after he'd landed a job with health insurance. This was after the NBC News brass had overturned my *Dateline NBC* boss's approval to work a four-day-a-week schedule. Fourteen years after leaving that job, when I'd appear on the *Today* show as a guest for *The Red Book*—the same day, I should note, Ms. Death Panel Myth* herself, Sarah Palin, co-hosted—the producer pre-interviewing me over the phone had said, "Wait, did you used to work here? Your name sounds familiar."

"Yes," I said. "From 1994 to 1998."

"Oh my god! Did you have a somewhat . . . spicy exit interview?"

"Yes," I said, suddenly alarmed. "How do you know that?"

Neal Shapiro, my enlightened boss at the time, had approved my four-day-a-week proposal at four-fifths pay without hesitation. He knew I could do the same job in less time, he'd pay me fewer dollars, I'd see my toddlers more, my childcare costs would go down, I'd get to keep my family's health insurance, and he'd retain a dedicated employee: win-win-win-win-win-win. But the NBC vice president whose job it was to formally approve this arrangement—a woman with children of her own—said a mother had to choose: You either worked ten to twelve

---

* Palin invented the lie of the "death panel" during the 2009 debate over healthcare legislation, falsely claiming that it would lead to U.S. citizens being judged as to whether or not they were worthy of healthcare.

hours a day, five days a week and on weekends, or you could go home and be a mommy. Which had been the unstated but understood policy at both NBC and so many other white-collar American corporations: To work a corporate job, particularly if you were on one of the lower rungs of the ladder, meant to be owned by your company every hour of every day, fifty weeks a year and sometimes during your two weeks of vacation as well, depending on the news cycle. (Back then, before cellphones, we all wore beepers.) This serflike system favored—still favors—parents with spouses at home to pick up the slack. It also discouraged removing your mouth from the health insurance–equipped NBC teat. Go free-lance and actually get paid for every hour you work, then if you get in a car accident or come down with a serious illness, you are screwed.

For a country founded on the ideals of freedom, liberty, and justice for all, having affordable health insurance tied to full-time employment is an ironic and often fatal prison of our own making. Not to mention an obvious hindrance to that other pillar of American pride, entrepreneur-ship. How many new ideas and cures and inventions have we missed out on because some cog in the wheel of a giant corporation couldn't risk taking that leap of faith without a parachute of health insurance for them and their family?

My request for a temporary four-fifths schedule, while my kids were toddlers, also came in the middle of an ongoing era of misleading jour-nalism: cover story after cover story on mothers "opting out" of work, framed as personal choice rather than a result of corporate and govern-ment policies—or rather, the lack thereof—that forced them out. Eight years later, in 2006, Joan C. Williams, founding director of the Center for WorkLife Law at the University of California, Hastings College of the Law, would publish a groundbreaking study on the false framing of the opt-out narrative that had been foisted upon American women since the mid-twentieth century. "Our review of these articles finds that the Opt Out story predominates in American newspapers, which focus overwhelmingly on psychological or biological 'pulls' that lure women back into traditional roles, rather than workplace 'pushes' that drive them out," she'd write.

When it dawned on me that the NBC vice president had decided to veto my boss-approved request, and that nothing I could say or do would sway her, I looked her straight in the eye and said, loud enough for the other C-suite executives to hear, "There are currently a dozen pregnant or soon-to-be pregnant women on my floor alone. All of whom have been paying close attention to this request and its approval process. It is not an exaggeration to say you will lose nearly every single one of them if you keep pretending that their children do not exist. Do you really want a newsroom filled only with men with wives at home to pick up the slack and childless women? How is that in any way representative of the world we actually live in and its concerns, including the monumental barriers still in place for families with two working parents?"

Some new mothers at NBC, where six weeks of paid maternity leave had been the norm and was considered generous, were coming back to work before their episiotomies had healed, or when they still had grape-sized hemorrhoids, or complications from cesareans. Or they were, like me, going into credit card debt taking extra months of unpaid leave to bond with their infants during those scientifically proven crucial first three months of infant brain development.

My maternity leave with my second baby, who was not close to being weaned, was suddenly cut short when Princess Diana died, and I'd been asked to hop on a plane so quickly, I hadn't had time to procure a travel-sized breast pump. My daughter wound up screaming and refusing the bottle for the majority of the ten days I was gone. I wound up manually expressing my milk, whenever engorgement became too painful to endure, into whichever Parisian toilet I could find. Upon my return, I greeted a baby who had learned, in my absence, both to crawl and to open my bottom dresser drawer, from which she would steal my nursing bras and wear them decoratively around her neck. I also ended up paying my babysitter more money in overtime than I'd actually earned during that week and a half abroad.

Many of my colleagues, shocked by how quickly overtime childcare costs ate up their own income; by how exhausting it was staying up all night with a screaming infant before working ten hours a day; by how unsanitary and chaotic it was to have to sneak in breast pumping sessions in toilet stalls, would simply quit soon after their too-early postpartum returns to work. The babysitters weren't happy with this state of affairs either. Yes, they earned more money when we worked more hours and traveled for our jobs, but they didn't want to work more than ten hours a day either, which they were often forced to do when the non-traveling parent—more often than not the father—wouldn't or couldn't pick up the slack.

"New parents not only want to work, we *need* to work and keep our health insurance now that we have the added expense and illnesses of kids!" I practically shouted at the vice president, pointing my finger straight at her. "But the way this job is currently set up doesn't work for two-parent working households or their kids. Part-time is an excellent solution! Job-sharing is an excellent solution. You'll get more work for less pay! You won't have to retrain new employees! Babies grow up! You'll get their parents back full-time soon enough. Even from a corporate profits point of view, why would you not support this?" On my way out, I'd slammed the door of her office, feeling like a deranged Nora Helmer in a rayon power suit.

"Oh my god!" the *Today* show producer squealed, a decade and a half later. "Half of us at the *Today* show work part-time because of that exit interview! Thank you!"

I choked up upon hearing that. Not only because I felt moved by the fact that the sound waves from my slammed door had reverberated into the future, but also because, having been denied those same rights as a young mother, I'd had to rely on my husband's job for health insurance when I switched to writing, which had bound me even tighter to my increasingly troubled marriage. How many untenable marriages in America, I wondered, stayed together for the sake of health insurance? It was a story I might have pitched and produced at *Dateline NBC*, had I not felt pushed out of my health insurance–equipped job when my kids were small.

At the same time, it must be said: Handing over the reins to my husband for procuring a full-time job with health benefits—I'd previously supported him over the first six years of our relationship through his various unpaid and underpaid incarnations—was what had finally allowed me to take the leap, at thirty-two, into full-time writing, which ended up bringing in more money while simultaneously slashing our babysitting costs in half. They're only small once, I reasoned. I wanted to be around for some of it.

Now my first child, no longer a child but—abracadabra—a young man I'm driving to his first year of college, stirs in his sleep, switching from reclining in the passenger seat to folding over his knees, which is how I would often find him in the mornings before school. "How is that comfortable?" I'd ask. He'd shrug his freakishly flexible tiny shoulders. It just was. And somehow it stayed comfortable even after those shoulders broadened overnight.

My husband's various jobs over the next several years were not steady, nor did they cover our family's growing expenses or COBRA hiccups between his jobs without my writing income. When we did have health insurance from his corporate gigs, it provided a safety net for our family that citizens of every other first world country take for granted as a right, not a privilege. However, on the day I am driving our son to college, September 15, 2013, my spouse has been out of a salaried position long enough for our COBRA coverage to have both eviscerated our savings and to have come to a screeching halt.

I've been on the road promoting *The Red Book*, which had landed on *The New York Times* bestseller list for two weeks before falling off with a quiet kerplunk. This has given me the right to call myself a *New York Times* bestselling author but zero in the way of extra cash, since I'm still earning out the book advance. Obama has passed the Affordable Care Act, but the open exchange to purchase health insurance won't begin for another few weeks for coverage that kicks in on January 1, 2014, three and a half months away. Can a boob lump wait three and a half months to be seen by a doctor?

The question is moot. Of course it can. Because it must. Plus it's enough just to deal with the simultaneous end of my marriage and first-born's flight from the nest on this particular morning without creating a third event on today's calendar. Besides, I tell my expert-in-denial self, I have lumpy breasts. I always have, particularly since childbirth. The official name of this is fibrocystic breast disease, which is a misnomer. It's not a disease. It's a condition, and approximately 50 percent of all women between the ages of twenty and fifty have it. I'll just assume that this new lump, though unusual in its placement, falls under this benign umbrella and is nothing nothing nothing. It has to be nothing. Because I don't have the time, money, infrastructure, healthcare coverage, or emotional reserve right now for something.

I palpate it again. It is not nothing.

The windshield wipers, set to intermittent, mirror the motions of my left arm, which reaches up periodically to wipe away tears. The gray scale Pennsylvania landscape stretching ahead is tedious and symmetric, a perspective drawing by a lazy artist who couldn't be bothered to sharpen his pencil or fill in the details. I glance over at my son, grateful that he's been asleep to give me this silent, private moment of processing the simultaneous loss of both him and my marriage.

Look at him: this big hunk of solid flesh folded over his knees like a marionette with slack strings. Yesterday, he was a ravenous refugee from the dark warm inside me, sucking sustenance out of my aching breast with the kind of force that draws blood. Today, I'm driving a car packed so full with extra-long college linens and man clothes, I can't see out the back window.

Earlier this morning, at around 7 A.M., I'd been cruising uptown to Harlem from the Hertz office in Midtown to retrieve him and his stuff and set off for Chicago, a twelve-hour drive under the best of circumstances, if you don't stop to pee or get gas. At that exact moment, my husband was waiting outside with two suitcases for a car that would whisk him off to JFK and out of our lives. His plan is to move to San Francisco to start a ride-sharing company that, unlike newcomers Uber and Lyft, would match carpoolers with other carpoolers, so they can get to and from work both cheaply and more sustainably in the HOV lanes: a noble and environmentally sound idea I support in theory but privately worry, with good reason, will be logistically too challenging to pull off even if he'd had proper seed money instead of the last of our marital savings. Which weren't even savings at all but rather the final remains of a loan from my mother, after my husband's company went bust after my hysterectomy, and COBRA costs strangled us—the first and last time she could ever help us out, she said, on her small retirement budget.

What I don't know, at this point, is that my husband—now ex—will lean on my solo parenting for the next three years and my nearly full financial support of our kids for the next six. Or that he'd taken out credit cards in my name. Or that his ultimate business plan is to win back my love, which explains why he's refused to sit down with me to tell the kids that we were getting divorced. "I'm not ready," he'd said, and left it at that, still not understanding that it was a lack of empathy that doomed us, not money.

"How will I explain it to the kids if I start dating?" I'd said one night, a week prior.

He'd shrugged. "Just keep it a secret."

"What about my friends?" I'd said. "I can't not tell them we're splitting up."

"Tell them what you want, as long as they don't let it slip to the kids."

"But then I'm asking everyone to lie to our kids! I'm not comfortable with this. I don't want to have to sneak around or hide the truth from our friends or children."

And now here was a photo of his face, on the last day of our marriage, popping up on the screen of my cellphone with an incoming call. "I have to go," he said. "The car's here."

"I'm eleven blocks away. St. Nicholas and 135th. Please. Can you ask the driver to wait for a few more minutes? It feels wrong to end our marriage over the phone." The line at Hertz had been long, his patience was short, but I convinced him to wait. Then he called again when I was two blocks away and said he couldn't wait any longer. Before I finished begging him to stay, I was already double parked in front of the apartment.

"Okay, bye," he said. We hugged for the last time as nominal husband and wife. His hug felt perfunctory, performative, proffered out of a combination of annoyance and duty because his wife had insisted on the symbolic, in-person punctuation mark. And yet suddenly, when he was pulling away, actual tears pooled in his eyes. I'd previously seen him cry only twice in our twenty-three years together: once after his best friend had committed suicide; the other at the end of *Schindler's List*.

"Are you okay?" I said.

"I'm going to miss my son growing up," he said, breaking down. Our little one, the caboose child, was seven years old.

"You don't have to move across the country to start a business," I said. "You can stay here in New York. Find a regular job. Co-parent."

"No. I have to do this," he said. California, he became convinced, like every prospector before him, held the golden keys to his future. He was tired of the East Coast tech scene, of middle management sales jobs and their tepid compensations and volatility, of constantly answering to others. He wanted to be one of the new kings of Silicon Valley. His own boss.

I'd considered uprooting our lives to be near his dreams, even though we were separating, since my sister lives in the Bay Area and could have provided a cozy beachhead of warmth and familiarity while my life unraveled, plus nearby cousins for my kids. But Silicon Valley real estate had become more expensive than New York's, plus my daughter was entering her junior year at Bronx Science, a good public high school where she was doing well and enjoying her final years with her posse of friends: If I moved, she announced, she'd simply move in with Louisa, her friend and classmate, and stay in New York. Geraldine, Louisa's mother, had already approved of this plan, but I could not abide by it. My entire friend and community infrastructure lived in New York: women and men I'd known for decades who would be allies, I hoped, as I rebuilt my life. The remaining media jobs were in New York, too. Meanwhile, my little one and his best friend had just landed two rare spots in the second grade at a progressive, arts-based public elementary school farther north in our district in Inwood, after struggling for two years at a brand-new public school within walking distance of our Harlem home, with high hopes pinned on its success.

The new Harlem school was a deal that had been struck between Columbia University and its northern neighbors, after the former's eminent domain land grab for an expansion into the heart of the neighborhood. The carrot that had been dangled to our mostly Black, Hispanic, and low-income community—where nearly every public school, measured by every metric, was considered to be failing—was that Columbia would be involved in the new school's formation and oversight, and therefore it would be a beacon of hope, light, and progressive learning that could spread to other schools in the district.

Alas, loud whistle-blowing became the disciplinary norm in its hallways and cafeteria, even though it had only two inaugural classes of fifty well-behaved, eager-to-learn kindergartners, all of whom, like my son, had won a neighborhood lottery to attend.

"What's with all the whistles?" the parents started whispering to one another during morning drop-off. I brought up my son's fear of the whistles with the school principal, who seemed to have gone completely rogue from Columbia's pedagogical methods and oversight, and asked her if she might consider switching to less harsh methods of maintaining order. She looked me icily in the eyes and told me that, because of my privilege, I could not possibly understand why this specific population of children needed whistles to control them.

"Could we please try the clapping method of getting the kids to be quiet?" I said. "Even just for a day?" In all the other schools my older children had attended, this method had worked well for kids of every color, creed, and background. It had even worked to quiet their much noisier parents at back-to-school nights.

"No," she snapped. This was, of course, her prerogative as school principal, to discipline her students the way she saw fit. I tried to see myself through her eyes, as a clueless, white annoyance. Nevertheless, it wasn't just my son who experienced those whistles as a daily form of torture. All of his friends did, too.

"Why don't you stick to writing books and I'll do the principaling around here," she said.

"Fair enough," I said. We'd migrated fifty blocks north to Harlem (61.7 percent Black, 18.4 percent white) from the Upper West Side (7.8 percent Black, 74.6 percent white) in 2009, in order to cut down on our housing expenses and get more space for our growing family. Our little one was turning three that year. Every time I told white friends we were moving to a rental in Harlem they'd ask, "But what will you do about kindergarten for him?"

"I'll send him to a local public school," I said.

I am a product of public schools. I grew up in Potomac, Maryland, just outside Washington, D.C., during Jimmy Carter's presidency. The day I went bra shopping for the first time in White Flint Mall, Amy Carter was doing the same two stalls down, only with the Secret Service guarding her door. Carter was the second and thus far only U.S. president since Theodore Roosevelt to send his child to the White House's zoned local public school, and a predominantly Black one at that. White flight from urban public schools, Carter knew, had done more in the Southern Strategy wake of *Brown v. Board of Education* to maintain the segregation of races in the U.S. educational system and to thwart opportunities for minority advancement than any official racist policy or political attempt to maintain segregation since. How could he stand up for the principles of equality for all in which he so firmly believed if his own family was excused from them?

Like Carter, I've become a proponent of putting my body where my beliefs are. We can talk about much-needed education reform in U.S. public schools until we're blue in the face, but it's all sound and fury if our kids are exempt from attending them. Take it from me, the hypocrite.

I was as guilty as the next egalitarian-minded parent of worrying about sending my kid to a struggling public school when it came to choosing a kindergarten for my first child, the son I was driving to college. Of course, I'm not alone in my hypocrisy. Kenneth Clark, the Black social psychologist whose pioneering work on the self-esteem of Black children was crucial to swaying the Supreme Court on *Brown v. BOE*, moved his own family from Harlem to Westchester when his kids hit school age. Why? "My children have only one life," he said.

So at the urging of both his preschool teacher and his bubbly summer camp counselor, the latter whose mother, it turned out, was the admissions director of a highly sought-after New York City private school, I applied and subsequently enrolled my first child in that private school, lured by a generous financial aid package; by their clean, state-of-the-art facilities; by its reputation as a place chosen by artists and writers for its progressive education (but today unaffordable to that same subset of families); by what turned out to be false rumors of the subpar education available to him at our zoned public school; by my son's own particular educational interests and needs; and by the alleged leg up in the college admissions game he would get.

Did he get a good education with individualized attention and excellent teachers in significantly smaller classes than those in public schools? Yes. Was it demonstrably better academically than his younger siblings' urban public school education? In some ways yes, specifically with regard to how to write clearly, think critically, and do independent research, as well as by providing adequate funding for the arts and science labs. Were the private school teachers better than those in public school? In some cases yes, in some cases no, but what my son's private school had that his younger siblings' public schools sometimes didn't was consistently good teaching across the board in every class, every year.

"Why am I pink?" said my youngest, crying, when I picked him up on his first day of kindergarten at the public school in Harlem. "Everyone else is brown." This was a bit of an exaggeration. Of the fifty children in the inaugural class at this new school, five were pink, forty-five were brown.

"You have different skin pigment than most of your classmates," I said. "Underneath, you're all the same."

"Oh."

I immediately second-guessed my response. Should I have delved deeper? Not whitewashed our history of Black pain? He was too young, I'd decided in that split second, for me to try to explain the entrenched caste system in America. To teach a five-year-old about the unfair privilege his pink pigment provided in keeping him alive and out of jail. Those lessons, I realized, needed to (and would) come soon enough. But even in his ignorance—and in my choice to keep him that way for just a little while longer—he was privileged. The parents of his classmates did not have the luxury of waiting to tell their young children hard truths. They needed to know now, for their own safety and psyche.

"Conversations about racism and discrimination will look different for each family," UNICEF explains. "While there is no one-size-fits-all approach, the science is clear: the earlier parents start the conversation with their children the better."

And while I obviously cannot fix our systemic problems of race or change the U.S. educational system by sending my pink child to a nearly all-Black school, I can tell you what I've learned from dealing with the system's inequalities from several different data points: suburban public (me), urban private (eldest child), test-in public (middle child), traditional low-income public (youngest child), and progressive low-income public (also youngest child). And one of the least discussed issues in this Game of Schools is this: Many parents send their kids to private schools not only for the better-than-average education for their kids, but also for the ways in which being part of the school's parent community can be of personal and professional benefit to them.

Send your kid to a well-reputed private school in a city like New York, and you can practically guarantee you'll be sitting in tiny chairs at back-to-school nights with members of the financial and cultural elite. In my eldest's private school, his classmates included the children of an Oscar-winning director, a world-renowned opera singer, several bestselling authors, scions of boldface families, and leaders of banks and businesses.

Did my son, the scholarship kid, constantly feel "poor" in his private school, and did he get a completely skewed view of what's normal? Absolutely. He entered kindergarten in 2000, when the CEO-to-worker compensation ratio in the U.S. was 344 to 1. This was also the beginning of the single largest rise in income inequality this country has ever known. By 2019, CEOs of the U.S.'s 350 largest companies earned an average of $21.3 million a year, with Sundar Pichai, CEO of Google, topping the charts at a whopping $280,621,552 a year. Meanwhile, the average worker in 2019 earned just $41,442 a year. Which means your run-of-the-mill, average CEO, earning $21.3 million a year, makes $10,240 an hour—that's $170.67 every *minute*—while the average worker is struggling to make ends meet on $19.92 an hour, and that's assuming they're working only forty hours a week, a large and perhaps laughable assumption. Google's Pichai (I had to check my calculations three times when I saw this number, because I couldn't believe it was true) earned a whopping $134,914.21 *every hour* in 2019. By the time he made a few phone calls, sent out a few emails, and drank his first cup of coffee, he earned more than five times the annual minimum wage salary of the barista who made it.

What does the disparity between $134,914.21 an hour and a middle-class income look like on the ground? Pull up a chair, folks.

As my family struggled to keep up with ruinous rent spikes and medical bills, I watched the wealthier families in my son's school—fund managers, bankers, business tycoons, the offspring of already well-established pockets of family wealth, and other one-percenters—go from run-of-the-mill rich to private-plane rich between the first day of kindergarten in 2000 and our children's graduation in 2013. Families that had previously employed both a full-time nanny and a full-time housekeeper suddenly had the means for a separate nanny for each child, a laundress, a house manager, a cook, a driver, a personal assistant, a trainer, a masseuse, and god knows who else was hanging out in all of those newly renovated rooms acquired by purchasing and then breaking through to contiguous apartments, but sometimes I'd pick up my son from a play-date at an apartment twenty times the size of ours and see several household employees scurrying around doing the tasks the rest of us do on our own every night between work and sleep.

I remember, in particular, as we were heading into yet another two-week private school break, during which I'd had to scramble once again for extra childcare so I could keep working, the buffed-to-a-Botoxed-shine mother of one of my son's classmates complaining at school drop-off about how hard it had been to pack for a spring break that would include one week in the Caribbean, another at a ski resort. "It was such a nightmare!" she said, without irony. "I had to FedEx all of our ski clothes to Gstaad." Then there was the bar mitzvah held at the top of the Mandarin Oriental hotel, with giant Warhol-inspired paintings of the boy's face hanging on every available wall, and a room off to the side where party planners had set up a make-your-own-skateboard station. Then there was the time, right after we moved to Harlem in 2009, when my eldest threw an end-of-year party in our new home, before which I received dozens of calls from his classmates' white parents expressing their concerns about the safety of our Black neighborhood, which, as I pointed out to them, was statistically identical to theirs with regard to crime: specifically 0.8 crimes per 1,000 residents in our Harlem neighborhood versus 0.8 per 1,000 residents in the wealthiest blocks of the Upper East Side.

A bunch of girls from a different private school had shown up drunk to that party, one of them in such bad shape she needed immediate medical care. But when my husband and I carried her outside to rush her to the hospital, suddenly we were surrounded by two giant SUVs filled with Ron Perlman's security detail, whose job it was to safely deliver his daughter and seven of her friends—including the dangerously drunk one—from my son's party in Harlem to Perlman's house in the Hamptons.

"We've got this," said a bodyguard, grabbing the girl. From the other SUV emerged a well-dressed, don't-fuck-with-me Clarice Starling–type, who rounded up the other seven girls inside with such military precision and swiftness, they didn't have time to collect their leather jackets or cellphones. The next morning, at 8 A.M., one of Perlman's drivers rang our doorbell, having been tasked with making the six-hour round trip journey between the Hamptons and Harlem to fetch them.

Even if I'd had the money to send my second two children to private school—which I did not, even with scholarships—I didn't want that for them. My public school–educated daughter, it should be noted, was admitted to the same college as her private school–educated older brother, so the argument that private school offers a boost for college admissions did not hold water, at least in my family. Today, if you ask my older son if all that money we paid for his private school education was worth it, he'll say—having watched his sister and little brother learn and thrive in public schools, without having had the added burden of being considered lesser for having less—no.

But, yes. The Harlem principal was absolutely right: Being white in a predominantly Black school in a low-income neighborhood—or anywhere in the U.S.—conferred immense privilege on us. Of course it did and still does. But the prisonlike discipline, subpar teaching, emphasis on standardized testing, and lack of safe outdoor space had become such an issue by first grade that other parents—Black and white—had started to pull their kids out and enroll them elsewhere. When I heard from one of them that a spot had opened up in a more progressive, whistle-free, playground-equipped, super diverse public elementary school farther north, in a predominantly Dominican neighborhood called Inwood (9.1 percent Black, 15.1 percent white, 72.4 percent Hispanic/Latinx), I took it.

His new public school, in which he would thrive, actively discouraged its culturally and financially diverse population of parents from allowing their children to take the statewide standardized test biased against them, which, every year, did little to actually assess student performance or intelligence in low-income neighborhoods such as ours. "Opt out," we were told, a growing rallying cry in New York City public schools, where teachers were growing tired of teaching to a test geared toward white, middle-class children with personal experience with words such as *fireplace* and *lawn mower*, neither of which many low-income Black or Latinx kids had actually seen with their own eyes, instead of teaching children of all colors and socioeconomic backgrounds actual skills, literature, and history. The fact that our son had landed a coveted spot in a racially diverse public school that had both these principles and an empathic principal felt like a miracle.

My husband understood this, as well as his daughter's desire to finish her last two years in her beloved high school in the Bronx. I understood that his move across the country might come to naught. And so all the theoretical talk of uprooting the family for the sake of his Silicon Valley dreams was quietly dropped.

"You sure you can't come to Chicago with us?" I said. The sight of his tears had softened me, reawakened the love that had forged us, our kids, a life. "Delay your departure by a day or two or even drive with us and leave from O'Hare?"

"No," he said. "I can't. I have to go."

Our college-bound son had planned to take a gap year between high school and college, but at the last minute—as in six days earlier—he'd had a change of heart. It had been a scramble to get him re-enrolled and assigned a dorm room; to find a hotel room near the campus for move-in day; to pay his first semester's tuition out of an empty bank account; to enlist friends back home in New York to feed, house, and get my little one off to second grade in his new school the three mornings I'd be gone.

"You can just change your ticket," I'd said to my husband, once the new plan had taken hold. But our finances were in such shambles that he did not want to spend the money to change his one-way ticket to San Francisco. Plus he was, by nature, averse to sudden changes in plans. Six days had not been long enough for him to get used to this new reality: His firstborn son was leaving home.

"Okay, so . . ." I said. "Take care of yourself." Our twentieth wedding anniversary had come and gone, unnoted, three days earlier.

"You, too." My husband—no, from now on I would have to refer to him as my ex—turned away and hopped into the back of the car, with its easy-to-remember telephone number—777-7777—emblazoned across the back window. As the lucky numbers blocking the back of my no-longer husband's head disappeared up St. Nicholas Avenue and over the horizon, I felt unlucky. And sad. And pathetic. *Is this how you end a two-decade marriage?* I wondered, choking back tears.

Love is not a light switch. Whatever alchemy draws two humans together in marriage cannot suddenly be extinguished as the curtain falls on that union, however troubled. Love is a dimmer, vacillating up and down between blindingly bright and barely perceptible, sometimes several times within a single hour. At the moment of my own marital implosion, I could actually feel love's light expanding, spilling out beyond the event horizon, brighter than it had burned in years. Then again, the memory of a star is not a star. It's an illusion of a former twinkle seen from light-years away.

My eyes bulged with pressure seeking immediate outlet, but I could not allow myself to release the floodgates yet, because then I'd have to explain my tears to our son, who'd just emerged from our front door toting two guitars and a box of linens, oblivious to what had just transpired between his parents.

"Dad *left*?" he said.

"He told me he'd already hugged you inside," I said, tossing the linens and instruments into the trunk. "Where's your suitcase?"

"I'm not done packing."

"Of course you're not." Parenting teenage boys has taught me much of what I know about patience and surrender.

A little over an hour later, after much sorting through piles of clothes and the squeezing together of zipper teeth until they yielded to our weight and grunts, we were finally on the road.

My son took control of the music. He put on Kanye's new album, *Yeezus*. It was loud and discordant: the antithesis of my Fleetwood Mac feelings. The words *Fuck whatever y'all been hearing. Fuck what, fuck whatever y'all been wearing* erupted from the car's speakers, but then the lyrics turned to Black dick and hoes, and I bristled.

"Seriously?" I said. "Black dick and hoes?" I felt like my parents must have felt when I blasted Prince in the family station wagon on the day we drove to my first year of college. Which felt like three weeks ago, not three decades. My father had packed and repacked the car several times, squeezing in my typewriter between milk crates full of record albums until he was satisfied with the placement of each object. Or maybe it was a way for him to prolong the transitional moment. While he was sad that I was leaving home, as he'd told me countless times, he was also giddily excited to drive me to my next stage of life.

Now I was bristling not only at Kanye's lyrics but also over the fact that my son would have no memories of his father dropping him off at college. "Does he have to use the word hoe?" I snapped, seeking a substitute outlet for my anger.

"Mom, please. Open your mind to new music. Stop judging a song by its lyrics. You can turn it off when I fall asleep," he said, balling his sweatshirt into a pillow. But the back seat was too stuffed for him to fully recline in his chair.

A few minutes after that—before we'd even crossed the bridge to leave the island of Manhattan—the kid, who'd stayed up all night doing whatever it is eighteen-year-old boys on the verge of flying the coop do on their final hours at home when they're supposed to be packing instead, collapsed over his knees, dead asleep for most of what would end up being a fourteen-hour drive.

I turned off Kanye at the next red light and searched for "Landslide":

Time makes you bolder and children get older, indeed, I thought, allowing each successive version of the song to play one after the other. First Fleetwood Mac then the Dixie Chicks[*] then The Smashing Pumpkins then onto lesser-known bands. Give me all the "Landslide" you got, Spotify. Because fuck whatever y'all been hearing.

The next morning, eating breakfast in the hotel with all of the other freshmen and their parents, we are the only ones sitting at a table for two. Everyone else is seated in groups of three—mother, father, child, or in one case mother, mother, and child—whether in booths or at four-tops. The families around us all seem joyous, carefree, engaging in gentle ribbing and inside family jokes born of eighteen years of cohabitation and history.

It isn't until we arrive at my son's dorm that I will meet another single mother: his roommate's. Though at this point I can't tell her I'm a day-old member of her club, since my son doesn't know this yet, I'm dying to ask her a thousand questions right now, beginning with the most obvious: "How do you manage the loneliness?"

She seems strong, resilient, a hearty cauldron of midwestern values dressed in practical, can-do flannel and mom jeans. As I watch her lift a small fridge up onto a wooden platform above our sons' beds, I say, "Wait, let me help you," and she gracefully accepts my aid, even though she clearly doesn't need it. If she's at all sad about being on her own, after moving her only son into this dorm room, she hides it well. The four of us decide to have lunch together, which immediately answers my unasked question about how to survive the solitude—you bond with other single parents—before heading back to the dorm, unpacking more stuff, and saying goodbye.

The sharp ache in my chest, after exchanging my final *I love you*'s with my eldest, now mixes with the dull ache on the outside curve of my left breast until all I am is pain and the desire to expel it. But I can't collapse yet. No. First I have to drop off the rental car and fly home to New York, surrounded by other humans, then head immediately to pick up my little one at my friends the Sylvesters' house. With four kids of their own in three different schools, they already had the infrastructure in place to get mine back and forth to his new school in Inwood plus the

---

[*] Renamed The Chicks in 2020.

kindness and grace to have offered. Then I have to meet my daughter back at home, where she's been staying alone, and make dinner for her and her brother while pretending everything's fine. I can't cry that night alone in my bed, either, because the kids share a bedroom next to mine. I can't lose it on the packed subway to my son's school the next morning or on the more crowded return trip home.

By the time I walk in the front door of my home after school drop-off, minus a marriage and my firstborn, both my sorrow itself and its desire for outlet have been building up for so many days, I don't even make it halfway up the stairs before I collapse with a plaintive, animal-like wail.

It's guttural. It's loud. I'm worried the neighbors will hear it through our shared wall, but it's all my body can do for now, this geyser of grief, so I just let it erupt, snot gushing, as the sharp angles of the wooden stairs dig into my rib cage, arms, the sensitive lump on my breast. I finally drag myself into my tiny writing studio, where I collapse onto the rug and cry some more. The pain flattens me. I'm unable to stand up. The desire to chuck it all and hop on a plane to anywhere feels overwhelming. But I cannot eat, pray, love my way out of this marriage, nor do I have the means to run away even if I didn't have two children still living at home and relying on me for shelter, succor, shoes. The baby hasn't even learned to tie his laces yet. Thank god for Velcro.

And, ew, what is that smell? I sniff the area rug: a 3' x 5' gift to myself during a literary festival in Vermont, where I'd been invited to speak after my first novel was published. Ugh. The dog must have peed on it again, because the stench is so overwhelming, it finally forces me to peel myself off the floor, roll up the rug, blow my nose, and take a seat at my desk.

Okay. I have to work. Now.

With tears still falling, I open up the file of the novel I've been writing for nearly a year to try to make sense of it. It's about an extramarital affair. The relationship has been saving my protagonists from their troubled marriages in different ways (him from ennui, her from abuse), but I can't figure out the ending. Yes, it's too-obvious wish fulfillment in the form of fiction—my way of coping, while writing it, with the end of my own marriage—but where these two end up has me completely stumped.

If they end up together, their kids and ex-spouses will hate them, plus he will eventually grow bored again and leave her, the same way he left his wife. If they end up staying in their marriages, he will mature past his inability to fully commit to real love, but she'll remain in a dysfunctional situation that will leave her more suicidal than she was at the beginning of the novel. And I refuse to throw her under the bus, either literally or figuratively. She has to live, to leave her husband, to work through her issues alone, to forge a new path as a single mother, but how?

The me writing these words today knows exactly how, if not several perfectly acceptable versions thereof, but back then I couldn't see a clear path for either myself or my protagonists. I have — in every way possible — lost track of the narrative: my characters', my own, their kids', my kids'. "What the fuck happens next?" I say out loud, starting to cry again.

I toss the sixty-thousand-word file into the trash. It had been a struggle to write from the start: never a good sign, plus I know in my heart it's not good, I don't know how to make it better, and I need money now, not when I turn it in a year from now, maybe longer.

I consider writing a YA novel. A few publishers have reached out over the years to offer an advance for one, if I can figure out a good premise and submit a proposal. J.K. Rowling wrote and sold *Harry Potter* after she was suddenly thrust into the role of single mother. Now she's the multi-millionaire author of the most successful children's series of all time. Sitting there at my desk, I suddenly come up with a story I'd like to explore: a first kiss, during a summer vacation on the Delaware shore, between a thirteen-year-old girl and a seventeen-year-old boy and the repercussions that follow. I was a rabid Judy Blume fan growing up. Her books dealt with previously taboo topics and feelings not only near and dear to my utterly confused teen heart, but no one else back then was talking about them.

Plus I had plenty of raw material from which to draw: That summer at sleepaway camp, on the bus back from Kings Dominion in 1979, when the much older boy I had a crush on took my prepubescent, thirteen-year-old hand and stuck it down his pants. "I think he peed on me!" I cried to my friend Nancy, who shook her head at my naïveté and helped me rid my shaking hand of semen. Or that night in seventh grade, when everyone else paired off in Adam Glickfield's basement and started to make out on the couches and floor, and that red-haired boy and I were — literally — the last two standing. "So, I guess you and I should . . ." he said. *Should what?* I wondered. How did everyone else know what to do?

"Sure," I shrugged. We lay down. He shoved his finger up my vagina, answering my question.

Yes! I think. That's what I'll do: the first kiss book. I'll put together a proposal, hand it in, get started right away. It will be both fun and exorcistic to write, and I'll get paid immediately instead of having to wait until the book's finished.

But, oh, right. Duh. Judy Blume was married during her most prolific years — albeit unhappily, on the verge of divorce — to a lawyer, whose job presumably provided health insurance. Rowling had Great Britain's cradle-to-grave welfare state, which provided public assistance, however minuscule, and their excellent, taxpayer-funded National Health Service. Ambulance rides, emergency room visits, mammograms, cancer care, long-term hospital stays: all paid for by the NHS, no matter your income.

I have an American passport and a breast lump. A bad combination when you earn your living as a writer.

Other authors I know rely on family or spousal support to keep writing without worrying about maintaining their health insurance. Or they deal with the issue by becoming college professors, a position for which I tried getting hired multiple times as well, but I kept getting told that, without a master's, I was unemployable in academia, never mind my published books and frequent visiting lectures at universities across the U.S. I also don't have the time or financial runway to get one. Some authors I know join the WGA — the Writers Guild of America — by writing film and television scripts on the side. If you earn approximately $35,000 a year (in 2013) so doing, you become eligible for excellent, low-cost WGA health insurance, but you can't join the WGA until you get assigned a script by a legitimate WGA signatory, and a legitimate WGA signatory will not assign a script to a writer who's not in the guild: a catch-22 that many writers get around by working their way up the ranks of the male-dominated TV writers' rooms in Los Angeles straight out of college, first as interns then as writers' assistants. But try to get your foot in that health-insurance-providing door as a middle-aged woman, I've been told, and they will laugh-track you right out of Hollywood.

I open a new file on my computer and create a list of immediate and pressing concerns:

1) I need a corporate job with health insurance, stat. In anticipation of my separation, I'd already been searching for months, with a couple of positions asking me back for multiple rounds of interviews, but I'd yet to get an offer. I'd recently been interviewing for a position at Facebook I was fairly confident would be mine, since the company's COO had recruited me, plus it had a photojournalism angle. Moreover, I'd been one of the last two candidates in consideration; the other candidate was a younger man with less experience and fewer qualifications; and *Lean In*, the COO's wildly popular new tome, had just been published a few months prior. But after several more rounds of interviews with one young male employee after another, all of which I thought I'd nailed, I lost out to the dude. Not surprising, considering that, statistically speaking, men like to hire other men. And they are particularly biased against older women.

2) I need to rent out my son's bedroom to make up for the 43 percent rise in my rent, from $3,500 a month to nearly $5,000, at the exact moment I'm suddenly in charge of paying for all of it. New buyers, a large real estate conglomerate, have recently purchased the Harlem brownstone I call home from my landlords. The new owner's goal is to force us and our downstairs neighbors out with crushing but somehow legal rent hikes, so they can do a much more substantial renovation and then rent it out for more money.

3) I need to transform my 6' x 8' office—my beloved and rare proverbial room of one's own, in which I wrote and edited my last two books—into a bedroom for an au pair, if a single bed and dresser will even fit in it, so I can get a job outside the home without worrying about my salary being eaten up by babysitting overtime. And I need to find an au pair without paying exorbitant rates to an agency to procure one. Childcare math, when you crunch the numbers, doesn't actually add up, particularly when the children are not yet in school. During those first years, you need a minimum of fifty hours of babysitting a week to work a forty-hour week, which includes an hour of commuting on either end of the day. If you pay your babysitter $20 an hour—the current minimum going rate in

urban centers like mine—that comes out to $1,000 a week before you even pay employer taxes and your sitter's benefits. That's $52,000 a year, out of pocket, of which you're allowed to declare 35 percent of only $3,000 a year on your taxes, which is less than the cost of most summer camp programs, which are not an optional indulgence for many families but rather a necessity for working parents. Which means you have to earn a low six figures just to break even. Daycare costs less but is much less flexible if you're a single parent with a job that requires working late or travel, as many white-collar jobs these days do. An au pair is a good solution, since they're seeking housing and experience in a foreign country as well as a little spending money, but you need an adequate spare bedroom, which is its own added expense, plus there's the au pair agency fee, I hear, which I've yet to look into.

4) I need to send out an email to a choice group of friends, to tell them I've separated from my husband, but please don't tell my kids, and by the way, if you hear of any available jobs or men, please let me know.

5) I need to start looking for new, cheaper digs for when my lease is up in nine months.

6) I need to move.

7) I need to find the money to move.

8) I need to figure out how to get a low-cost mammogram, if that even exists near me, and I need to pray this lump is nothing, because I won't be able to afford it if it's something.

9) I need to pay off the mid-five figures in credit card debt that has been placed in my name, only half of which I'd previously known about.

10) I need to find a way to extricate myself from risk of further credit card debt being placed in my name by getting divorced, but how do I do that without paying a divorce lawyer a $30,000 retainer to get the ball rolling?

11) I need $30,000 to get divorced. Minimum, as I understand it. Many friends and acquaintances of mine going through divorce, particularly if their cases had to go to trial, were suddenly on the hook for multiple times that amount. One friend of mine was paying her divorce lawyer $700 an hour. $700 an hour!

And oh, shit, I think, opening up my calendar and seeing a work event to which I'd said yes before knowing it would take place on my first weekend as a solo parent:

12) I need to find someone to watch my seven-year-old this coming Saturday from 7:30 A.M. until 3 P.M., while my older daughter takes the SAT, so I can speak on a 9 A.M. panel at the Brooklyn Book Festival, an hour away.

I check my bank statement. Paying a babysitter to watch him, if I can even find one willing to show up that early on a Saturday morning, will eat up a good chunk of my current reserves.

The book festival, as absurd as this sounds in retrospect, is the minor task, once I write it down, that breaks me: the too-much thing, the I-can't-do-this thing, the I-give-up thing. I'm suddenly struggling to breathe. I clutch my chest, in full-on panic attack. Yes, I needed to extricate myself from my marriage, and I'm relieved that the first step has been taken, but I'm just now realizing the implications: I'm on my own. Completely. No more, "It's your turn to throw out the trash." No more, "If you run his bath, I'll do the dishes." No more, "I have to fly to Houston this Thursday to give a lecture, I'll be back Friday," which means no more speaking fees to tide me over between books, right at the moment when magazines, my other source of income, are entering their death spiral. No more spending my days as a writer, after fifteen years of both defining myself and earning a decent living thus. No more sex. Wait, seriously, no more sex? Yes. No more sex. Because how can I justify spending $20 an hour in babysitting to meet a man who might not even show up, and even if he does, and our fleshes actually hit it off, then what? A quickie at his place before rushing home to relieve the sitter and walk the dog? My other separated and divorced friends plan their dates during their evenings and weekends off, when their exes have their kids and pets. I won't have nights off. Or the money to pay a lawyer to fight for child support. Or any family nearby with whom to drop him off when weekend work situations arise. Never mind *any* situation I haven't even considered that might arise.

"Pull it together!" I say to myself. "Stop crying!"

I palpate my breast lump again. Fuck. It's still there.

Chiaroscuro

DECEMBER 2008

Pull it together! Stop crying!" said my mother, dragging me by the armpit into a nearby kitchen with a door that shut. "Everyone can hear you!" Suddenly I was on the floor, my back up against a refrigerator.

"What the fuck?" I said, shocked. I was, I should add, forty-two years old. I'd just stepped out of the hospital room where my sixty-seven-year-old father, dying from pancreatic cancer, had told me he loved me and wanted to make sure I understood this, because he wasn't sure he'd be able to say it again, which he wouldn't.

A few minutes earlier, my father's doctor had followed me into the hallway, where I'd escaped to pace the floor and maybe look for a sandwich, since I hadn't eaten in . . . I wasn't sure. A day? Two days? Hospital time is different from regular time. Both faster and slower. You look up, a day is gone, while the seconds tick by in slow motion. Dad's liver was shutting down, said the doc, as were his kidneys. It was only a matter of time — twenty-four to forty-eight hours, give or take — before the rest of his body would follow. And so hearing this news had made me cry. Okay, loudly.

"You are bothering the other families!" said my mother. There were no other families in the hallway. They were all in their loved ones' hospital rooms, saying their own goodbyes. Could they hear me? Sure.

Probably. Had I heard the same lamentations dozens of times in those same hallways? Yes. Every day.

"But this is a terminal cancer ward!" I said. "I'm pretty sure the other families will understand."

"You're scaring them!"

"I'm not scaring them, Mom! Death is."

"You will stay here and compose yourself until you can be quiet!"

"Oh, for fuck's sake. My father is dying. If I can't cry in public now, when can I?"

I have countless memories of my mother caring for me—bloodied knees bandaged, doctors visited, food cooked, shoes purchased, carpools driven, school supplies bought, front-row seats to the school play saved, she was nothing if not responsible, always early, and on the ball as a parent—but what I craved was comfort. Her hugs, quick and contrapuntal, had to be rationed out between towels folded or dishes loaded. Meanwhile, breastfeeding was still frowned upon when I was born back in 1966, so I have no preconscious memories of the comfort of her breast either. I don't blame her for not breastfeeding me or my sisters. At all. I blame the industrial revolution. I blame bad science. I blame a society that not only told women that breastfeeding was kind of icky, indecent, and strictly for those in the lower classes who couldn't afford formula, but that also frowned upon a woman breastfeeding in public without providing any viable alternatives.

My dad, on the other hand, while incapable of care or even of the organizational skills necessary to do so—he never even had his own ATM card, my mother so firmly took charge of every aspect of family logistics and child schlepping—provided comfort. It wasn't until I was a mother myself that I understood that being the sole caretaker of children could sap one of the energy, time, and patience required to provide simultaneous comfort and care. Comfort was a luxury for the unfrazzled. And Dad took full advantage of the hours and mental space he was given, by never having to think about folding, rinsing, meal preparation, or care, to provide comfort to his four daughters. An expert hugger, his was the lap into which I'd collapse.

And now that lap was hours away from growing cold. And I was on the kitchen floor of the hospital, losing precious moments of his final hours.

I composed myself, blew my nose, stood up, and returned to my father's room to sit with him, my mom, and my three younger sisters, for however many hours we had left. Dad was passed out in a Dilaudid haze after having mustered enough energy to sit up and sign his hot-off-the presses book to my sister, Jen, who'd just arrived from California. "Dear Jen, I love you so much. We have said what we needed to say last night. All my loe always. Love, Dad," he wrote on the title page, leaving off a *v* in one of the three *loves* in his short message—as clear a sign as any that though his heart was as expansive as ever, his normally tack-sharp brain was contracting.

Target Culebra was his first and only book. He'd been an international lawyer, representing the government of Puerto Rico, and the book described his years-long, pro bono legal battle against the U.S. Navy to persuade them to stop bombing the inhabited island of Culebra and using it as target practice. Apparently, "People live here" wasn't good enough.

Because his law practice was fairly intense, at one of those white-shoe Washington, D.C., law firms that requires its partners to bill many hours on top of whatever pro bono work they've got going on, it had taken Dad the better part of his life to finish that book, on weekends, nights, whenever he could squeeze in a minute to work on it. Some of my earliest memories, in fact, involve the sound of his typewriter on Sunday mornings. And no, the parallel has obviously not been lost on me that to write the book you're now reading, while holding down a full-time job and two other gig jobs as a single mother, I've had to do the same. It's 5 A.M. on a Sunday morning as I type these words. It's always 5 A.M. as I start typing these words. Understanding the fragility of the human body, on a personal and cellular level, has had its generative upsides.

While other kids played hide-and-seek, my friends and I played goin'-to-Culebra: You were either a good guy, trying to save the island from being bombed, or a bad guy in the U.S. Navy, trying to bomb it. We even had our own theme song, sung as you rocked back and forth at the top of the playground slide before gliding down and starting the game: "Goin' to Culebra, goin' to Culebra . . ." One day, a friend challenged me on the premise of my game: We pledged allegiance to the United States every morning at school. How could our own country's military . . . be *bad*? "Haven't you watched the news?" I said.

It was 1972. Nearly every night, Walter Cronkite presented images of American soldiers burning villages in Vietnam. "A country can be founded on good principles but act in a manner contrary to those principles," Dad used to say, as we watched the nightly horrors unfold: words I would revisit hundreds of times over the course of my life, whether while learning history in school or living through it as a journalist. *Target Culebra* was officially scheduled to be published two days hence, on December 9, 2008. And while Dad was able to see and hold the finished book in his hands as well as sign several copies to my sisters and me, I was hoping—in vain, as it would turn out—that he'd live long enough to wake up on his publication date.

"Please, Deb," he'd said, a few days earlier, when we were alone. "I'll need you to be my representative on book tour." I promised I would, not understanding that his book tour would culminate in a three-hundred-person banquet in his honor hosted by the former governor of Puerto Rico and the former mayor of Culebra in a massive ballroom at which I, his still freshly mourning daughter, would be the substitute guest of honor. During this formal dinner, they would show footage from an old *60 Minutes* story on my father's victory against the U.S. Navy, including shots of me, age nine, sitting on a dais erected on Culebra's famed Flamenco Beach, where Dad was giving a speech announcing the end of the bombing.

The camera first panned to then lingered on little Debbie smiling, clapping wildly, beaming with pride at her father's victory, which, even then, she understood had been hard-won. Present-day Deb, seeing these moving images of past her for the first time, would be unable to stop sobbing. She would end up having to excuse herself from the festivities, leaving the banquet a half hour earlier than planned, to wander the streets of Old San Juan in the pouring rain, until she found herself, at dawn, on her Jewish knees inside a Catholic church. "I get it!" she'll shout to a wood-carved Jesus. "You're suffering. We're all suffering. Now what?" A nervous breakdown, my doctor would later call it. "Meshugganah," my family would call it. This message has been brought to you by Lexapro.

My mother was now in the corner of the hospital room on her cellphone, periodically nodding and saying, "Mmm-hmm."

"Who's Mom talking to?" I whispered. My sisters shrugged.

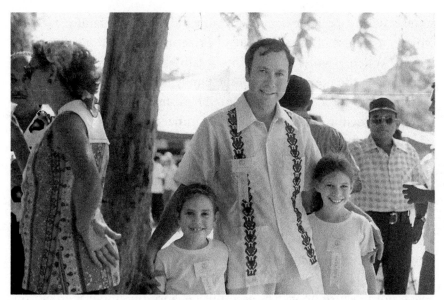

(L to R) Jennifer, Richard, and Deborah Copaken in Culebra,
Puerto Rico, 1975, © Margie Copaken

"Tomorrow at 8 A.M.?" she said. "Yes, good, I'll be there. Thank you."

"Wait, where will you be tomorrow morning at 8?" I said.

Mom held up a finger. "Yes, of course. If anything changes, I'll let you know."

"Who was that?" I said when she hung up.

"The funeral home," said Mom. "We have a meeting tomorrow morning at eight. I want one of you to come with me."

"But . . ." I was at a loss. How to respond? Psychologically, I understood my mother's need for control during a moment when the entire idea of control is shown to be illusory. But practically, I wanted no part of this delusion. I wanted to be able to sit with Dad as he did the hard work of dying. To remain by his side until he was gone. I whispered the obvious: "But Dad's not dead yet."

"I have to meet with the funeral director," she said, "so we might as well do it now."

"But funeral homes are used to getting calls after the fact," I said. *"That's their entire business model."*

My sisters bit their lips. The oldest of four, I'm considered the troublemaker, the truth-teller, the one who ends up calling things by their names without whitewashing or soft-pedaling, frequently at great personal cost and periodic exclusion from the bosom of family. Czesław Miłosz, recipient of the 1980 Nobel Prize in literature, once famously wrote, "When a writer is born into a family, the family is finished." I would argue the opposite: When the family is finished, a writer is born. Writers don't suddenly drop from the womb fully formed. They're planted as seedlings, nurtured in soil fertilized with family secrets and false fronts, until they emerge from the darkness into the light and suddenly notice the difference.

A few months earlier, much to everyone's consternation and disapproval, I'd said, "Why put Dad through chemo right now if he's stage four? If he wants to go on a cruise through the Greek isles, let him go!" I knew better than to suggest he forgo chemo altogether, which would have been my choice given the same diagnosis, not Dad's. But Dad had seemed oddly okay at the moment of his diagnosis, which had been made not because he was in pain but because my uncle Stan, an oncologist, had noticed two things when he and my aunt were having dinner with Mom and Dad: My normally plump father had lost a massive amount of weight without trying; and both he and his eyes were yellow.

After his diagnosis, followed immediately by a prognosis of four to six months, Dad started looking into the cost and logistics of the cruise: a trip he'd been meaning to take with my son but kept putting off. When I suggested that night at the dinner table—we'd all gathered in Bethany Beach, Delaware, for what would turn out to be our last family vacation with Dad—that he throw caution to the wind and just go, I was shut down. "No, we can't take the risk that he'll get sick on the boat." Which I countered, less than generously and more than imperiously, with "For fuck's sake, *he's already sick*! So what if he dies on a boat instead of in a hospital!" But families and death sentences are tricky bedfellows: It brings them together then tears them apart. Rationality in the face of a loved one's terminal illness is not always the most tactful approach. And it is all-too-frequently replaced with magical thinking: If he undergoes chemo, maybe he'll beat the odds and live. Even though we were told his odds of living more than six months were nil.

In the end, the chemo did shrink the tumor a bit, as promised, but with the cancer already having spread elsewhere, he would die on schedule anyway, exactly four months from the day of his diagnosis. Meanwhile, nearly half of every week of the last four months of his life was spent not out in the sunshine or at his easel, where he was painting the last in his series of abstracts, but in bed, in agony from the side effects of the poison that had been pumped into his bloodstream.

"I don't care if that's their business model," my mother was now saying, growing upset. "I'm going to the meeting with the funeral director at 8 A.M., and I want one of you to come with me."

"But it's supposed to snow tonight," I said.

"Light flurries!" She would not be swayed. "I need one of you to come with me," she kept saying. Her husband was dying, and people with dying spouses get a pass on irrational behavior, so it was decided that I would be the one to accompany Mom from Baltimore back to my childhood home in Potomac, Maryland, an hour away. My sisters would stay with Dad at Johns Hopkins. "Just promise me," I said to my little sister, an orthopedic surgeon, "that if it looks like we're getting close to the end, you'll call so we can be here."

"I promise," she said.

I kissed my father's still-warm forehead. I told him I loved him and would be back tomorrow, and off we went.

Five minutes into our silent drive home, both of us lost in our own thoughts, Mom finally spoke. "I'm worried about Bart Dibble," she said. Not the sentence I was expecting. But as I was quickly learning, terminal illness brings out the odd and unexpected. Bart was my parents' financial advisor. It was December 7, 2008, the white-hot center of America's worst financial crisis since the Great Depression. Bart was moving his practice from one large bank to another, which meant Mom and Dad had to sign a bunch of papers to move their savings—which had taken a massive hit just like so many others' that year—into the new bank as well.

"Don't," I said. "He's fine."

But Mom had suddenly become convinced that Bart Dibble had lost his job, and she would soon go bankrupt. "How do you know he didn't lose his job?"

To be fair, my husband had just lost his job, as did so many others that fall. Banker greed and speculation were to blame. "Because he didn't," I said. "These guys get million-dollar bonuses to hop from one bank to another. He's fine. The paperwork is just standard banking stuff." She'd had my dad sign all the necessary papers in the hospital. Everything was kosher on that front.

"I'm worried," she said.

"I know," I said, softening. It was so much easier, I understood, to replace her fears over her husband's death with fears of losing her life savings. Of not being prepared for a funeral. Of a dying man dying on a boat halfway around the world instead of in a sterile hospital room near home. "But of all the things to be worried about at this juncture in time, Bart Dibble's career is not one of them."

By 4 A.M. the next day, the front yard of my childhood home was covered in snow still fluttering out of an ink black sky, and my sister the doctor was on the other end of the phone, saying calmly but firmly, "Come now."

I woke my mother. "We have to go," I said. "It's time."

"Okay," said Mom. "I just have to take a quick shower."

"You don't have time!" I said, growing agitated. "She says we have to come now. And it's snowing!"

My mother's face scrunched into that don't-mess-with-me look I know too well. "I will not be dirty for the death of my husband!"

Reframe, I thought. Don't get angry. She hasn't showered in three days, which in her worldview is unthinkable, but also she is not being rational. It's not about getting clean. It's about pushing off the inevitable. "Okay," I said. "I'll meet you downstairs in the kitchen." I absentmindedly poured myself a bowl of cereal but couldn't eat it. I flipped through a *People* magazine on the counter but couldn't read it. "NEVER GIVING UP HOPE" the cover announced in all caps, over a photo of Parkinson's-stricken Michael J. Fox. This, I thought, is what's wrong with American healthcare. Not for Parkinson's—who was I to deny Michael J. Fox his hope for a cure?—but rather for end-of-life care.

Hope is not a plan when a patient is actively dying. It's a mutually agreed upon delusion.

What if, instead of remaining passive, I'd gone full metal jacket and insisted everyone just shut the fuck up about shrinking tumors and trials and let Dad sail off into the Aegean? Did I fail him as an advocate and as a child? Or was this the death he actually wanted: on a dark and snowy predawn morning, in a nondescript hospital room an hour's drive from home, holding on as best he could until his wife and eldest daughter arrived?

"Let's go!" I said firmly, when Mom finally walked down the stairs, freshly showered, but instead of heading out immediately, she started putting the paperwork for Bart Dibble into a FedEx envelope. "What are you doing?" I took a deep breath. Then another. It was all I could do not to lose it.

"We have to drop these papers into a FedEx drop box before Daddy dies."

"Wait, what?" *Reframe, reframe, reframe. This is not about the FedEx drop box, it's about being mortal.* "No, you don't! Dad already signed and dated them! The envelope itself doesn't have to be time-stamped."

"But what if it does? You don't know that!" Mom was starting to cry now. She looked like a little girl, not like a sixty-six-year-old grandmother of five.

The snow continued falling. I wanted to hold out my hand to my mother and help her across the icy bridge to her husband's death. But I also selfishly wanted to run across it to be there with my father when he took his final breaths. "No," I said, even more firmly now. "We're not going to the FedEx drop box. We're going straight to the hospital."

"But it's on the way!"

If I've learned one thing from being my mother's daughter, it is this: Resistance *is* actually futile. So as my father lay dying in his hospital room in Baltimore, we drove to the nearest FedEx drop box in a strip mall. In a snowstorm. My boots crunched the first tracks into the pristine white coating of the streetlight-lit parking lot as I raced across it, my feet shouting with what felt like indecency, "Look! I am here! I walk this earth!" I slipped the carefully sealed envelope, addressed to Bart Dibble, into a drop box that was not exactly on the way to Johns Hopkins, but whatever. Each of us processes grief in our own way. Me? I wasn't processing anything for the time being. I was too busy worrying about getting to the hospital before Dad's last breaths and answering two constantly ringing cellphones, Mom's and mine. "Where *are* you?" my traumatized sisters kept shouting. "What's taking you so long?"

I started enumerating the various hold-ups: "Mom took a shower. Then we had to drop off an envelope at FedEx . . ." It was as if I were speaking a foreign tongue. *What?* They kept saying. *WHAT?* "Never mind. Don't ask. We're on our way."

Outside the car, it was still dark. As we drove, we were privy to periodic updates. One sister, Julie, was too upset to speak. Jen could speak, if barely, but my brain couldn't process what her eyes weren't able to process either. My surgeon sister, Laura, who would never so much as pilfer a candy bar from a drugstore, had taken it upon herself to swipe another bolus of fluids from the hospital storage, to keep Dad alive until we got there. "I can't keep propping him up with liquids," she said. "How close are you?"

We were still on the beltway surrounding Washington, D.C., before the turnoff to 95 north. "Pretty close," I lied. I didn't want her to worry about the timing of our arrival on top of everything else she was managing.

When you're the sole person with a license to practice medicine in your family, and you're all of thirty-six years old on the morning your sixty-seven-year-old father is in the final throes of dying from pancreatic cancer—but really he's dying from everything else that was shutting down his organs that morning, after his belly filled with ascites on Thanksgiving day—you are put in the unfortunate position of having to be both the newscaster explaining the carnage to your family as well as their go-between with the oncologist. Laura, in other words, was not given the chance, as her father lay dying, to be the grieving child. She had to be capable, on top of things. Keeping her father alive until her mother and sister could get back to the hospital after their ill-conceived detour.

Mom and I made it to the hospital, parked the car, zoomed up the elevator, and sprinted down the hallway to Dad's room. He was still functionally alive, if barely. His death rattle was pronounced, a hideous, gear-stripping struggle to pull in oxygen and push out carbon dioxide. His tongue was hanging out of the right side of his mouth. His chest rose and fell out of sync with his periodic gasps for air. *Make it stop!* I wanted to scream, at the same time I was begging whatever deity might have been listening for one more crack of Dad's crooked smile. I was used to movie death scenes: The soft music swells as the patient quietly says his meaningful goodbyes and slips away. This, however, was a horror film. My father's lungs were filling with fluid. He was literally drowning in front of our eyes.

His vitals on the monitor were fading: low numbers, long valleys between heartbeat mountains, a barely perceptible pulse. My mother, walking in on this scene, was clearly and quite visibly unnerved. Her husband had gone from slightly cogent, when we'd left ten hours earlier, to barely of this world. Mom, either trying to crack a joke to lighten the darkness or maybe she was experiencing a trauma-induced psychotic break, poked Dad in the upper arm and said, "So, Dick, did you hear? Bart Dibble lost his job."

Dad's vital signs visibly spiked. His rattle grew more intense.

"Mom!" we said in unison, followed by a distinct choking on our own chuckles. Scientists who study the hows and whys of humor refer to this as "relief theory," a release of psychic energy during moments of extreme tension. I prefer to think of it as the Bart Dibble theory, which is closer to Schopenhauer's theory of incongruity: Humor, according to Schopenhauer, is what happens when we violate expectations, like when sixty clowns crawl out of a tiny car or, as linguists will add, when nonsense words in Dr. Seuss make us laugh. Was Mom's joke inherently funny? No. Was its timing, during a hideous death scene, an unexpected comic gold gift of untold value? Yes. Now, whenever I remember the unspeakable pain of my father's last hour, it is counterbalanced by the Seussian sound of that double B followed by an L (may Bart Dibble, too, rest in peace) and Mom's spurious report of his job loss.

"Dad, we're all here now," said Laura, bringing us back to the macabre task at hand: watching the man we loved die.

My father, who was born in 1941, had been raised as a latch-key kid in Kansas City by a married pair of lawyers with their own two-person firm—Copaken and Copaken—and rock-solid humanist principles. Their specialty was representing the indigent, who otherwise would not have been able to afford legal services. My grandparents accepted everything from sacks of potatoes to homemade pies as recompense for their services, meaning money was as absent in Dad's life as love was present. His father, a Jewish refugee from Kiev, had one arm that didn't function. It hung limp by his side, ragdoll-style, shorter than the other. Its bones had been shattered by Cossacks who, while ransacking his family's home, had lifted him out of his crib and smashed his infant body against a wall. Dad's mother, whose Jewish parents had also fled persecution in Eastern Europe—Vilnius, in her case—was one of the rare female lawyers in America of her generation. She sewed her own clothes, wore sensible flats, and eschewed makeup and artifice of all kinds. She was gentle, calm, brilliant, achingly sweet, and both a prolific letter-writer and great listener, but she also had no time or patience for the roles culturally expected of her, particularly housework. This had been a source of secret shame for Dad, who—though he loved his parents deeply—felt he couldn't invite friends over to his unkempt home after school.

My mom, born in 1942, was raised in the Bronx by a comically gifted if culinarily challenged housewife, who believed ketchup was a perfectly acceptable condiment on pasta, as well as by an emotionally distant, sometimes volatile army doctor, who would apply his leather belt to his children's skin whenever he felt it was warranted. When Mom told her father she wanted to be a doctor like him, he told her there wasn't enough money for a girl to go to medical school. My grandfather's mother, from whom he was estranged, had stolen every dollar he'd saved and hidden under his mattress, which he'd planned to use to go to medical school. He then became a postal worker for several years to afford his tuition.

So while money in my mother's home was also tight—an army doctor's salary barely covered their two-bedroom, basement apartment, in which he and his wife slept on a pull-out sofa in the living room, to give their three kids, two girls and a boy, the two bedrooms—my grandfather's pronouncement that whatever was left would be wasted on a girl wanting to become a doctor was uttered just as Mom's older brother, my uncle, was finishing up his studies to become the oncologist who would, years later, discover Dad's cancer.

Subconsciously or not, like many married couples, my parents had each chosen the other, I've come to believe, as a salve to heal past wounds. He would have a sparkling clean suburban home and a wife who would forgo her own career to look after the children. (The song they chose to dance to at my wedding was "Wind Beneath My Wings.") She, after a lifetime of living below ground level, would have a skylit roof over her head, a baby grand Steinway—she'd been a gifted musician, a Music and Art graduate who played piano, flute, and cello, and had once conducted at Carnegie Hall as a teenager—and enough tuition for her kids' college education, no matter their gender.

My parents married young, at twenty and twenty-one, during an era when an unmarried twenty-four-year-old female was already considered an "old maid," and college-educated women with master's degrees like my mother were expected to become homemakers. How could these two have possibly understood, on their wedding day in 1963, what it might be like, decades hence, for one of them to have sacrificed their dreams for the other's? Or maybe both of their dreams were subsumed into ours. Dad was a weekend painter. He built an art studio onto our house. He would retreat there to throw paint on a giant canvas, à la Morris Louis, which he sold and exhibited here and there. Though he rarely complained and claimed to enjoy his job as an international lawyer in a white-shoe law firm, my hunch growing up—and particularly toward the end of his life—was that, had he not had to support four daughters and a wife; had healthcare been a national right instead of a privilege; had choosing art as a career been as acceptable in his circles as choosing law, he might have happily spent every waking hour in that art studio, making a professional go of it.

Or maybe I'm just projecting, knowing how euphoric I'd felt during my twenties as a photojournalist based in Paris, creating images that also paid my bills while relying on France's excellent free healthcare; or between my midthirties and early forties, spending every day, from dusk till dawn, in the mentally challenging but giddy flow of composing income-generating sentences. I tried talking to him about all of this before he died, but he quickly shut me down. "No, I've loved every second of my life," he said, ever the optimist with that constant, crooked smile, "and I wouldn't change a thing." But it's telling that he spent nearly every hour of the last two months of that life, whenever he was not in pain from the chemo, with a paintbrush in his hand. He even managed, with my sisters' help, to put together a final show of his new work within a month of his death.

I was on a twelve-city book tour during Dad's show. "You cannot renege on your responsibilities to your work," he'd said. "I'll be upset with you if you come home for my show." To say I still regret missing that show is an understatement. I look at the photos that were taken that day and feel a deep ache. What was so important about selling a few extra books that I missed out on my dad's final moment of glory?

As we girls grew up, and as my parents' traditional gender roles began to chafe, Mom lashed out with words and silences, Dad with secretly gobbled sweets—he contracted type 2 diabetes in late middle age and was less than stellar with compliance—and impulse purchases: sports cars, cameras, top-of-the-line stereo and video equipment. Could he afford these frequent indulgences, on top of his art supplies, food, clothing, four college tuitions, two weeks of summer vacation every year in the little cottage in West Harwich, Massachusetts, and the extra mortgage to build the art studio onto the house? Yes. Sort of. But all of this meant that our modest kitchen, which Mom had always hoped to renovate and expand to fit our growing family after my twin sisters were born, would remain too small, in her eyes, for the six of us to sit there comfortably during dinner, until years after her daughters were already out of the house: a symbolic rebuke, she felt, to the role she'd taken on as homemaker.

One time, at that kitchen table, Mom stood up in the middle of dinner and announced, "Girls, if I'm not here when you wake up tomorrow morning, you'll know I've finally left your father." At the time, I was mortified. And seething, just under the surface of my adolescent skin, with a hidden rage that I lacked self-awareness to process or understand. During our one attempt at family therapy soon thereafter, with Mom's therapist, I hijacked the last fifteen minutes of that session with a string of wrath-filled expletives I could hardly believe were erupting from my mouth, but there they were. Out there. Naked. I begged for more sessions, but no one else in the family wanted to uncover *that* can of worms again. So we never went back.

Decades later, after having experienced similar frustrations in my own marriage, only with the added burden of having been the primary wage earner on top of the outmoded expectations that I would take on all the responsibilities of house and home, I not only understood my mother's threat that night to leave her husband, I was the one who ultimately followed through on it.

Why didn't my mother do the same? Part of it, I'm sure, was a lack of wage-earning options for women of her generation who'd left or never entered the workforce, as well as the social stigma of divorce. But also there was the undeniable fact of my parents' palpable bond of love.

Yes, it could often be plagued by what psychologists call the four horsemen of the relationship apocalypse: criticism, contempt, defensiveness, and stonewalling. And those horsemen would one day gallop straight into my marriage and turn me into an oft-raging monster: a trauma my own children, in turn—particularly the older two, who were teenagers for the worst of it—must now process in their adulthoods. (I am ashamed of this, but it must be noted.) At the same time, there was also the way my father told their origin story with still-sparkling stars in his eyes; the way he always told my mother, whenever she was feeling down about herself, that she was the most beautiful woman in the world; the *I love you*'s he sprinkled like fairy dust, often and freely. Mom's language of love resided firmly in selfless acts of service, which she performed dutifully and daily, making sure Dad's shirts were ironed, his doctor appointments were booked, his meals were cooked, his social life was organized. Whenever he traveled for work, she'd make countless round trips to the airport. And she would blush like a girl and say, "Oh, Dickie," whenever Dad presented her with one of his homemade cards, each festooned with one of his signature smiling birds atop his cartoon characters' heads and filled, inside, with words of love and admiration.

"Oh, Dickie . . ." said Mom, starting to tear up again. Looking even more lost and scared: How do you summarize a lifetime of love, with all of its ups and downs, in the few minutes you have left? With her four daughters looking on, Mom grabbed Dad's hand. "Well, Dick," she said, massaging his knuckles with her thumbs. "We've been together for forty-five years." She froze, stuck at this setup of fact. Now what? Ask anyone who's watched a loved one die, and they'll tell you that trying to say something meaningful and cogent in the last hours of someone's life can feel not only performative and uncomfortable, it can also devolve into farce. As when Mom finally found her Borscht Belt–delivered punch line: "I can't say they've been the happiest years of my life, but they've been years."

"Mom!" I said, snorting at her valiant if failed attempt, as unintentionally hilarious as it was true.

Mom sputtered, unable to form sentences. "I just . . . how do you . . .

I can't . . ." She finally settled on the only words that made sense: "I love you," she whispered, multiple times into Dad's ear, before we moved her down to Dad's feet to massage them as each of his four daughters grabbed an arm or a leg to do the same. How lucky, I remember thinking, to have four daughters and four limbs. Being on right arm duty, near his right ear, wanting to assure him that all was well, I leaned over and whispered, "Dad, Bart Dibble did not lose his job. Mom loves you. We all love you. We're all here now. All five of us. You can go." Each of my sisters reassured him of the same: We were all in attendance. He could stop struggling. Soon thereafter the room, with the exception of one long steady beep of the EKG flatlining and five women's simultaneous sobs, grew silent. No more soul-shattering death rattle. No more breaths in or out. No more pulse beeps or blood pressure or brain waves.

At that exact moment, the first rays of sun shot through the hospital window, illuminating my father's still-warm body and turning the tableau of our newly pruned, mourning family into a chiaroscuro. The photographer in me wanted to put a camera between the pain and my overflowing eye and shoot this. The newly fatherless daughter in me had lost her ability to take action. She stood inert, broken. For the next several years.

Dad had told each of us that whenever we needed to speak to him, he'd appear as either a sunrise or a rainbow. And while we knew our father was just trying to make his transition to nonexistence easier on us— since every day there's a sunrise, and rainbows are cool—you have to admit it was an inspired idea to claim two natural phenomena as his own.

On his cancer blog that morning, I posted a final photo of him staring out at the sun rising over the ocean a couple of days after he found out he was dying. "Dad died at 7:02 A.M. . . . ." I wrote, ". . . four months to the day from his diagnosis." He'd spent every morning of that final vacation on the Delaware shore waking up in time to watch the sunrise, sharing it with whichever grandchild he could convince to join him, which they knew meant not only watching the magical fireball rise in the sky with their grandfather but also hearing him expound on photosynthesis, on the speed of light, on Einstein's theory of relativity, on why the moon causes waves, on the parabolic arc of earth's rotation, on why we have seasons, on seeing Simon and Garfunkel play in a tiny venue, before they were famous, on art, on evolution's punctuated equilibrium, and on the vast mysteries of the universe as yet unknown and forever unknowable. To this day, whenever I see a sunrise or a rainbow, my father feels both physically present with me and comforting in ways I find difficult to describe. "Oh, hi, Dad," I'll say, just as I did that morning he left his body and reappeared as the sun.

Yes, and . . .

SEPTEMBER 2013

My father's last hours became both catalyst and fuel. I did not want to reach the end of my life unable to conjure anything but pain and years. Dad's death also became a constant reminder to tune in to the mechanics of my own body, a flawed system designed to expire but also to prevent its own cells from mutating, dividing, and conquering itself during our approximately 28,835 days on earth.

I palpate the breast lump again: a nervous tic now. Fuck.

Step-by-step, I tell myself, sitting at my desk, staring at my to-do list. Take it step-by-step.

The Brooklyn Book Festival seems the most easily solvable problem, plus I cannot cancel since the panel was provoked by an essay I'd written in *The Nation* entitled "My So-Called 'Post-Feminist' Life in Arts and Letters." I'd composed the essay quickly, in a slow-simmering rage, after *The New York Times*'s obituary for Yvonne Brill, a renowned rocket scientist and winner of the National Medal of Technology and Innovation, led with "She made a mean beef stroganoff, followed her husband from job to job and took eight years off from work to raise three children. 'The world's best mom,' her son Matthew said."

The lede, after readers revolted, was later reworded online—"beef stroganoff" was removed, "brilliant rocket scientist" was added, it's the little things, really—but while it was still up there, in stark black-and-white, it reminded me of similar sexist belittlements leveled at me.

"After two years of painstaking work to produce the book," I wrote in the essay, "nearly every review refers to me as a stay-at-home mom. One such article is entitled 'Battlefield Barbie,' which calls me a 'soccer-mom-in-training*.' I look nothing like Barbie. My kids don't play soccer." I'd tried finding one instance in which a male author was called a stay-at-home dad, full-time dad, or soccer dad. But no. They were just called authors.

In the essay, I'd also pointed out that I was worried that the act of writing such an essay would ultimately be judged and punished. "It's career suicide, my colleagues tell me, to speak out against the literary establishment; they'll smear you. But never mind. I'm too old and too invisible to said establishment to care. And I still believe, as Carol Hanisch wrote back in 1969—when I was having my then three-year-old feet forced into stiff Mary Janes—that the personal is political."

For six years after the essay's publication—hard as I tried—I could not sell a new work of literary fiction or nonfiction. To anyone.

The essay was also inconveniently posted online while I was on a flight to Ohio, heading to a college visit to Oberlin with my son. By the time we landed, my phone was buzzing with notifications. At one point, before deciding to simply turn off the phone for a few days, I had to duck out of the college tour to speak with several reporters who had been hounding me with emails, DMs, Facebook messages, texts, and voice-mails. The next day, headlines such as "Women's Prize for Fiction nominee Deborah Copaken Kogan lifts the lid on sexism in publishing and the arts" appeared in English-speaking publications in both the U.S. and abroad. A Hollywood arts organization published a story calling me "Heroine of the Day." A pull quote from the story became its own meme: "This is what sexism does best: it makes you feel crazy for desiring parity and hopeless about ever achieving it." And of course there were the requisite abusive, misogynist tweets and DMs from trolls, the kind that every

---

* The term *soccer mom* has gone from descriptor, when it was first used in 1982, to sexist trope. Like other descriptors such as *mistress, working mother, slut, Karen,* and *spinster,* it has no male counterpart: usually as good a sign as any that those slinging it are using it more as insult than identifier.

woman who uses her voice receives on a regular basis and often contain recurring words and phrases such as *cunt, ugly slut,* and *i wanna cum on your face.*

A Wikipedia troll who went by the handle Qworty and spent his days vandalizing women writers' biographies, went to town on my biography as well, after which he was permanently banned from the site. How did he vandalize mine? Not with insults and name-calling but with erasure. He removed all of my books. He edited out my Emmy. He erased the film in which I acted, my photojournalism career, even the monologue I'd once performed on the New York City stage in honor of one of my heroes, Anita Hill. He removed my name from all professional writing and photographer categories, to make it unsearchable in those data-bases. The only Wikipedia categories in which he left me were 1966 Births and Living people. In retribution for publishing an essay about female erasure, he did to me exactly what *The New York Times* had done to Yvonne Brill, which is what had sparked my essay in the first place.

I was proud of that essay and of its wildfire spread through various literary and feminist ecosystems, but how was I going to talk about all of this and sign books on a Saturday morning with a seven-year-old, no co-parent to stay home and watch him, and no wiggle room in my budget to pay a sitter? (I was not getting paid to speak on the panel. It was yet another one of those things we writers are urged by our publishers to do in the name of exposure.)

I'll have to bring my son with me, I decide. But then I realize I can't speak frankly about rape, name-calling, slut-shaming, and internet trolls who say they want to cum on my face in front of a second grader. I also can't talk about the way the word *mother* has been subverted into an in-sult hurled at professional women, who are either blamed for not being mother enough or derided for being too maternal. He might somehow misunderstand the discussion and feel bad for having been born. Plus let's not forget he'd just turned seven: too young to sit still for an hour-long panel on misogyny and sexism in the literary world at 9 A.M. on a Saturday morning.

I google the address of the festival and zoom in on the map: It's a few blocks from my friends Tad and Amanda's apartment. Great! I call Amanda and ask if my son and I can have a sleepover the night prior at their apartment.

I'm not used to asking for help. It feels wrong, even shameful to have to say, "I can't do this on my own. Please help." But there is grace in asking for help and, as I will discover, grace in receiving it. Tad is one of my oldest friends, the senior I met on my first night of college as a freshman, back when I was just starting to make a string of bad choices in love, to which he bore compassionate witness. Amanda, Tad's wife, is a balm in human form. I played an enthusiastic if secondary role in igniting their coupledom through our mutual friend Jennifer, who had the inspired idea of setting them up on a blind date. Their twins have been my son's friends since birth. Our little ones even look slightly like triplets when the three of them are together. We've shared Thanksgivings and New Years, brunches and tears. They are, in other words, my chosen family.

"Of course you can stay with us," says Amanda. They'll blow up the air mattress and await our arrival. My son can sleep with the twins in their bedroom, no worries. I can sleep in the living room. Tad gets on the phone. "We're here for you," he says, and I can tell he means it. When I hang up, I smile through a new kind of tears: the kind that spring forth each time I encounter these small acts of kindness I see as gigantic impositions, until I learn to accept that asking for help from people you love is not shameful or wrong but—welcome to my TED talk—an opportunity for transformation and connection.

With one action item crossed off my to-do list, I'm emboldened to try to knock off a few more, so I google "free mammogram Harlem" and find that, right here in my neighborhood, Memorial Sloan Kettering offers free screenings at the Breast Examination Center of Harlem to women like me who've lost their insurance. I pause, wracked by shame once again. Is it wrong for me to use a charity health service when there are probably so many other women in my neighborhood with suspicious lumps who are in straits more dire than mine? Then again, I remind myself, I have less than next month's rent in the bank, no health insurance, a mid-five figures in credit card debt, and a lump in my breast. That counts as dire-ish straits, right? Plus if I'd stayed in Paris I wouldn't even be asking myself this question. I would, no matter my income, find the nearest breast-screening office near my apartment and get a government-mandated free mammogram every two years. In fact, I would first get a letter every two years from the French government health office, politely reminding me to come in for my free screening. Then I would get my free screening.

I call the Breast Examination Center of Harlem. The woman on the phone asks me a bunch of questions, to see if I qualify. I do. Their next appointment is in two months. I take it.

Next, I compose an email to friends, alerting them both to my separation and to my job search. Then I contact my friend George, to see if he still wants to rent out my college son's bedroom. Yes, he says. He's in. But first we have to see if our dogs get along, and he'll be moving in with two cats as well. The idea of this large menagerie moving into my apartment gives me pause, since I find caring for one poorly house-trained dog trying, but I love George and would rather share my home with someone I know than someone I don't. Plus we can take turns with dog-walking duties.

George and I had recently reconnected at our twenty-fifth college reunion the previous May. He was still reeling that weekend from the suicide of his husband seven months earlier. Zhang, a chemist, had been raised in China. Prior to marrying George, Zhang had yet to come out to his parents, who were still living in rural China. After the wedding, however, feeling emboldened by love, Zhang sent a photo of his wedding day to his family, along with a note explaining the circumstances of its having been taken: He'd married a wonderful man; he was happy and professionally flourishing; he hoped to have their blessing. The photo showed the beaming couple at City Hall, along with their beagle, Elvis.

His parents never responded. His sister sent a letter containing only one sentence: "Are you going to eat that dog?"

After receiving this, George said, Zhang seemed to grow increasingly despondent. Five weeks after the wedding, he mixed himself some cyanide, rented a hotel room, and inhaled it.

Several months after our college reunion, I read a Facebook post of George's, written with palpable grief a few days before what would have been his first wedding anniversary. I reached out to him in a long email, suggesting he move in with us. "We can feed you a hot meal every night," I wrote, "you'll get that comfort of living in a home with kids (good kids, I promise), it'll be a radical change of pace, away from the place where you and Zhang shared a life, and we can, well, heal each other. This will be a rough year. Might as well share it . . ."

To which he'd responded saying he'd love that and would get back to me. Now he was getting back to me, and the plan was a go. He was an adjunct professor of English as a Second Language, helping immigrants adjust to the rigors of taking classes in a different language from their mother tongue. His hours were such that he'd be a presence in the home, often enough, when my son arrived home from school.

In retrospect, I couldn't have known just how therapeutic his presence in our newly fractured home would be. That he'd bake bread in the afternoons, filling the apartment with curative aromas and our bellies with joy. That he would bring my son small additions to his Disney Infinity plastic figurine collection now and then, just because, and always be available not only to listen but to hear and to thoughtfully respond. That he and my daughter would bond over their mutual love of animals, and that the antics of his cat, a malodorous nuisance, would become a source of dark humor. That George's own dark humor—honed by years of improv, by growing up intelligent and gay in the Deep South, by tragedy, by grief—would feel essential each time the spinning plates over our heads would come crashing down. That I looked forward to talking to him after work and sharing the details of our days: the petty territorialism at the office, my latest lab results, some story I read somewhere about something; his struggling students and the financial indignities of adjunct life; his constant haunting by memories of Zhang. That our platonic domestic partnership would serve as a benchmark of what a romantic domestic partnership could look like, should I be lucky enough to find one. George and I wouldn't "heal each other," as I'd ignorantly Kumbaya'd in my email, so much as we would serve as compassionate witness and comic foil to the widening and deepening of each of our wounds during one of the hardest years in each of our lives.

After organizing a time for Elvis and Lucas, our dogs, to meet, I look into hiring an au pair to pick up my seven-year-old from school and bring him home every day at 2:45 P.M.: a time that was useful for turn-of-the-century rural parents, who needed their kids home before nightfall to help with the harvest, but that is not only not useful to modern-day working urban and suburban parents, particularly the single ones, it is the number one bane of their work-life existence. "But what about after-school activities?" you say. "Shouldn't they have time for sports and piano and all the rest?"

To which I say, yes, please! Build art and music and dance and debate and sports into the end of the school day. Officially and financially.

Provide time, space, and a helpful instructor or two for nightly home-work, to keep it from destroying the sanctity of the hour or so we actually get to spend with our kids at home, or, better yet, do away with home-work altogether, particularly when children are young. They've done studies. It's useless. And a school day that ends before the end of business hours means that every American family has to figure out how to cover those uncovered hours, a burden that falls predominantly on the shoul-ders of—you guessed it—women.

It's also, if you think about it (as I so often do), a hidden tax on women, much like the cost of feminine hygiene products or the monu-mental time suck/logistical hassle* and monthly cost of birth control pills: both, by the way, important tools in mitigating the mess of not being pregnant and limiting the number of children you have to pick up at school at 2:45 on any given day. The U.S. government does not recog-nize the reality of our childcare costs, since its own tax code assumes we only spend $3,000 a year in childcare expenses instead of, on average, more than three times that amount per child. In New York City, where I live, you can't even get bad daycare for under $20,000 a year, let alone any. Meanwhile, the Department of Health and Human Services sug-gests American families spend no more than 7 percent of their house-hold income on childcare when, if they'd taken the time to glance at the statistics, they would know that there is literally no state in the entire country where this is currently possible.

All of this is a roundabout way of saying that hiring an au pair, if you have a separate room for one, is the most economical way of being a solo working parent to a young child, since single parents end up spending, on average, 37 percent of their household income on childcare. By U.S. State Department law, if you house and feed a live-in au pair, the man-dated weekly stipend you must pay them is $195.75 a week: that's $10,179 a year, meaning the first $20,000 or so of pretax income goes directly to

* I've lost count of the number of times my daughter has texted me in a blind panic about her birth control pills, when some glitch in her prescription delivery service—now required by our health insurance, if we want them to help cover her pills—sends her scrambling to fill in the gaps with her friends' pills. (Her friends' pills!) She, like all Americans on the pill, must visit her doctor in person for a new prescription every year. This not only costs money, it costs time and effort, and then something always goes wrong anyway.

pay someone to pick up your child at school and watch them until you get home: a relative bargain.

The problem, I realize when I look into it further, is that the au pair agencies ask for $8,500 up front to match you with your au pair. Suddenly my bargain childcare solution looks like every other childcare solution: too expensive. I don't have an extra $8,500 lying around. Most of us don't. In fact, a 2019 Federal Reserve study found that roughly 40 percent of Americans, including yours truly at both this juncture in our story and for many years thereafter, would not be able to cover a $400 emergency. This is not because we are spendthrifts. It's because as wages stagnated, the cost of childcare, housing, healthcare, and food is now greater than our income.

I back-burner the seemingly impossible task of finding affordable childcare until I land a new job. Speaking of which, oh, look! Into my inbox pops a new email asking me to come in for a third round of interviews at a company called Health Today,[*] an online health magazine in search of an executive editor. I'd never previously heard of the publication or the company, but I'd won my Emmy with its COO, Rick, for a story about an Amtrak train crash when we worked together at ABC News.

Rick, unlike many others at ABC News, not only welcomed and honored the input of his female collaborators without even the hint of impropriety or harassment—back then, in the mid-1990s, the majority of men in my office were producers, the majority of women were their underlings, and sex and/or power imbalances between them were rampant—but he always insisted upon leaving the office by 6 P.M., whenever possible, to have dinner with his wife and to put his son to bed. This had left me in charge of editing our story by myself after business hours. It had also given me a road map for the kind of parent I wanted to be.

The job opportunity with Health Today had come about as a result of running into Rick at a school event the previous May. I joked with him about my fruitless search for full-time employment. Our Emmy, my books, decades of journalism experience on several continents in several

[*] Name has been changed.

mediums: None of it seemed to count, I told him, when you walked into an interview wearing middle-aged, female skin.

"I'm warning you, it's a viper's nest in here," he'd said, at the end of my first round of interviews, only half chuckling, "but they liked you, and we could use someone with actual journalism chops and ethics."

Viper's nest or not, I think—checking my bank statement, feeling my lump—I need a job. Now. I don't have time to wait for something better. There are too many former magazine writers looking for work ever since the internet blew up our industry and turned it into a musical chairs death match. I respond to the email and make an appointment to come in for another round of interviews the following week. It has been over four months since my first interview. This is a pattern I will see repeated: job tangos that stretch on for six months or more before you either get hired or ghosted.

As it will turn out, I'll land the editor job at Health Today that fall, but my health insurance won't kick in until just before Christmas—many companies these days make you wait a month between your starting date and getting coverage, which: why?—so I keep the late November free clinic appointment with the Breast Examination Center of Harlem to figure out what's going on in my boob, if anything.

As I twist myself into this healthcare pretzel to get a simple lump examined, I imagine citizens of Sweden or France or England or all the other first world countries in which healthcare is sewn into the fabric of society hearing my story and saying, no, it can't be *that* bad. Well, yes, I want to tell them. It can be. This is what it's like for us. People die in America because they can't afford insulin or because they must ration the insulin they have. Sometimes they can't even afford the cost of the check-up to let them know they need insulin to stay alive. Or their doctor, trying to maximize profits by seeing as many patients as possible in a single day, is too rushed to notice anything amiss or to order a simple test.

My first cousin, Jeremy Copaken—with whom I spent every Thanksgiving, many Passovers, and countless weekends as a child—will die in 2014, just after his thirty-ninth birthday, of undiagnosed diabetes. At home, alone, on his living room floor, halfway between his TV and couch, hours after visiting a too-harried doctor and saying, "I don't feel well."

In America, people in their thirties should not be dying from diabetic shock on their living room floors. It's a manageable, easily diagnosable illness. Jeremy was obese. Shouldn't some doctor somewhere at some point along the way have thought to test him for diabetes? It's a blood test. One fucking blood test.

In 1952, George Merck, the CEO of his eponymous pharmaceutical company, declared, "Medicine is for people, not for profits," on the cover of *Time* magazine, and his company subsequently donated $200 million worth of river blindness medication to Africa in the late '80s because it was the moral thing to do. Today's Merck is using its $6.2 billion in profits to buy back shares of its own stocks and to keep its shareholders and CEO happy. Merck CEO Kenneth Frazier received a 2019 pay package worth $22.6 million while also selling $54.8 million in his own stock between July 2018 and July of 2019.

Several smart economists studied the numbers in 2017 and all but named the pharmaceutical industry a Ponzi scheme. How do these companies get away with this? Well, in 2018, Merck spent $10 billion on research and development of new drugs. This seems like a lot of money to help fund new research until you realize that they spent 40 percent more—$14 billion—on share repurchases and dividends. Moreover, from 2008 until 2017, the company distributed 133 percent of its profits to shareholders. Let's pause to consider that number again: 133 percent of Merck's profits are handed out to its shareholders. (Yes, I had to read that number twice, too.) Even I, who was as pitiful at playing Monopoly in my youth as I am in understanding simple economics today, can tell you that a business that gives away more than 100 percent of its profits to shareholders is Bernie Madoff–level unsustainable.

What this means is that those of us in America who need drugs and healthcare—meaning all of us—have to make up the difference. Today in the U.S., George Merck's 1952 *Time* magazine quote would be flipped on its head: Medicine is for profits, not for people. And drug companies and private insurers are now incentivized, by their own business models, to save a buck over a life. It is telling that Frazier gets lauded in the press not for helping to save millions of lives with Merck's groundbreaking immunotherapy cancer treatment, Keytruda—a true breakthrough, let's all acknowledge that—but "for building Keytruda into a franchise that can be used to fight a range of tumors, navigating challenging political currents, and delivering strong returns for shareholders."

This push to keep shareholders happy means the pharmaceutical lobby is the most powerful lobbying group in the U.S. today by nearly a factor of two, pumping nearly $4.6 billion into lobbying efforts since 1998. Meaning every year they donate not just millions of dollars but rather hundreds of millions of dollars to those candidates and lawmakers who will protect their financial interests.

In 2017, U.S. congressman Raúl Labrador, whose campaign was partly funded by pharma-dollars, said, "Nobody dies because they don't have access to healthcare." Of course we know that this is not true. In fact, if we're getting down to the statistical nitty-gritty, one can reasonably argue that Chief Justice John Roberts, in his majority opinion in *National Federation of Independent Business v. Sebelius*, personally killed 15,600 Americans by creating the legal rationale that would allow states to opt out of the ACA's Medicaid expansion. According to a 2019 economic study, which looked at death rates since the Supreme Court's decision in 2012, those states that ignored the Supreme Court's decision and opted in for Medicaid expansion saw death rates drop, saving 19,200 lives over the course of four years. Had all states opted in, those 15,600 lives could have been saved.

Pre-Covid-19, that was a big number—a battlefront casualty number—these 15,600 dead Americans. And our brains are terrible at processing big numbers: 2,977 people were murdered on 9/11, but, even though I personally knew three of them, I had to read every single obituary in *The New York Times* "Portraits of Grief" to feel the gaping hole each left behind. We build monuments to those murdered in acts of war or terrorism, carving their names into shiny stone, but exterminate more than five times the number of people who died on 9/11 with corporate greed and political indifference, and deaths like my cousin Jeremy's remain an uncarved rounding error.

Or as that paragon of kindness and empathy, Joseph Stalin, once allegedly exclaimed: A single death is a tragedy. A million deaths is a statistic.

The London-based American actor Rob Delaney, of *Catastrophe* fame, lost his two-year-old son, Henry, to a brain tumor in 2018. He's so appalled by the absurdities of the U.S. healthcare system that he still lives abroad. "How to say this simply?" he wrote in a 2019 Twitter thread. "I lived in the US until I was 37 & had private health insurance most of my life. For the past 5 yrs I've lived in the UK & use the NHS. The NHS is a HUGE part of why I might never move back to the US. . . . Most critically the UK spends dramatically LESS per patient than the US. IT COSTS LESS."

The United States also lags behind the following countries, all of whom have nationalized healthcare systems, in healthcare quality and so-called "amenable mortality" scores—that's a number that measures the rates of deaths considered preventable by a combination of timely and effective care: the Netherlands (96.1), Australia (95.9), Sweden (95.5), Japan (94.1), Austria (93.9), Germany (92), France (91.7), and the United Kingdom (90.5). The U.S., which spends more on health-care per capita than any other developed nation on earth, only scored an 88.7 amenable mortality score: a solid B, okay, sure, but—call me picky—when it's a binary matter of life and death, I'd rather live in a country that gets an A when graded on its ability to keep me alive. Not needlessly dying due to a lack of timely and effective care for a prevent-able illness only 88.7 percent of the time doesn't seem like a reasonable score for a country with a higher GDP than the eight countries ranked above ours.

I wonder how long I'd have to wait to have a breast lump examined for free in the Netherlands.

It's important to note, too, that, as I sit here writing this, seven years after I needed that free breast exam, Title X, which was a landmark federal program aimed at supporting women's health for low-income Americans, has been all but dismantled. This means that a formerly free breast exam now costs $160. Pap smears, which test for cervical cancer, have gone from free to $264. And two of the most foolproof methods of birth control, which require a doctor's insertion—an arm implant and an IUD—have skyrocketed from zero to in some cases more than $1,000 a pop.

I sit at my desk, still staring at my to-do list, hyperventilating. I've crossed off the tasks that don't require financial solutions, but those that do weigh on my chest like lead aprons, one atop the other. My heart hurts. My lungs won't fill. If it were just "find cheaper apartment/move," I'd still be experiencing minor anxiety, sure, but combined with the rest of the list, it paralyzes me. I am the Little Engine Who Couldn't, a negative subversion of my favorite book as a child. *I think I can't, I think I can't, I think I can't.*

My office window faces east, into the bricks of a large apartment building on Edgecomb Avenue overlooking Jackie Robinson Park. Several musicians live in that building, and when I'm not trying to concentrate on crafting sentences, I'll open my window to let in their notes: Bach, Beethoven, jazz, ragtime, piano, a saxophone, an electric guitar: You never know which genre or notes will waft in from which type of instrument, but you're guaranteed to hear whichever they happen to be repeated multiple times, for many hours, until their creator gets them just right. It has given me comfort to know there were others like me nearby, sitting alone in their rooms, polishing their little offerings to the world.

On September mornings like today's, when the sun is still high enough in the sky, light infuses my office until it glows. It kills me to have to give up this room of my own. Yes, it's under six feet wide, and its floors are so sloped that the magnetic balls my son likes to play with after school roll from one end of the room to the other, but it fits my desk, a chair, and a narrow shelf, and it is the place in which I have done work that has fed me, both literally and figuratively. The spines of said work, translated into various languages, now line that narrow bookshelf, atop which ten copies of a new French translation are now stacked, waiting for me to find a place to store them. One of the reasons we'd moved to Harlem, back when the rents were still cheap, was so that I could have this home office. One of the reasons I stayed in my failing marriage for so long, aside from not wanting to hurt my kids, was to keep writing in it without worrying about where I'd get my healthcare.

I stand up. Lean my arms and forehead against the glass pane. Stare down at the sharp angles of my neighbor's patio below, then back up at the sun: *How do I do this?* I wonder, meaning the rest of my life. *Who am I without the work I do in this room?* The questions bring on a new eruption of tears. I consider jumping. Joining Dad. The crack of skull against slate. The blissful release of letting go. The definitive *no* and *I think I can't* and *fuck this shit, I'm done.*

I open the window. Poke my head out. Contemplate the impact of an object falling four stories. I'm terrible at physics. There's velocity, time, and gravity, but how do you calculate the actual force of a body in free fall? A shiver runs up my spine as I lean out too far. I readjust my center of gravity and pull my shoulders back in. The late summer air is already cooling. Soon ice and snow will cover the slate below. Branches will crack under its weight. One October, when the trees outside my office window had hit peak foliage, a freak snowstorm erupted. The combination of red, orange, and yellow leaves dusted in powdery white had thrilled my children. They'd all crammed into my tiny office to stare at the snowliage, a reminder that life could still hold unforeseen beauty.

Somewhere, a violin bow strokes the first few notes of "The Sound of Silence," the song my father insisted my son perform at his funeral. We'd all joined in to sing—my three sisters, our kids—while my son strummed his guitar, none of us able to move past the line about *silence like a cancer grows* without choking on our tears.

I cup my ear to better hear the tune. *Enough,* I think, imagining how Dad might react to my self-pity at a moment when resilience and strength are required. You can't kill yourself. Of course you can't. You have children. You can't do that to them. You wrote a whole fucking novel about how you can't do that to them, back when your marriage was disintegrating into toxic sludge, and ideations of suicide became the daily drumbeat of your hours.

You remind yourself that, in escaping your marriage, you've taken the first step toward a mentally healthy and tenable future existence. You knew it would be difficult, this whole starting over from scratch part, which is why you kept putting it off, and though you hadn't really understood just how difficult, you did understand, as every Nora Helmer had before you, that walking out the door of your marriage semi-intact was preferable to coming unglued inside it. You wanted this separation, you remind yourself. You made it happen. So count your blessings, motherfucker. You cannot kill yourself today. Nuh-uh. No way. *No!*

No. If it were possible to "command + F" a marriage, the most commonly used word in mine would have been *no. No, I won't. No, I can't. No, I don't like that. Stop it, please, no!* Is it any wonder, then, that the first phrase that strikes me at this first moment of its untethering is *Yes, and . . .*

Yes, and . . . is the basis for improv, which is when two people or more perform a comic scene together on the fly, without script or plan. So, for example, if your scene partner says, "Oh my god, I'm late for work, can you watch my pet hedgehog?" you cannot counter that with "No, I'm busy," or "That's not a hedgehog." You have to "yes, and" it, responding with something along the lines of "Yes, and I'll be sure to sauté him with some shallots and vermouth," because now your scene partner has something to work with: hedgehog Provençal.

Obviously, I'm not great at this, but good lord do I enjoy trying. Performing onstage, back in college, had always provided me one of the more pleasurable, illicit substance-free ways of both coping and staying present: a relief from the pressures of academia; a means of joining a supportive and judgment-free artistic community; a way of letting go and turning off those parts of my brain that either remained stuck in the past or worried about the future in order to live fully in the present. I also feel an almost compulsive need to laugh, or to at least find pockets of laughter . . . somewhere.

After a nervous breakdown, "The Lottery" author, Shirley Jackson, started keeping a journal, in which she admitted her desire to escape her painful marriage in order "to be separate, to be alone, to *stand* and *walk* alone, not to be different and weak and helpless and degraded." But even though she'd started writing a joyous new novel about a widow who sloughs off her married name and embarks on a new beginning, her fears of leaving her real marriage prevailed. She died of heart failure in her sleep at forty-eight, still married to her tormentor.

At this point in my own story, I am forty-seven.

Six months before Jackson's death, she wrote these final words in her journal: "I am the captain of my fate. Laughter is possible laughter is possible laughter is possible."

I impulsively google "improv classes NYC." All of the classes at UCB (Upright Citizens Brigade) are already filled up this late in September, but there's a $40 promotion for four introductory Level 0 classes with a few slots open at the PIT (Peoples Improv Theater). On a whim I can only describe as involuntary, I sign up for the class. Did I realize, before stepping onto this new stage of my life, that saying "Yes, and . . ." would be the thing that will save it? No, but it is there at my first class, held in a nondescript rehearsal room in the West 20s, where I will meet Brittany, the raven-haired, twenty-something aspiring actor who will eventually move into my former home office to become my seven-year-old's live-in au pair. During improv class one day, Brittany had told me she was having both roommate and rent issues. Two weeks later, in exchange for free housing, food, and a $200 weekly stipend, sweet Brittany from improv class, with her voice of an angel, will become part of the glue that holds my family together.

Yes, and!

Soon after that, sixteen-year-old Hannah, my daughter's best friend, will move in with us and sleep on a trundle bed in the room shared by my daughter and seven-year-old son. Hannah—blond, leggy, so dazzling she glows, but with dark undertones of my-alcoholic-dad-abandoned-me pain—has been skipping school every day, sleeping in until noon. Our home full of people getting up and going to work and school every day, her fed-up solo mother hopes, will be a good influence. "Yes, and . . ." I'll tell her mom. "We'll take good care of her, I promise." We've been Hannah's default second home for years at this point anyway, as her mom often has to travel for work as an event planner.

Which is how six of us, each at a moment of inflection—George from college, mourning the loss of his husband; Brittany from improv, trying to find her way in the world; Hannah from my daughter's class, struggling with chronic truancy; my daughter and son, adjusting to life without their father and older brother; and a forty-seven-year-old, newly untethered me, hoping for both a mammogram and transformation, in that order—begin living together under one roof, with my dog and George's dog and two smelly cats, in what we will from then on lovingly refer to as the Commune.

Yes, and . . . in fact, will become my new rallying cry and modus operandi. When a stranger randomly knocks on my door, wondering if she can pay us a thousand dollars in exchange for using my home as a holding area for the actors and extras in her film, The Mend, I'll laugh (I mean, come on, The Mend?) and say, "Yes, and I can cook them dinner as well." When a young student director asks me to play a Russian spy in his graduate film, The Super, I'll say, "Yes, and I can actually speak Russian at the beginning of the scene if you'd like."

When I receive a call from my Parisian friend Marion, who's wondering if her niece and two friends can come stay with us for two weeks before they head off to medical school, I'll say, "Yes, and I can ask if they can be extras in an American film as well!"

One night, during the shoot for The Mend, my friend Soman, a frequent dinner guest at the Commune and our honorary seventh member, shows up as I'm putting out snacks for the crew and spots my daughter

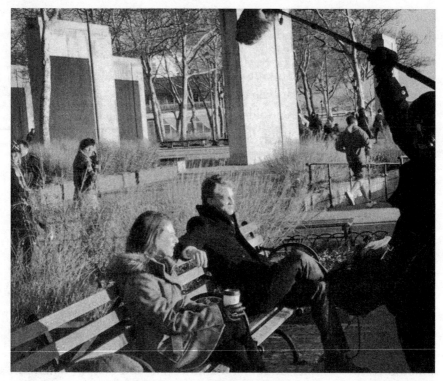

On set of *The Super,* 2013

doing her homework on the living room couch, surrounded by two dozen actors crammed into every corner of the room, including our three French exchange students, who were all thrilled to be asked to be extras. "What's going on?" Soman says, searching in vain for a place to sit.

"Don't ask," says my daughter. "Mom's saying, 'Yes, and' to every-thing."

Health Today

A couple of weeks before my new job as executive editor at *Health Today* is set to begin, my little one accidentally bumps his head into the lump on my breast, and I wince. I call the Breast Examination Center of Harlem to see if there are any cancellations. Miraculously, they have one a few days later, so I take it, after which I receive a call from Sloan Kettering's main switchboard, telling me they did not like what they saw on my scans. They want me to come into their Upper East Side office immediately for more tests: another mammogram, possibly an ultrasound, possibly a biopsy, depending on what they find.

I cannot afford these tests. I explain this to the accounting department at Sloan Kettering: that I still don't have health insurance but I will, at my new job, and it will kick in a month after my start date. They're not happy about waiting six weeks for a biopsy, but I'm not happy about spending thousands of dollars I don't have, so what else is there to say? Healthcare in gig-economy America feels like a constant game of Frogger: You can't hop to the next level until the logs line up with the turtles.

Eight weeks later, after I'm gainfully employed and safely afloat on a new healthcare log, the radiologist who does the ultrasound is not happy with what she sees either. It sort of looks like a cyst, she says, but she does not like that the fluid inside it isn't registering as pure black—meaning clear liquid—on the ultrasound. "See this here?" She points to a gray, fuzzy patch in the middle of the lump. "We need to get that biopsied and clip it. In case you need surgery."

I get the biopsy and the clip. Biopsies are painful. I did not know this. You need to lie down when you get home, I'm told, to recover. Ice and pain relievers will help. I do not yet want to tell my new employer or my kids what's going on inside my left breast, however, so when I'm back at the office later that afternoon following the biopsy or cleaning off Elvis's dog shit from my bed later that night while George and Brittany deal with the caked-on pieces of turd somehow caught in the wheels of my ex's desk chair, I suck up the pain, do my work, change the sheets, light a candle to mask the stench, and make us all dinner as usual.

(Elvis, George's beagle, is still getting used to living in the Commune. He sometimes deals with his anxiety by taking a dump on my bed.)

Three days later, Sloan Kettering calls with a diagnosis of "atypical ductal cells with focal atypia and foam cells," aka atypia. I have no idea what this means. Foam cells? Sounds like a boob latte. But over the course of the next forty-eight hours, I will learn that medical reactions to such a diagnosis vary widely. The first breast surgeon I visit, who's not at Sloan Kettering but is in network for my new health insurance, does her own diagnosis and says, no, it's not atypia, it's DCIS (ductal carcinoma in situ, aka stage 0 breast cancer because it has not spread beyond the ducts). She wants to put me on tamoxifen, an antiestrogen hormone therapy that will send my still-ovulating body into immediate menopause, kill my libido, wreak havoc on my sleep, dry out my vagina, and make it itchy. (Fun!) She mumbles something about possibly getting a mastectomy and definitely getting radiation and possibly chemotherapy.

Whoa! I think. What? I call my friend Ayelet to cry. Though we live on different coasts, she's always the first person I call whenever I need emotional release or advice, as hers is always sound and given with love and lack of judgment. She urges me, immediately, to call her friend Peggy Orenstein, who'd recently written a seminal story on the overtreatment of DCIS for *The New York Times*. Peggy, in turn, urges me to get another opinion, even if it's outside my insurance network. "Go back to

Sloan," she says. "They know what they're doing." This second, more expensive opinion, from a female oncologist at Sloan Kettering I found by watching videos on their website and choosing the one with whom I'd want to share a cup of tea, is more wait-and-see and measured.

This lovely, calm doctor—who will soon leave Sloan to become chief of breast surgery at a different cancer hospital in a different state— says she first wants to stick me into an MRI to make sure nothing else lights up before we do anything, and no, tamoxifen is not necessary at this time. I choose this less alarmist, more expensive oncologist outside my healthcare network, but I worry both about the co-pays and about missing another day away from the office so soon after the start of my job. Then again, it's better than having to go into immediate menopause as a result of taking tamoxifen, and to miss work every week for radiation and chemotherapy.

I'd arrived at work on my first day as executive editor of *Health Today* eager to write and assign stories about our healthcare system, various illnesses, and scientific breakthroughs in medicine. Health, I tell myself, is one of those topics that many of us like to read about. And while I would rather spend my working hours writing my own books, I feel grateful and lucky to have landed an editing job with benefits, covering a topic I care about, living, as we all do, in a dying body.

During my multiple interviews leading up to the job, I was told several times that I'd have a budget to assign and publish stories covering all aspects of health. "I find it offensive that publications such as the *Huffington Post* expect their writers to produce 'content' for free," I'd said to one of my interviewers, testing the waters to see if we were aligned on the issue of fee for hire. "Work is work. Writing is writing. It should be properly remunerated."

Free content—and those willing to produce and publish it—has decimated my profession and eroded trust in the news. Anyone with a laptop could publish any un-fact-checked, unedited nonsense they wanted to publish and push it out onto social channels. The Russians will make excellent use of this chink in our national armor during the 2016 elections, as we will learn all too well, but now, in the fall of 2013, I see this more as a pressing moral issue about the value of work and the obligation of those who financially gain from that work to provide fair compensation.

If I ask a carpenter to come to my home and build me a shelf, it's not okay for me to send him away without payment. Or to tell him, "Maybe someone else who needs shelves will come over to my house and see this beautiful one, and they will pay you to build shelves for them!" Similarly, I do not want to be put into a position where I'm asking people to write for free. This is my line in the sand, the same as my father's refusal to represent tobacco companies in his law firm. "You have to know where the line is," Dad told me often, starting on the day he turned down a giant sum of tobacco dollars for the sake of his conscience. "If you earn your money off the suffering or deaths or exploitation of others, that's not a moral income. That's blood money. And I'd rather see you be a waitress or a housekeeper than take blood money. Serving food and cleaning toilets is noble work, contributing to the greater good of society. Helping a tobacco company kill people is not. Do you understand the difference?"

I was six years old when he first said this, sitting shotgun in his beloved red Mustang, trying to chomp on a still-warm-from-the-oven egg bagel without my front teeth. "Yes, Daddy, I do."

The woman with whom I was meeting, a vice president of *Health Today*, nodded vigorously in mutual agreement. *Of course, of course, we would never expect anyone to write for free.* I'd spoken to another of my interviewers, one of the company's founders, about producing hard-hitting investigative stories about sexism in healthcare. *Great idea,* I was told. I talked about redesigning the site, to make it cleaner, more easily navigable. *Yes, that's exactly what we want,* everyone said. *Welcome to the team!*

None of my ideas, I realize by the end of week one, are possible. They've hired an editor from a different health magazine to be both editorial director and my boss, and she's been put in charge of the redesign, which I'm relieved about, knowing nothing about doing such things myself. She calls me, a few days before my start date, to ask me to have lunch with her, during which she announces that she's asked the company to push back my start date by two weeks, so that she can get settled in before I arrive. It's an odd power play, and I'll have to call both my landlord, to tell him my rent will be two weeks late, as well as Sloan Kettering, to push off my second round of breast tests by another half month, but I have no desire to make waves or to butt heads right out of the gate, let alone with someone to whom I'll be reporting. "No problem!" I say.

I just want to keep my nose to the grindstone, do good work, replenish my empty bank account, procure health insurance, and have enough time at the end of my workday to rush home—my commute will be over an hour each way—and sit down for dinner with my children and the rest of the Commune.

On the first day of my new job, my desktop computer won't turn on. So I ask my new colleagues what to do. The last time I'd held a corporate job that required me to go to an outside office every day, back in 1998, the internet was just getting started. I still shared a personal email address with my husband. I didn't yet have a cellphone. And our NBC computers were old clunkers. When they broke, as they often did, you'd walk down to the IT department and ask someone to come back to your office to help you fix it. Now, I'm told, I have to fill out a help desk request on the computer. Since my computer won't turn on, and no one else can fill out the request for me—it has to come from my specific log-in for record-keeping purposes—this is a conundrum. I look around the large open-plan room and spot what looks like the IT department off in the distance. "Do you know who can help me fix my computer?" I say to one of the young men sitting there.

"You have to fill out a help desk request," he tells me.

"I know. But that's the problem. My computer won't turn on."

"Have you checked that it's plugged in?"

"Yes."

He shrugs. "Sorry. I can't do anything without a help desk request."

"Can you help me load my work email onto my phone, so I can work off of that?"

"Again, that would require a help desk request."

Every minute of his day, I would soon understand, is being monitored for efficiency. How long does it take between the time a help desk request comes in and the person requesting it marks the issue as resolved? These were numbers that could be counted. If you were slow, you could say goodbye to your job.

"The turnover here is insane," one of my new colleagues warns me that first day. "One minute you think you're making a new friend at work, the next they're collecting their family photos and walking out the door forever." This would turn out to be an understatement. One day, an entire section of my floor is fired before I've even had a chance to figure out what that part of the room does. Or rather: did. Never before, outside a funeral or terrorist attack, have I seen this many grown men and women hugging and crying together in unison.

This fear-based management style, where every piece of equipment on every desk is logged and accounted for; where minutes must be filled with labor and then noted in a ledger; and where those in charge squeeze out every drop of worker sweat, has its roots in American slavery: "You report to someone," writes Matthew Desmond in *The New York Times Magazine*, of offices such as mine, "and someone reports to you. Everything is tracked, recorded and analyzed, via vertical reporting systems, double-entry record-keeping and precise quantification. Data seems to hold sway over every operation. It feels like a cutting-edge approach to management, but many of these techniques that we now take for granted were developed by and for large plantations."

"Low-road capitalism," the University of Wisconsin-Madison sociologist Joel Rogers calls our American style of capitalism, in which jobs lack flexibility of purpose; training pertains only to that one job in that one office—you can't take your skills with you to your next job because they won't transfer; bosses closely monitor and measure workers' rule-compliance and performance; hierarchies are rigid; wages are low; and workers are denied the chips of collective bargaining that could both get them out of this rut and keep them from getting fired without cause or severance.

In fact, the Organisation for Economic Co-operation and Development—an intergovernmental organization headquartered in Paris, with thirty-seven member countries all committed to democracy and to the market economy—places the United States dead last on a list of seventy-one nations ranked according to how difficult it is to fire workers. Meaning that every other country in this large and detailed study has much stronger protections for workers than the U.S. Here, firing people is literally as easy as saying "Goodbye, don't come back tomorrow." The invisible axe constantly hanging over American workers' heads feels like the psychological equivalent of war coverage: You do your job as best you can under fire, never knowing which pink slip bomb, if any, has your name on it.

On my second day on the job, I bring in my own laptop and plug it into the office ethernet. Success! I'm in the system. I fill out a help desk request, and an hour later someone from IT walks over and figures out what's wrong with my desktop: "It's broken," he says. He swaps it out for a working computer, at which I sit down and type up a list of magazine writers with whom I'd love to work. I email this list to the editorial director. Great list, she says, but you'll never get the budget to hire any of them.

My mandate, she tells me, is to manage and grow the company's current roster of sick and dying people—my bloggers, as they're optimistically called, though half of them are barely literate and some are barely alive—who've all volunteered to write, gratis, about what it's like living and/or dying with their various ailments. Specifically those ailments with pharmaceutical interventions, like type 2 diabetes, so that targeted pharmaceutical ads can be published next to their blogs. We're not interested, I'm told, in publishing stories about type 1 diabetes. There are no ad dollars in insulin.

It's all about the ads, I suddenly understand. There's gold in them thar pharmaceutical hills, and my company's business model is to mine it. This had also been true of my former industries (magazines, newspapers, and TV news) with one major difference: an established and long-standing firewall between ad sales and journalism. "Church and state," it was called, though like the pope and the president, the two would meet up now and then to unruffle feathers. Nevertheless, a legitimate news outlet could assign a hard-hitting series about the greed of Turing Pharmaceuticals CEO Martin Shkreli—dubbed "the most hated man in America" after he raised the price of the antiparasitic drug Daraprim from $13.50 to $750 per pill—and still have at some point accepted ad dollars from Turing. They could report on the American obesity epidemic, naming soft drinks as one of the main culprits, and still run ads for Coca-Cola. If a particularly harsh and revealing investigative story, such as "Fast-Food Nation," led to McDonald's pulling all of its ads from the pages of *Rolling Stone*, so be it. It's not a magazine's job to kowtow to advertisers. It's to report the news, however unfavorable to everyone's bottom lines, including their own.

At *Health Today*, this notion was reversed. The ads dictated the content; the tail wagged the dog. Put simply, the content I've been hired to edit is secondary to ad delivery: a bait-and-switch lure not unlike the plastic toy in the box of sugar cereal; the 15 percent off your purchase in exchange for signing up for another credit card you don't need; the free stay at the Vegas hotel tonight so you can lose all of your chips tomorrow to the blackjack dealer.

The writing itself, if you can even call it that, is simply a way to get people who type in search terms such as "Crohn's disease" or "fibromyalgia" or "COPD" into Google to see ads for pharmaceutical products targeted to those illnesses. The company has amassed a crack team of SEO (search engine optimization) specialists tasked with making sure ours is the first site that appears in such searches. I like the SEO dudes. They're the only ones, at first, who'll invite me to have lunch with them. While the rest of us sit in an open office, the five of them sit cheek-to-jowl in a private office built for one, a tiny anthill of young, already disillusioned men whose combined heat and stress forms condensation on the glass wall separating us from them. With the company on the verge of going public, the CEOs are not happy that our rivals consistently rank higher than we do in searches. More worrisome, because our main competitor has made a concerted effort to publish content consumers trust, the majority of their traffic is organic—a sustainable business model—while ours is purchased—an unsustainable model.

Every day at *Health Today* begins to feel like that scene in *I Love Lucy*, where Lucy is working in the chocolate factory, unable to process all the chocolates whizzing by. A new essay comes in, I'll rewrite it from scratch while fact-checking its claims, three more will come in, rinse, repeat. I don't mind the work—writing and editing are enjoyable activities for me—but each blog post begins to sound the same as the one before. There's no nuance. Nothing original. Nothing that makes me want to copy the link and share it with friends. And I don't feel comfortable asking my own friends who are writers to contribute work if I can't pay them.

At some point I'm telling all of this to an actor friend from college whose roman à clef I helped edit during the weeks after my marriage ended. He kept offering to pay me, but knowing his own financial burdens—a crushingly large alimony, calculated by the courts when he was at the peak of his Hollywood career, but now nearly impossible to keep up with—I kept saying no. Not only was the work saving me from self-pity during those difficult first post-separation weeks before my job began, this is what writers do for one another. We read one another's work and offer red-pencil guidance. It's part of the barter economy between underpaid wordsmiths. You throw the karma out there, because good books are a greater good, and it almost always comes back in some welcome and unexpected way.

Of course, I should also add that I had my first small, post-marital crush on this man, and I thought he might have a small crush on me. And after years of a bad marriage, I was desperate for affection. Like, any affection. And editing, when done well, can be an intimate act. And I suppose I thought if I did a good job editing his novel, maybe it would lead to us talking about our hidden feelings. Which it eventually did, but not in the way I'd assumed. We ended up talking for hours. And chastely hugging. And going on a long walk, hand in hand. And trading stories of our failed marriages. And sitting down for a meal, at which I realized my crush was wholly a fantasy of my own making: the romantic lifeboat I'd mentally conjured out of an old friend, who should really just remain thus, my fellow bobber, drifting along on our own separate currents into uncertain futures. In fact, had we made the leap from friends to lovers, not only would our friendship have most certainly ended, we would have probably killed each other. He was as unreliable as I was in need of constancy, as free to float on the wind as I was shackled to the ground by responsibilities, as certain of his inability to wholly connect as I was certain of my need for connection.

"I could write about my skin cancer for you?" the actor offers, when I call to complain about the terrible, unpaid prose I spend my days editing for my job. It's the least he could do, he says, after I edited his novel. (See? Karma.)

"Oh my god, that would be great," I say. The actor is not only a good writer, he has more than a hundred thousand Twitter followers plus a hit show. One tweet from him, linking to his story, could not only prove my worth to my company, it could help them see that if we actually pay decent writers for decent work, it will pay off handsomely in organic pageviews. It's also an excellent public service announcement. Whether we like it or not, we Americans are highly influenced by our celebrities, and an actor on a hit TV show writing a story about the small spot on his forehead that turned out to be life-threatening cancer might be just the kick in the pants others need to get their skin checked.

The story is a hit, giving me a win at work but still no budget to commission more. In the meantime, I've had to come up with other clever ways to barter for better writing. I ask Brittany, our new au pair and hilarious Commune chanteuse, if she'll write about her Crohn's disease in exchange for dinner out and a night off from work. Meaning, technically I'll be paying her out of my own pocket, but public school teachers in this country pay for classroom supplies out of their own pockets all the time, so who am I to complain?[*] Plus I need to keep my job, by any means necessary. Crohn's stories, I'm told, are pharmaceutical ad bonanzas.

"Yes, and . . . !" says Brittany, always game. Her story, infused with her quirky brand of self-deprecating humor, describes her constant need to know where the nearest bathroom is at all times. It not only cracks me up, it also does well on our site. Next, I work with our video team to produce a story about the benefits of yoga to counterbalance depression: my own, in the wake of my father's death. The video will also garner many views, which means more eyeballs will see more ads for SSRIs. In other words, things seem to be going well at work, with *well* being defined as: creating professional-looking, high pageview content to pair with pharmaceutical ads.

Then I go in for my MRI, and my house of cards begins to collapse.

I receive the call with the results while I'm sitting at my open-plan desk, with co-workers all around. Seven more masses have been found, I'm told, three of them highly suspicious. I need to come in immediately for more biopsies. Tomorrow, if possible. I don't handle the news as gracefully as I would have hoped. In fact, I immediately burst into tears at my desk and run downstairs without a coat to regain composure. It's January of 2014, the middle of the polar vortex, but to retrieve my coat from the staff coat closet would have meant having to pass by a dozen more co-workers with tears streaming down my face. These tears freeze on my cheeks as I pass through the lobby and out onto the street. I take a right on the next block and lean into the frigid wind from the Hudson as I wail, but the cold gets the best of me, and I head back inside. I will myself to stop crying in the elevator back up to my floor. I cannot show weakness.

The office has become a pressure cooker. We're going public in less than three months, and those in charge are looking to trim fat to boost our numbers. A crying and newly appointed executive editor, as thin as she might appear right now from stress, will definitely be seen as trim-

---

[*] A joke. Public school teachers in the wealthiest country on earth should definitely not be paying for classroom supplies out of their own pockets.

mable fat. In fact, studies have shown that women who cry at work are viewed as less competent in the workplace. Most women don't need a study to know this is true.

"Where were you?" says my boss, the editorial director, when I walk back in. I've been gone for five minutes. "I need an update on your 30/60/90."

A 30/60/90 report is a new concept to me but not, apparently, to everyone else in the corporate world. The idea, as I understand it, is to lay out a clear course of action for the next thirty, sixty, and ninety days, written by the new employee herself, but A) I've never written one before; and B) I'm not sure how to fill in the three buckets. My job, as I see it, is to edit bad prose and make sure it's not poorly spelled malarkey. To figure out how to hire better bloggers without paying them money. To write stories myself with any extra time available. I don't understand how ninety days later this situation will be any different.

"Sorry," I say, "I had to run out for a second. I promise, it won't happen again." I sit down and, using my best corporate speak, with terms like *leverage, growth, SEO,* and *KPIs,* I try to map out subtle differences between my first, second, and third months on the job. In the ninety-day slot—meaning right after the IPO—I write that I'm hoping by then we'll find the budget to hire a few good writers to pen personal stories about health, as well as to pay the bloggers we already have, even if it's a small honorarium tied to pageviews. Some of these bloggers, I note, have crushing doctors' bills they can't pay. Or they require expensive home health aids. Or they have terminal cancer and young kids. Nearly every day, one of them writes to ask me whether an accounting system has finally been set up—apparently some of them have been promised this?—to provide a sliding scale payment tied to the number of eyeballs their blogs garner. It feels immoral to keep asking them to work for free; to keep dangling the false carrot of a possibility of future payments without a plan in place to make this happen.

"Wow," says the radiologist at my next visit. "There's a giant party going on in your breasts!" She shows me the films, the masses that concern her and those that don't. A few days later, I meet with my surgeon. We schedule more biopsies, during which a new radiologist overseeing them says that my MRI films were so unusual, he was hoping, with my permission, to use them later that week at his teaching hospital, as a case study in abnormality. "Your films can really teach us a lot about the variations in disease presentation!" he says with enthusiasm. "I've never seen anything like them."

"Sure," I say, "knock yourself out." I feel slightly vulnerable and confused with my naked breasts exposed, being poked and prodded with more biopsy needles, wondering who'll take care of my kids if I die. Will their father move back east? Will they have to move out to California? How will he support them and also make sure our little one's fingernails are neat and trimmed? And what does it mean, my breasts "were so unusual" or that the doc's "never seen anything like them"? After the second needle goes into suspicious new lump number two on my right breast—*oh, god*, I think, wincing, *I'm going to be in serious pain tonight*—they try to biopsy the lump on my left, attempting to reach it from two different entry points, but it's located too far back in the chest wall. It's also the largest of the three and the most worrisome. They'll have to cut me open, they say, to yank it out.

I photograph the aftermath in the changing room—once a war photographer, always a war photographer—and meet my surgeon in her office for a consult.

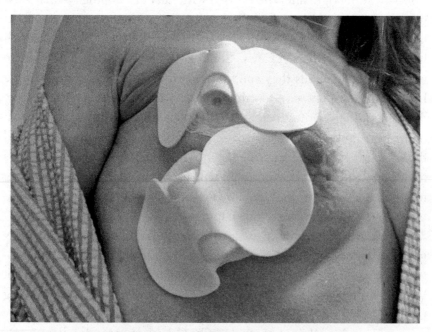

After the biopsy, 2013, © Deborah Copaken

"I'm sorry," I tell her. "I can't have surgery this week. I've already been out of the office three days in the past two weeks. Things are just too stressful right now."

Rick, our COO and my ally, had called me into his office earlier that week to tell me that the young VP with whom I'd met during my interviews—the one who'd promised me a budget to hire writers—was upset that I kept asking for money to pay writers, particularly now that I'd officially written it in my 30/60/90, which others could read. He urged me to suck it up and apologize to her. "I'm sorry," I said to the VP later that same night, after everyone else had gone home. "I'll stop asking for money to pay writers or putting it in writing." As I left her office to head home to the Commune, I could hear my dad's words echoing in my ear: *You have to know where the line is. If you earn your money off the suffering or deaths or exploitation of others, that's not a moral income. That's blood money.*

Worried about further angering anyone else, I schedule my lumpectomy for a month later.

Because all of these doctor visits, tests, and scheduled procedures have been taking place during business hours, I've had to level with the editorial director about my situation. Sloan Kettering, I explain, has excellent WiFi, so I can just edit the blog posts during my time in the waiting room between procedures. She's fine with this, she says, but her eyes speak otherwise. The axe has been falling hard all around us, and her boss, the aforementioned VP, has been put in charge of further wielding it pre-IPO. The talented producer of my yoga and depression video, who'd survived a serious bout with breast cancer and gave me reams of notes and words of encouragement, had recently been told one morning, without any warning, to gather her things and leave. She'd been less than fully productive during her months of treatment, but still: She got her work done eventually, and it was brilliantly executed. "Fuck this place," I heard her say under her breath. Then she was gone.

It was dangerous to be unhealthy at *Health Today*.

Meanwhile, with exactly one month between now and my surgery, I suddenly have an intense desire both to have my breasts photographed for posterity as well as to put them to good use before they're disfigured. No one aside from my oncology team has touched them or even glimpsed them in nearly a year.

This must change.

In Flagrante Delicto

The questionnaires for dating sites such as OkCupid and eharmony are so long and detailed (this is a year before Tinder fully entered the zeitgeist, going from five million swipes a day in December 2013 to over a billion a day the following year) that by the time I've done the dinner, bath, and bedtime story hustle, I fall asleep with my laptop open on my stomach, having left most of the questions unanswered. Do I care if my future partner smokes marijuana, yes or no? That's not a binary question. I wouldn't want him to smoke every day, but a quick hit now and then before sex, I mean, no? There are no boxes to check for that level of subtlety.

I have no idea what I'm looking for, what I believe in, or what I want from my next relationship after twenty-three years with the same man. I just know my body needs sex with an aching thrum not unlike hunger and thirst, and I don't know how, as a middle-aged solo mother, to get it.

A newly divorced dad in my son's school who also happens to be a professional photographer has been flirting with me, however, so maybe I can address both the physical and photography desires simultaneously. Or rather, I *think* he's been flirting. It's been so long, who knows?

Santi and I met manning the photo booth at the school Halloween fundraiser. He's eight years younger, one foot taller, olive-skinned, and movie-star handsome, with black ringlets framing searing brown eyes and the gentle manner of a shepherd who moonlights as a yoga instructor. An immigrant from Mexico, he arrived in the U.S. as a tourist a decade earlier, fell in love, overstayed his visa, started a family. His ex, also an immigrant, has managed to obtain a green card, but he has not. Instead, he constantly worries about being deported and separated from his children, who, having been born in the U.S., are officially citizens. Because he cannot get hired to shoot for American newspapers or magazines without a Social Security number, even though several editors have expressed interest in tapping into his talents, he shoots private family and individual portraits for cash and takes the odd job now and then to make ends meet.

In other words, he's not my usual overconfident college grad with self-esteem issues masked behind thick horn-rims and pointed quips type, but my usual type has gotten me here, so maybe it's time to reconsider those factory settings. Kindness and empathy, I've decided, are the sexiest attributes a man can have. And Santi has both in abundance. I also once caught him sweeping his own floor when I dropped off my son for a playdate: If a greater aphrodisiac exists, I do not know it. So one morning, in front of our kids' school, lit by the fire of knowing my left boob is about to be sliced up if not at some point maybe even sliced off, I tap into my new improv-trained powers, take a deep breath, and go for it. "I'd like to hire you to shoot nudes of my breasts before my surgery," I tell him, using the same neutral tone I might have used to ask for his help folding the programs for the second grade play.

His chestnut eyes widen. His eyebrows arch up. "Wonderful!" he says, smiling. "Let's do that."

We settle on a price and make a date to do the shoot the following Friday after I get home from work. But when Friday rolls around, the brown-and-yellow biopsy bruises on my breasts still look hideous, so we decide to push off the shoot until they heal and go to see a movie instead: An actual first date, I realize, my first in a quarter century. Santi tells me to choose the film, so I pick an early screening of *The Great Beauty*, an Italian film about a man who emerges from sixty-five years of aimless wandering into a moment of transformational awe: Something I'm hoping will happen to me one day. Before my sixty-fifth birthday.

In the days leading up to our date, I make sure the Commune will be empty when he drops me off, so we can have some privacy if it goes well. This takes major operational planning. I schedule a sleepover date for my son at his friend's. I help my daughter find a babysitting gig, which will get her home, she says, just after midnight. I suggest to Hannah that she visit and stay with her mom, since she doesn't have to get up for school the next morning. George makes a Grindr date. Brittany will head to a rehearsal for her one-woman show. I've been joining her on stage for that show from time to time, strumming "Take It Easy" on the guitar while singing it as a duet, once even right after a biopsy.

The song, because we often rehearse it at night, has become both the Commune's theme song as well as my earworm: *Come on baaaaaaaaby, don't say maaaaaaaybe, I gotta know if your sweet love is gonna saa-aaaaaaave me* . . .

Santi and I arrive back in Harlem after seeing the film and downing tacos and beer at a Mexican joint that reminds him of home. He has not hugged his parents, he tells me, in years. We head to my room and sit face-to-face on the love seat across from my bed: an Ikea Klippan, the two-person couch of college co-eds everywhere, which is what I suddenly feel like as we start to chat, awaiting a signal from the other. The moment the tips of his fingers reach out to touch mine, I evaporate into molecules. We start kissing. Which is to say I lose track of where my mouth ends and his begins. It's a revelation, human touch. I hadn't exactly forgotten, but I had blocked out my needs for so long, it feels as if I'm learning anew what they are. In the midst of this still-clothed euphoria, I break away to give him fair warning: My daughter will be home sometime after midnight. It's 10 P.M. He needs to be gone no later than 11 P.M., just to be safe. Understood, he says.

It's been thirty years since I've had to worry about anyone barging in on me in flagrante delicto. Because my daughter has not been told her dad and I are getting divorced, I have to be just as careful as I'd been back in my teens, if not more so. I can't even speak freely in front of her about what's happening. I'd recently called her father to say the situation has become untenable. While he's living his best life in San Francisco, going out on dates and bringing them home to his bachelor pad unimpeded, I'm trapped in Harlem in his lie of omission. He has to find a way to sit down with me to tell the kids we're getting divorced, I told him. We have to present a united front. *Together.* All the books and articles I've read on divorce are insistent on this particular point: The way you impart the news to the children is critical for their future emotional health and well-being. Too many close calls have slipped out already, what with friends, my Commune roommates, and all of my family members knowing the marriage is over but forgetting that my children don't and nearly blurting it out in front of them. Please, I begged. I'm not okay with gaslighting my own children or asking others to do so as well. Let's sit them down and get this over with.

No, he'd said. He wants to wait. *Until when?* I wondered. We'd known we were separating for over a year at this point, and we'd been physically separated with a whole country between us for five months. At some point, the kids are going to figure it out on their own, whether or not we ever tell them. And that would be worse than sitting down to tell them, because then we will have broken their trust.

Santi and I continue kissing. Our clothes start to come off. We move to the bed. I am—my body is—desperate for this affection. For any affection. He touches my still bruise-covered breast, releasing a sudden flood of oxytocin into my bloodstream I can actually feel as it shoots out and courses through me.

This bonding hormone is physiologically identical to the one released during breastfeeding. Homo sapiens are the only members of the animal kingdom who engage in breast and nipple stimulation during sex, and scientists are starting to hypothesize that the subsequent release of oxytocin, which promotes both social bonding and empathy, might have been one of the factors, along with face-to-face copulation, that led to our advanced communication skills and cognition. I wonder whether I'll opt for implants if my breasts have to be removed. My gut says no, but how does one give up this incredibly pleasurable part of the sex act? In fact, researchers now believe that *not* engaging in the occasional nipple stimulation can actually be detrimental to women's health, as it decreases the risk of in situ cervical cancer, endometrial cancer of the uterus, ovarian cancer, and breast cancer.

The moment I snap off the bedside light and start to relax into this oxytocin-induced haze—we're not having sex yet, but we might be heading in that direction—I hear the dogs bark. Someone else from the Commune has come home. Brittany, probably, I think. Or maybe

George's date went south? It can't be Hannah, my son, or my daughter, but I lock my door just to be safe.

"Mom?" I hear. My daughter jiggles my bedroom door. Then she knocks. "Mom? Are you there? They came home early." Meaning, the parents down the street for whom she'd been babysitting. "Mom! Your door is locked."

I feign sleep. Fuck. This is not how I would have wanted this to go down. At *all*. In fact, I can't imagine a worse way. *You are a shitty parent!!!!* I chastise myself. *How could you have let this happen?* She's sixteen years old. She's been told her dad just moved away to start a business, not that her parents' marriage is kaput. Why did I agree to perpetuate this lie? Why didn't I insist her father sit down with me and tell her the truth before he left last year? It's not healthy, I've read, for only one parent to tell the story of marital rupture. There's an agreed-upon dual script you need to follow: "We're getting divorced," I wanted to tell her, with her father sitting next to me, "but we both still love you, and we are united in our desire to get along for your sake, to be here for you whenever you need us, to make sure you're okay as you navigate this new reality."

Never did I imagine her discovering it this way. I start to panic. What do I do? My bedroom's on the third floor, too high for Santi to jump out the window. My daughter's bedroom is next to mine, off the same nineteenth century–constructed hallway with the creaky floor. I'm paralyzed with fear, not knowing how to proceed. Where's the script for this scenario? I wonder. I didn't read about this one in the divorce books. "Get dressed!" I both mime and mouth to the man in my bed, whose presence now fills me with shame. "Now!"

"What do you want me to do?" he shrugs.

I shrug back, on the verge of tears. "Just don't move," I whisper. "She'll fall asleep at some point. Then you can sneak out and leave by the front door."

The hour that passes between her knock on my door and Santi's silent exit feels like a lifetime, during which neither of us moves. I stare straight up at the ceiling, its surface periodically aglow with the light from passing headlights. A couple argues on the sidewalk below, screaming obscenities. A car honks. Rap music thrums out an open window. Whatever oxytocin had been flooding my arteries has now been replaced by cortisol. Who is this stranger I invited into my bed, jeopardizing everything I hold dear: my children's trust, their love? I spend the rest of the night, after Santi escapes, fretting, awake, trying to figure out what to say to my daughter the next morning. My bedroom door these days is never locked. And the only times it had ever been thus was when her father and I needed privacy. She's too smart to see this as anything but what it is.

The sun rises. A new day begins, whether I like it or not. My room faces west, so I can't see the sun, but I can see its fire turning the clouds purple then pink, now warming the top half of the buildings across the street, first red, then yellow, now white, infusing my room with reflected glow. "What now, Dad?" I say, "How do I fix *this*?"

My father was vehemently opposed to divorce. "You stick it out," he always said. "You make it work for the sake of the children."

"But what if the children would be better off with their parents apart?" I sometimes countered, never referring directly to us kids and his marriage, but he knew what I was saying.

"They never are," he said, certain of his opinion. The man was completely judgment free, except on this one topic: He judged anyone who got divorced as bad, selfish. "You don't do that to kids," he said. "You just don't."

I never brought up my marital problems with him. Not once. Not even when he was dying. I didn't want to worry him, for one, but I also knew what his response would be: Work it out. I don't care how bad it is, just work it out.

Now I'm suddenly angry about this. What if only one person in the marriage wants to solve its problems? What if conflict and derision have replaced love and compassion? What if the children of dysfunctional relationships carry that dysfunction into their own partnerships, and the cycle keeps going? Shouldn't somebody somewhere along the way stand up and say, *No, time out! We're not going to do it this way anymore?*

Or maybe I'm just angry at myself for not mentioning to my own father my one real and crushing secret for fear of disappointing him. I'm angry that I didn't make it clear to him, after putting in years of fruitless work trying to save my marriage, that every marriage is unique, and that some marriages are so untenable, they become detrimental to one's physical and emotional health and well-being. "No!" I suddenly whisper-scream at the sky, five years after Dad's death. "You're wrong! Sometimes you have to cut your losses and give up!"

"Mom," says my daughter, sitting on my bed. "Mom, what's going on?" The look of hurt and betrayal on her face will enter my brain permanently. She demands answers. I give them to her as succinctly and as honestly as I can. It is my nadir as a parent, and we both know it. It might take years for her to recover from this moment, if not the rest of her life. My guilt over this feels crushing, suffocating. I make arrangements to fly to Chicago the following weekend with her little brother to tell both him and her big brother together. Their father will not meet me. It's too expensive, he says, to fly out and get a hotel room for the night, plus he's angry with me for letting the cat out of the bag. I offer to help him with the cost. The boys need to know we're getting divorced. Now. We can't ask our daughter to keep that kind of secret from her own siblings. Plus my surgery's coming up, my job is stressful, and, yes, okay! Fine! I fucked up! I know I fucked up.

I just wanted someone to hold me.

With only enough money for one night in a hotel and two plane fares—thank god for Spirit Airlines, with their $50 round trip specials between New York and Chicago—I fly with my seven-year-old son to Chicago early Saturday morning to tell both boys together that their father and I are getting divorced. It's an inopportune weekend to do this, as my eldest is in the undergraduate musical, with little time to actually sit down and chat. He can have a late lunch with us on Saturday, he says, but only for an hour or so, as he has to run back to the theater right after. I try to get him to come up to my room after dessert, but lunch has taken longer than expected, even though the restaurant is practically empty at this hour, and we've run out of time. His little brother and I are leaving the next morning. It's now or never, I tell myself. You have to do it here, in this restaurant. Ugh. After some loving if confusing throat clearing, I say it plainly: "Your dad and I are getting divorced. I'm so sorry. We both love you so much, and that will never change . . ." The two brothers burst into tears and hug each other tightly, but only the little one will allow me to comfort him. Over the next few months, my texts, calls, and emails to my college freshman go unanswered. I've lost him forever, I fear. My friends say, no, don't say that. He'll come around. Every child processes these things in their own time, on their own schedule. No, I think. I really fucked this one up but good. He will eventually forgive me, but it will take years.

My daughter, too, gives me the cold shoulder when I come home. I find her a therapist. Apologize profusely. Hope for the best.

This, I think. This hideous pain I have now inflicted upon my three kids and my disconnection from them for being the cause of that pain is why I and so many others put up with untenable marriages for so long. And yet I am also highly aware of the ways in which high-conflict marriages can leave equally noxious fumes within the adult psyches of grown children, particularly when they are forced to pretend to the outside world that everything is peachy inside it. My hope is that, by opting for radical honesty with my kids—saying no both to the poisonous atmosphere within the home and to the concomitant necessity for keeping the truth of that poison hidden inside it—I will have taught my children lessons about boundaries, honesty, self-respect, and mitigation that they can carry with them into the future.

Or at least that's what I keep telling myself in order to make it through each day.

Santi calls and texts daily, wanting to know how he can fix what he's broken. You didn't break anything, I tell him. I did. Some weeknights, after cooking dinner for the Commune, putting my son to bed, and trying to make things right with my daughter, I override my crushing guilt and exhaustion from work and make the round trip subway journey to meet Santi sixty blocks north. I meet him for sex, yes, but also to spoon, even if only for a few minutes before I have to head back home to my empty bed. Eros consumes me. Human touch—and the soothing hit of oxytocin it releases—feels like the sole antidote to my shattered life: a necessity, not a desire or diversion.

Santi lives in a tiny, dilapidated apartment with few possessions aside from his cameras, his computer, a gallery of photos from his last show, and a couple of paintings by his father, a Mexican artist who was once celebrated in his country but is now apparently struggling to stay both solvent and relevant. I bring my new lover sheets for his bed, dinner leftovers from the Commune, the occasional bag of groceries. Without a means to work legally, he lives below subsistence level poverty. His one pair of shoes have holes. With my new *Health Today* dollars, I buy him two pairs. Some nights, when the rice runs out, he goes hungry.

The bruises on my breasts have now healed, and he offers to shoot them gratis, but I insist on sticking with the deal we struck before we started sleeping together. I have a salary now, I tell him. Please let me pay you for the work I've asked you to do as planned. You need the cash. I need to feel, after spending every day not paying my sick and dying bloggers for their work, that I'm not exploiting anyone else in the world. We plan the shoot for the night before my surgery, which is dumb. I try to relax into it, but in each photo from that night my expression is marked by the tension of a woman hours away from going under the knife. My surgery is scheduled for 7 A.M. It's now 11 P.M. I have to go, I tell him, but as I'm about to get dressed and leave he says, "No. Stop. Before you put on your clothes, I have an idea. Lie down here, in a fetal position." "Here" is a large green trash bag he places on his floor.

"What? Why?" I say.

"Please," he says. "Just trust me."

Trust me: I override my doubts that the male species is actually trust-worthy and do what he asks, scrunching myself into a fetal ball and clos-ing my eyes. He circles hawklike around my coiled body, shooting off frame after frame from this angle and that. A few minutes into this, I picture what he pictures and feel tears splashing onto the green plastic below.

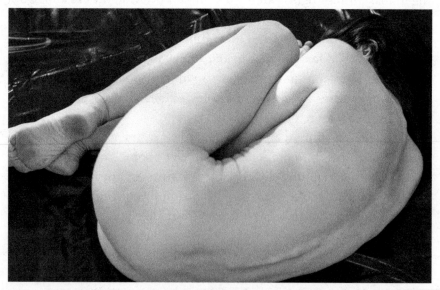

February 6, 2014, the night before surgery, © Cristobal Vivar

Yes. Of course. Here I am, eight hours pre-op, a discarded body atop a body bag, awaiting rebirth. Will that rebirth come? Or will the bag cover her fetal corpse before she has a chance to unfurl? The bottoms of my feet are dirty, I think, from walking around barefoot on the living room floor. I wish I'd taken the time to clean them. Ice coats the New York City sidewalks outside. The salt and sand tossed onto it, to keep us from face-planting, are impossible to keep out. The world creeps in, no matter how diligently you sweep it out. Looking back on the image now, years later, it remains the most brutally honest portrait of me anyone has ever taken, before or since. I feel seen during this particular moment in time: known, understood. And my dirty feet are what make the photograph.

You Won the Lottery!

FEBRUARY 2014

On the morning of my lumpectomy, I change into a hospital gown before dawn and watch a nurse stick a line into one of the arteries atop my hand before covering it with tape. The anesthesiologist arrives next, to talk me through his plans. Next, my oncologist arrives to tell me that I'll be put in an MRI first, so that a wire can be threaded into my lump, to help her locate it during surgery. You won't be in there for long, she tells me. After the MRI, someone will come get you and bring you into the operating room.

Breast MRIs require lying face down with your boobs dangling through two holes. I don't usually mind the enforced entombment of MRIs. In fact, I often fall asleep in them, despite the noise. But on this particular morning, with the operation looming, my mind is racing and unable to find peace. The minutes stretch on, longer than I'd assumed, and I start to panic. What's going on? She said I'd only be in here for a little while. This feels closer to an hour.

When I finally emerge from the tube into the light, the radiologist smiles. "You'll never believe this," she says. She is—what?—giddy? Giggling? Everyone in this room, in fact, seems to be smiling. "The lump is gone. Completely gone. You won the lottery. This only happens once or twice a year, if that."

"What?" I say.

"Your mass is gone. You don't need surgery."

"I don't . . . *what?*" I stare down at my hospital bracelet, at the yellow I'm-a-fainter bracelet, at the line in my artery. I can't process this information. Part of me, writing this today, still can't process it. You go into a hospital one morning, expecting to be sliced open, chunks of flesh removed, but suddenly the bad cells inside you have retreated, and the woman pulling you out of the tube has become . . . Emily Litella? *Never mind.*

Wait wait WHAT?

I put my hospital gown back on, and make my way to the MRI anteroom, where my scans are put up on the computer. On one screen, dated January 7, 2014, sits a left breast with a clearly visible mass next to the chest wall; on the other, from today, February 7, 2014, a completely normal-looking breast. "I don't get it," I say to the radiologist. "It just . . . *disappeared?* Where did it go?"

"Who knows?" she says. "Sometimes—like I said, not often—these things just happen." My surgeon, she says, will have to ask me a bunch of questions about any diet, exercise, or behavioral changes between the film on the left and the film on the right: These disappearing masses, rare as they are, are useful. They might one day provide important information about the body's own ability to combat abnormal cell growth.

I wander, dazed and in shock, back into the pre-op room to get the line removed, put my street clothes back on, and meet my surgeon. We go over the thirty-one days that have passed between the MRI with the lump and the one without it: Has anything changed between then and now? Diet, exercise, work? I wrack my brain, trying to come up with anything of note. I've kept the same diet, the same daily regimen of either at-home yoga or walking, the same crushing work schedule and childcare responsibilities. The only thing that has changed this past month is that I went on that ill-fated date with Santi on January 8, 2014, the day after the first MRI, and I've been having frequent sex with him ever since.

She smiles and asks if I plan to keep seeing this man. I'm not sure, I say. He's kind and loving and an ace with a broom, but I don't see us working out long-term. He's already been hinting at wanting to get married for a green card, but I'm not divorced yet, not even close, and if I do end up getting married again, I want it to be because I am loved, not because I'm useful. The doc seems disappointed by my answer.

"What?" I say.

"Nothing . . ." she says. That *nothing*, I think, is definitely something.

"Wait. Hold on a sec. Are you suggesting I fucked my way out of a breast lump?"

"No," she says, laughing. She would never suggest that. We don't have the data to support such a theory. As with most things concerning the female body, there's a lack of adequate research. But of course oxytocin *is* a powerful hormone. We're still learning about its effects on cancer.

"So, are you saying he's my chemotherapy?"

"I would never say that," she says, all business.[*]

"Then what are you saying?"

"I'm saying we still know so little about what causes or inhibits abnormal cell growth, that's all."

"I'll keep seeing him," I say. "For you."

"Don't do anything on my behalf," she says, but I can tell by her smile she's pleased. She'll need me to come back in six months, she says, for another MRI, to make sure the breast lump is gone for good. Someone from her office will call me to set that up.

My daughter, who has taken the day off from school, arrives in the pre-op room, her mouth agape. "Wait, what? I don't get it," she keeps saying. "So you *aren't* getting surgery? What'll I tell my friends?" Her

---

[*] Later at home, I will do some research and find only one old study from 1994, suggesting that oxytocin could play a role in breast cancer reduction, but I could find no further follow-up. Then, just as I was wrapping up the final edit of this book, a new article appeared in *Oncogene*: "The oxytocin receptor signalling system and breast cancer: a critical review." It's the first article I could find that addresses the possibility of oxytocin's role in breast cancer reduction of the *non-lactating* breast. As with most studies of women's bodies, there's been a dearth of data. "The effects of OT [oxytocin receptor] on non-lactating mammary gland remains poorly explored since most studies have focused on OT's role during pregnancy and lactation." In other words, though we know women who breastfeed their children have a lower incidence of breast cancer than those who don't, no one has actually studied the effects of the oxytocin triggered by sexual arousal and sexual activity on neutralizing cancer cells, but perhaps they should. Especially since a study in Sri Lanka of the incidence of breast cancer in sexually active women versus celibate women, all of whom did not have kids, thereby removing lactation from the data set, showed that "breast cancer incidence was lower in the sexually active group than in the celibate group."

phone is vibrating with dozens of text messages from classmates, wanting to know how the operation went.

I shrug. "Tell them your mother doesn't have cancer," I say.

"I love you," she says, hugging me.

"I love you, too," I say, tearing up. It's our first step back to who we were before that fateful night when she came home early. For my birthday, a month later, I will come home from work to a cake she and George have baked from scratch, replete with pink frosting and a phoenix she's made out of strawberries.

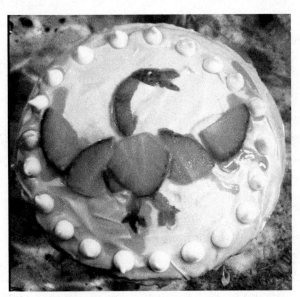

My daughter's and George's birthday cake,
March 11, 2014, © Deborah Copaken

Back at *Health Today*, I ask an oncologist—an old acquaintance from high school who is happy to trade her unpaid writing for exposure—to write a weekly column on breast cancer, and it does well. I've made it through nearly five months of this game of musical chairs, and then I make it through the IPO and its self-congratulatory celebration at City Winery as well, and though I have no shares in the company—others with bigger jobs do and are suddenly rich, in no small part off the labors of unpaid sick people with pharmaceutical-ad-friendly illnesses—I start to breathe easier. I don't love my job, but I'm putting everything I have into it, and that has to count for something.

On the Monday morning after Friday's IPO, I head to the apartment of one of our newest bloggers to interview him about his multiple sclerosis and take dictation, as he's not feeling well enough to type. He's the husband of one of my oldest friends, who said he'd be happy to help me out and write a column. That morning, he recounts a disturbing story of disability discrimination. I shoot off a few frames of him with his wife and kids as well, to go along with his post, and then I head back to the office just before noon to download the images and edit the text down to a manageable length. As I sit down to do this, I see my boss, the editorial director, walking over to speak with me. She looks angry, but I'm not immediately concerned by this. These days her face is nearly always pinched into a scowl, and I'm excited to tell her about our new contributor. "Oh my god," I tell her, "wait till you read the new blog post I'm editing. That man with MS I told you about, he has a *doozy* of a story about—"

"Where have you been?" she snaps, cutting me off.

"Taking dictation. From a blogger with MS. He can't type. I told you this on Friday. Then I sent you an email about it over the weekend to remind you."

"Oh, right," she says. "Well, they've been looking for you. You better go talk to them." Her eyes are oddly averted.

"Who's been looking for me?"

"HR."

"HR? Why?" I'd spoken to someone in HR a month earlier, to alert them to my upcoming surgery. Just make sure you get your work done while you recover, he'd said. This isn't the most opportune time to be absent, what with the IPO coming up, plus he'd heard from the vice president that I'd been asking for money to pay our contributors, which had upset her enough that she'd filed a report. We don't pay for blog content, he reminded me. I know, I know, I'd said, choking on the apology. I'm sorry for pushing.

"I have no idea why they want to see you," my boss lies.

"Am I getting fired? Please, just tell me, so I can prepare."

"Just go talk to them." She quickly pivots and walks away.

The editorial director and I have actually become friendly over the past few weeks since my aborted surgery, or so I thought, going out to lunch together and sharing stories of single motherhood and postmarital dating. Her ex is in the picture, though, and sharing custody, so she's able to spend part of the week with her boyfriend. That must be nice, I'd said, not having to jump on the subway and sneak in affection between *Harold and the Purple Crayon* and Jon Stewart. It is, she said, except her new boyfriend is kind of a dolt. Why stay then? I'd wondered. The same reasons we both stay in this job, she said with a shrug: inertia, need.

The ground under me drops out, as in a Gravitron, as I make my way to the HR department and take a seat. I can't stop staring at the neck of the man who meets me there. It's so thick, it spills out over his shirt collar like mozzarella tied with string. He's the head of human resources, and he's pointing at me, menacingly, his face frothed into a red frenzy. "You've been absent so often, we couldn't even find you to fire you!" he says.

I remind this massive man with the finger in my face that in the hours after the company went public, which is when he says he first couldn't find me to fire me, our computers had crashed from the sudden interest in our brand, and all of us in editorial were told to go home and finish working on our own computers. I remind him that my sole other absences—aside from this morning when he said he wanted to fire me, when I was taking dictation from a new blogger with MS—were spent at Sloan Kettering. I show him those well-documented absences, nine in all, mostly half days, blocked out on my calendar between December 2013 and February 2014, when I would edit from the hospital waiting room instead of from my desk. Never once, I tell him, did I shirk my responsibilities. Despite my absences, my work was never late. I made sure of that. And I grew our contributor base and organic traffic all the same. Surely a health organization understands that workers sometimes have to go to a doctor when they get sick. I ask if I will receive severance. He shakes his head no.

I start to beg. I'm a single parent, I say. My family's sole wage-earner. Please. Just a month or two of severance, so I can have time to find a new job and still pay rent and my son's college tuition bills. There's also a growing stack of bills from Sloan Kettering I've yet to pay off. *Please!*

No, he repeats. You have fifteen minutes to gather your things and leave.

PART IV

HEART

2014–2015

Inwood

MAY–AUGUST 2014

The palpitations begin their nocturnal visitations every night at around 3 A.M. Which is just so dark-night-of-the-soul cliché that I refuse to believe they've become a daily feature of my life until they've been striking for several weeks.

I am not, by nature, anxious. When I was four years old, I got stuck alone in an elevator and, certain all would be straightened out soon enough, I sat on the floor picking a scab off my knee. While getting mugged at gunpoint, I asked the mugger if I could just hand over my cash instead of the whole wallet because, you know, what a hassle at the DMV. When my older son's toddler forehead collided with a broken bottle on the sidewalk, I stepped into an ambulance cradling his skull with the shard of glass still protruding from its center, telling him, softly, "You're okay. It's okay. Everything's going to be fine," having just handed over my baby daughter, who was not allowed in the ambulance,* to the super.

---

* This is a really stupid rule, by the way. What if my building's super hadn't been around to watch and feed my little one while my son was sewn up? Also, I should note: I did not call the ambulance. My son was bleeding so profusely, bystanders did. That ride, which I did not order, cost me $1,200. The rest was paid by insurance.

But being a forty-eight-year-old, suddenly unemployed, severance-denied solo parent in need of expensive medical tests in a gig economy has shattered any claim I've ever had on innate calm.

The nightly awakenings are more than rude, they are sweat-soaked and terrifying: a nightmare that only worsens when you open your eyes. I can't catch my breath. I clutch my chest, inside which my heart makes its normally quiet and obedient presence *known*, motherfucker, like a prisoner banging a tin cup against my rib cage.

PVCs—premature ventricular contractions—I'll later find out they're called. But not for another two years, when they become so insistent, I'll collapse at work. For now I just call them my beat-skipping thing.

Anxiety is one of the four major risk factors for PVCs, which are harmless when they happen occasionally, but when they become a chronic feature of your heart's mechanics, they can lead to permanent damage from cardiomyopathy and arrhythmia. I try to will myself to breathe through these nightly episodes but end up pacing the floor instead, perseverating. The accompanying brain swirl, during these nightly awakenings, is always the same and always as maddeningly circular as my floor-pacing, in the way all money panic spirals down through the catch-22 funnel of not having any:

My lease is up in two months. I should really move to cut down on my rent. I can't rent a new place if I can't show monthly income or at least cash in the bank. It took me six months to find the last job. I'll be homeless at that rate. I have to let go of Brittany. Then she'll be homeless. Plus how can I go to work, once I find a new job, without Brittany?

The Commune has two new members: a fellow middle-aged, newly separated mother, introduced to me by a friend, and her son. The woman moved into my older son's room after George grew weary of the lack of privacy and noise of communal living. Her teenage son floats in and out of my tiny once–writing studio formerly occupied by Brittany. Brittany now sleeps on the floor of the family room.

This brings human membership in our commune up to seven. In a three-bedroom apartment, in the top half of a narrow Harlem rowhouse. The newly separated mother, already thin, is shrinking thinner. Hannah, after several months of spotless attendance at school, has started to backslide in other ways. So now my brain swirl has drawn these other souls into its vortex as well, picking up speed and draining down through my heart.

How can I tell a woman who's in the middle of her own moment of inflection that I can't afford to keep paying this noose of a rent, even with what she's paying to live here, so she'll have to find new digs, too? That's not fair to her or to her son, and it's a betrayal of her trust. I promised her safe harbor while she figures out her next move. I've promised Hannah, who's a truly good kid at heart, the same. They are counting on the Commune as a place of refuge. The woman actually went out and bought new furniture for her room and made it adorable and cozy. How can I tell her that, now that I'm out of a job and can't find a new one, we all have to leave? How can I tell Hannah she has to go, when she's made so much progress living here? I'm a monster, I'm a monster, I'm a monster . . .

And then, as the internal winds intensify, all the normal concerns of marital rupture rear their delightful heads: debt, destitution, desolation, darkness, depression, day-to-day survival, and the divorce process itself, as yet uninitiated. And once that D-bag of distress gets sucked into the maelstrom of circular thought, my brain short-circuits into sparks and smoke.

I need an MRI, to make sure the breast lump's gone. MRIs without insurance are $6,000. COBRA's $2,000 a month. Where will I get the extra $2,000 a month? I have to find a way to control these panic attacks, maybe with medicine? Talk therapy? Shrinks in New York cost $300 a session. Oh, well. Another college tuition payment is coming up soon. How will I pay for it plus a second college tuition in a year? I need to stop the clock and get officially separated from my husband so we can disentangle our joint credit cards and shared bank account, from which he continues to draw down my cash, but how do I do that without hiring a divorce lawyer? Can I just take out the meager remaining balance from the account and start a new account, or are there legal ramifications to that since money I earned from my job is still considered his joint marital asset? And where will I find the $30,000 retainer to pay a divorce lawyer to help me sort out all of this? Or the $4,000 to move? Or the $39,000 to pay off the debt? Or even $200 for next week's groceries? Plus the kids need shoes, haircuts, field trips, therapy, school supplies . . . aaaagggggghhhhhhhhhh-hhhhhhhhhhhh!!!!!!

I research "mindfulness," to help quiet my thoughts. I take advantage of an offer for one free meditation class, then another. "Notice and accept your thoughts without judgment," they tell me, "and focus on your breathing. It's all just brain chatter anyway: irrational fears coming to the fore." No! I want to shout between breaths. These are not irrational fears. They are real, and they are destroying me. You cannot meditate away an empty bank account when you're the sole human in charge of the health and welfare of three children. That's an actual problem requiring immediate attention.

Sometimes, when the anxiety-triggered palpitations strike during the day, I faint. I've always been an occasional fainter, but my fainting episodes are becoming regular enough now that I'm constantly gauging my environment for sharp angles. "Mom's down again," I hear, upon coming to, followed by the upside-down head of one of my offspring shouting above me: "Mom! Mom! Can you hear me?"

I call ADP, the company managing my COBRA account, and ask if I can pay my bill quarterly instead of monthly: If that money is sitting in my account, I will spend it on food, and right now health insurance is more important than food. No problem, says Christy, the nice woman on the end of the phone. I send ADP a check for $5,292.87 for the quarter. ADP cashes the check. Then they immediately cancel my COBRA coverage. Apparently, the check arrived in their office a few days late. I appeal. My appeal is denied. Without any money left over to hire a lawyer or file a second appeal, this is the end of that. It takes another month to get my money back.

Sloan Kettering calls to set up the MRI my oncologist ordered, to make sure the lump is still gone. I tell them I'm sorry, but I don't have insurance anymore, and I can't afford the $6,000 they charge out of pocket. I need to keep that money in my account to apply for a new apartment.

I take advantage of this tiny pocket of time with the cash sitting in my bank account to search for an apartment closer to my son's school, located in what has been called "Manhattan's last affordable neighborhood": Inwood. After a dozen unsuccessful visits to dark, two-bedroom hovels in my price range with either mouse droppings, no closets, awkward layouts, or one-bedrooms listed as having two ("You can just turn the living room into a bedroom!"), I talk my way into a brand-new building, still under construction and not yet listed, which has just gone up directly across the street from my son's school.

"$4,500 dollars a month! For a tiny two-bedroom!" I'm yelling into the phone to Santi, after visiting an apartment with brand-new appliances but barely room for beds and definitely no room for dressers. "In *Inwood*! Can you believe it?"

I'm yelling this loud enough to be heard by the fifty-or-maybe-sixty-something man sitting on a bench in front of the bar next to the coffee shop where I often go after school drop-off to scour the latest job listings and write cover letters. "You lookin' for an apartment?" he shouts, running to catch up with me. His accent is pure Bronx. He's out of breath from the half-block sprint. His pale skin bears the marks of the ghost of teenage acne past, and his slicked-back hair is bottle-dyed black. He snuffs out a cigarette, standing close enough that the stink of morning booze is unmistakable. "I gotta three-bed, two-bath just around the corner. $2,300 a month. Wanna come see it?"

When you've been mugged and assaulted as many times as I have, the amygdala's don't-fuck-with-me wall immediately goes up the minute any stranger enters your airspace. "Excuse me?"

"Who's that?" says Santi, still on the phone.

"This dude who just stopped me in the street claiming he has a $2,300-a-month three-bedroom to rent . . . No, I'm not kidding . . . I'll be there in a second," I lie. I want to show the stranger that someone will notice if I don't show up.

"Sorry," says the man. "I didn't mean to butt in to your conversation. I just overheard what you were saying, and there's this beautiful place around the corner you should see. Wanna come see it?"

"Are you a broker?" I say. "Do you have a card?"

"Um. . . ." He pats the pockets of his pants several times to no avail. "Hmmm . . . I'm not really a broker," he says. "I just help out the landlord. You know, to find tenants."

"Isn't that the definition of a broker?"

"Do you want to see the apartment or not?"

I've seen enough police procedurals to know that this scene will not end well for the woman playing me. "No, thanks," I say. "I'm in a rush."

"Well, take my number anyway," he says. "In case you change your mind." He holds out the sole crumpled business card he's finally located in his jacket pocket. It has no name. Only a phone number and the name of a company I've never heard of.

I hesitate. Then—I mean, $2,300 a month for a three-bedroom in Manhattan—I take it. These days, the average rent for a one-bedroom Manhattan apartment is $4,208. (Yes, I know, this is crazy, but this is the city where most of the media jobs and companies who might hire me have their offices.)

Santi, having overheard all of this, thinks I should go check out the apartment, why not?

"Are you crazy?" I say.

"It could be life-changing for you and your kids."

"Well, yes," I say. "That's one definition for getting murdered."

After several hours of sitting in the coffee shop typing yet another cover letter to yet another job listing that seems vaguely in my field, curiosity wins out. I call the number on the crumpled card. It's the same Bronx accent as before. "Okay," I say. "Show me the apartment."

The man meets me near the building on the corner of Seaman Avenue and West 207th Street. He has a key to the lobby. This seems promising. He's affable, even friendly now that I've agreed either to be shown an apartment or cut up into tiny pieces. The apartment, on the third floor of a down-at-the-heels, six-story art deco building abutting Inwood Hill Park—its windows look out over the trees of an actual forest I never knew existed, with hiking trails—has three decent-sized bedrooms, two bathrooms, and a small galley kitchen with room for a tiny breakfast nook. Sure, the oven is from the 1950s and coated in grease, the fridge is small with two broken door shelves, the black-and-white checkered tiles on the kitchen floor are the stick-on kind with caked-on dirt between them where grout should be, there's neither a washer/dryer nor a dishwasher nor room for either one nor permission to have one installed, the cabinets are crumb-strewn and sticky to the touch, and I spot several dead roaches in two of them, but the bones of the living and sleeping areas are good. More than good. The living room is sunken with decent afternoon light, and the master bedroom is flooded with natural light all day, plus it has its own tiny bathroom with a miniature shower stall. "What's the catch?" I ask the not-really-a-broker.

"No catch," he says.

I ask him if I can have my friend Caroline come by and look at it. Sure, he says. Caroline is a no-bullshit, independent film producer. If anyone can sniff out a scam, she can. The next morning, we are sitting on the floor of the living room. "You could put your dining room table right there. It would probably fit," she says, pointing to a narrow space between the front door and the kitchen.

"Maybe. It'll be tight," I say. "So you think I should take it? It's not too good to be true?"

"I mean . . . it *is* too good to be true. But if it's even halfway true, you've still scored. Plus, what other options do you have?"

"None," I say. I've now seen all of the listings in and around my son's school. Three bedrooms are rare, and after a year of living communally and cooking for seven, I'm aching for family privacy and one-pan meals. Plus brokers have once again been traipsing in and out of the Commune with potential buyers. The writing's on the crumbling limestone walls: The new owners, an Australian real estate conglomerate, plan to renovate and flip the house now shared by two rent-paying tenants into a single family home for a buyer wealthy enough to afford all of it.

Meaning, not me.

I impart the news to my children and fellow Commune members that the lease on the house is up in a month, and I don't have the funds to renew it. The kids and I, I explain, will be moving up to Inwood by ourselves. I promise Brittany that I will find her a new au pair situation in a new home, and I do. We will remain friends to this day. Hannah moves back in with her mother before heading off, a year later, to college. My younger son, while sad to leave his childhood home and our weekend walks in Jackie Robinson Park, is excited to be closer to his school, on the same street and within blocks of two of his best friends. My daughter has only one more year at home before she goes to college, her family has already blown up anyway, she'll have her own room for the first time in seventeen years, and she'll be closer to her high school in the Bronx, so it's all good, she says, except for the name of our street. "*Seaman* Ave? I'm never inviting a friend over ever again," she says, then laughs even harder when I tell her it's near the corner of Cummings. The newly separated mother in our midst, however, while completely understanding of and empathic to the necessity of the move, is also quite reasonably upset over losing her new home barely three months after having moved in. My guilt over this remains.

And yet I also know that I'm not solely to blame for her woes or mine. The Commune's formation as well as its demise can be traced straight back to the rotting fruits of unrestrained American capitalism: laws and policies favoring landlords over tenants; a deliberately inflated housing market; the 2008 recession; a 40 percent rent hike; the for-profit divorce racket; a for-profit health insurance industry; the outrageous cost of an American college education; the gig economy; private equity takeovers, which stomp on workers like so many underfoot ants; historic levels of income inequality; and a government too corrupt, incompetent, and mired in partisan acrimony to keep dog from eating dog.

"Try not to get sick or hurt," I tell my kids as we're packing up to move to Inwood, using every penny of my meager savings to cover the cost of the movers and the first and last month's rent. "We don't have health insurance right now, and we have no reserves to cover anything serious."

"When will we have it?" my daughter asks. "And what about birth control?" Her birth control, she knows, costs around $480 a year without insurance. I don't even have $480 in the bank right now.

"We'll have it soon," I say. "And don't worry about birth control. I'll figure out a way to cover it until I get health insurance." I've started looking outside the journalism job boards for work, applying for positions in other industries, including as a holiday greeter at The Container Store, just to have those three months of health insurance while I continue looking for a job in my field. In the meantime, I've been taking on whatever freelance work I can find, but with magazines now often offering a flat $200 fee for work that used to pay between $3,000 and $10,000, depending on the number of words produced, these efforts can feel futile.

I've also been writing and trying to sell a forty-page proposal and first chapter of a memoir I'm calling Yes, And . . . , about the curative powers of saying, "Yes, and . . ." to a world that's constantly telling middle-aged women no. True to its themes, after a bunch of initial responses from editors expressing some version of Yes, and . . . !, it gets a bunch of No, but . . . rejection letters from every major publisher, with some version of "Sorry, our marketing department doesn't really see a market for a middle-aged woman's memoir, but we love the writing and hope it finds a good home elsewhere."

This is in 2014, five years before The New York Times will announce, in the wake of #MeToo, that older women are in vogue again. "Ageism is one of the last acceptable biases in our culture, but it powerfully intersects with sexism," a University of Michigan professor quoted therein will say. "Older women are now saying 'No, I'm still vibrant, I still have a lot to offer, and I'm not going to be consigned to invisibility.'" I will read these words and this article, having finally sold the book in your hands to an enlightened male editor in late 2018, with a mixture of elation and rage.

I hand the not-broker broker a deposit check and fill out the rental application in a questionable-looking office at the foot of the George Washington Bridge. If it is a scam, I tell myself, I'll stop payment on the check. Spoiler alert, the apartment is legit, but at each baffling new personal-information-revealing step along the way toward signing the lease, I'm sure I'm being scammed, even on—no, *especially* on—the day I sign it.

"Who are these people here?" says the landlord, a gruff, elderly orthodox Jew pointing dismissively to the names of my children on the lease under the part that says, "Other Occupants." We are signing the final papers atop what will soon be my very own Formica kitchen counter, part of which is peeling off. ("You'll fix this?" I ask him. "Sure," he lies.)

"They're my kids," I say.

"Who said anything about kids? You can't put your kids on the lease. We never agreed to kids living here."

My heart is doing its beat-skipping thing again. I feel on the verge of fainting, but I grip the peeling Formica and feign strength instead. "Why would a mother of three rent a three-bedroom by herself? I have kids. They come with the package."

"No, sorry. No kids."

If I were standing here with my husband, this would not be happening. I've learned, as a solo mother, that the terms of a deal are more malleable if you say, "Hmm, I need to speak to my husband about this. That sounds a little off." But I'm screwed on this one. He knows there's not a proprietary penis standing between him and me.

"You can't be serious. You cannot tell me I can't live with my kids. That's absurd. And illegal," I say, even though I'm not certain about the latter. Can a landlord forbid children from living in an apartment?[*] I try

---

[*] No. Thanks to the Fair Housing Act of 1968, it's illegal for a landlord to refuse to rent to a family with children.

googling the question, but the cellphone reception in the kitchen is nonexistent. Is that why we're signing the papers in here?

"Do you want the apartment or not?"

"Of course I do! But not if my children can't live with me. That's nonnegotiable. Their father lives elsewhere. I am the only parent taking care of them. They either come live with me or I can't sign the lease."

The owner stomps dramatically into the living room with the non-broker to have a private discussion. Ten long minutes later, they step back into the kitchen. "Fine," says the owner, "but you have to sign this, too."

In all my years of renting apartments, I've never once felt like I needed a real estate lawyer to help me sign a simple rental lease. "What is this?" I say.

This is a pages-long rider that somehow gives my landlord—no, let's call him what he is, a slumlord—the right to transform my low-income, rent-stabilized, government-subsidized apartment into market rate after I leave. (I think. Even now I'm not sure, as I was never given a copy.) So the whole you-can't-live-with-your-kids drama, in retrospect, was most likely a ruse to disarm me and make me sign anything to keep the apartment, once I'd jumped through so many hoops—yes, many more hoops than normal—to rent it. "It's nothing," he lies. "Just a precaution. Because no one told me you have kids."

"That's ridiculous! I told the broker I have kids. When we were walking through the apartment I said things like, 'This bedroom will be my daughter's room, and this will be my sons'.'"

"He's not a broker."

"Whatever!" My frustration is now palpable.

"You're not a lawyer, are you?" He looks at me suspiciously.

"No," I say.

"A journalist?"

A *bad one*, I will later think, because had I done a little more digging, I would have discovered that the umbrella organization of the real estate firm I'm dealing with—which has its own easily googleable complaints, including mold, roaches, and entire months of no heat—is actually the Death Star of crooked New York City slumlords. They send private investigators to spy on rent-stabilized tenants they want to evict. Their multiple one-star Yelp reviews ("Beware!"; "This company is a scam!"; "Considering legal action"; "STAY AWAY FROM THESE CROOKS!!!!") describe dozens of illegal, corrupt, morally suspect, and racist business practices.

I avoid answering the "Are you a journalist?" question and redirect. "I'm a Jew," I say pointedly, hoping that the fact of our shared heritage of abuse will make him less abusive. (It doesn't.)

He takes the bait. "You go to shul?"

"Of course," I say, leaving out the whole part about not having been since my father died six years earlier. Our family used to go to synagogue (aka "shul") on Rosh Hashanah and Yom Kippur every year without fail, but when Dad was given his death sentence, and I called him to ask if he wanted me to join him for Yom Kippur services down in Maryland, my Kansas City–born and bred father—whose most virulent curse prior to this moment was either *gosh darn* or *golly*—said, "Fuck Yom Kippur. My fate has already been sealed. I'm going to the beach."

We finish signing the papers, with the caveat that my kids cannot take over the lease should I die, which I'm sure is illegal, but at this point I don't care. And I don't plan on dying before leaving this place, which is shortsighted, considering I nearly do from excessive blood loss three years later. I just need an affordable home—now—and this one looks decent enough. The landlord hands me a set of keys and leaves, and suddenly I'm alone in the new apartment I will officially dub my "divorced-lady apartment" because "separated-and-still-in-divorce-limbo-lady apartment" seems too cumbersome.

I walk through the still-empty rooms of my new home, be it ever so humble, feeling a sense of pride and wait . . . is that? . . . yes . . . *joy*. Pure joy. I did it. I left a bad marriage. I got myself out of the outrageously high Harlem rent. I found a place overlooking a forest with actual hiking trails. It's three blocks from my son's school, so I've just bought myself an extra half hour every morning to linger over breakfast instead of commuting with him on a crowded subway, plus in two years, when he turns ten, he'll be old enough to walk by himself. It's half the rent I've been paying, so I no longer need to live with boarders to survive. And my bedroom has its own bathroom and tree-filled windows. I'm literally surrounded by the kind of Edenic green that, were this a novel instead of my life, an editor would remove with a "Too on the nose."

I will live in my divorced-lady apartment on Seaman Avenue for the next four years, during which I will walk nearly every morning through Inwood Hill forest, my daily Thoreauvian act of reclamation. This simple practice of putting one foot in front of the other will serve as a new baseline. Whatever comes next in my life—whether a job or love relationship or a new home or life situation, if any—I want it to feel like this at its root: grounded, shade-providing, leaf-crunching, oxygenated, sun-dappled, quiet, calm, forward-moving, and verdant, no matter how steep the hills. (There will always be hills.) During these daily hikes, as I watch the leaves turn from green to red to gone to snow-covered and back to green again four times, I will ask myself what I want from this second half of my life, and this daily questioning and awareness of both the self, its evanescence, and time's passage through the seasons will eventually act as catalyst.

But not yet. At this point in our story, I'm still at the bottom of the hill, where each morning several paths present themselves. The climb, every day, shows me what's possible. You choose a path. You stick to it. Sometimes you lose your bearings or trip over an exposed root or slip on a patch of ice or get scratched by an errant branch. But eventually, like every Dante, Hansel, or Gretel before you, you find your way through the forest into the light.

While the trees of northern Manhattan provide an unexpected, hyper-oxygenated boon, the apartment itself will have its unexpected, well, let's call them challenges. Gradually, or sometimes in great geysers of sludge, "the catch" of my new home, on the edge of Inwood Hill Park, will reveal itself. Or rather themselves, I should say, as there are many. I will love my new home, let's be clear, and I remain grateful to it today for its sudden appearance—literally—out of nowhere, but while living in it I will also be inundated with roaches (and I mean thousands of roaches, not just a few); sickened by mold; and frozen on multiple consecutive subzero days by a lack of heat and hot water. My bathtub will emit noxious, brown, poop-smelling sludge that shoots straight up from its drain. The drinking water will constantly turn brown or stop running altogether. Rain will leak through loosely installed windows, transforming two of my windowsills into moldy, paint-flaked pulp that, no matter how many times I inform the management

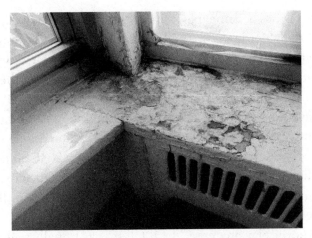

Living room windowsill in Inwood, © Deborah Copaken

with photos like the one above, will not only never be fixed, they continue to worsen.

The pilot light on the stove shuts off every day, so I'll often come home to an apartment reeking of gas. The broken door shelves in the fridge will be held together by duct tape. The elevator will often stop working, sometimes when I'm in it. Only three out of the five communal washing machines in the basement will work at any given time.

All of these scarcities and inconveniences are classic slumlord ploys aimed at enraging rent-stabilized tenants enough to force them to leave, so they can jack up the rent for the next tenants. In response, the tenants in our building have created a private listserv, which urges us to call 311 en masse each day, every day, whenever the no heat/no hot water situation goes on for more than a week, or whenever the tap water looks as if it's been tinged with human feces.

Security will also be an issue. The building has no doorman, and our buzzer intercom delivers unintelligible static instead of a human voice. One of my neighbor's more troubled psychiatric patients will get buzzed into the building, despite warnings sent via the listserv not to let her in. She will squirt lighter fluid onto his doormat, light a match, and nearly burn down the building. Burglars will find their way into several apartments through windows with busted locks. Another neighbor will be attacked in the unlit area in front of our building after the tenants begged for a light for years. The list goes on and on.

Minor issues become major quality of life hassles as well, particularly after my daughter leaves for college, and it's just me and my still-young son. I will spend an hour most nights scrubbing our dishes by hand, often with cold water when the boiler is once again on the fritz. Yes, I realize this sounds petty and entitled, since 25 percent of all U.S. households have no dishwasher either, never mind the rest of the world, but this nightly hour of cold-water dish-scrubbing after a long day at work, instead of the ten to fifteen minutes it used to take to do dishes with a dishwasher in Harlem, means I miss out on four crucial years of post-dinner hanging out with my eight- (then nine- then ten- then eleven- then twelve-) year-old, who already feels abandoned.

"We never play anymore," he'll tell me, as I finally collapse into his bed to read him a book. Since I can't afford takeout, I institute a weekly cereal-for-dinner night, just to have time for a couple of rounds of pick-up sticks together or snuggling on the couch watching TV before bed.

One sunny Saturday morning, a few months after having moved into our new home and still searching for a full-time job with benefits, I head to the Inwood farmer's market on Isham Street to buy apples. After weighing the apples on the stall's hanging scale, I quickly log in to my bank account's mobile app while standing in line, to make sure the freelance payments I'm owed and have been hunting down by email have finally been deposited, as I've been promised they would. Not one of the four payments I'm owed has hit my account, which has $18 left in it. Meaning the $6 worth of apples I'm about to buy will slash my current cash reserves by a third. I dump the apples out of the bag and walk home, fruitless.

Back home, my heart palpitations now at DEFCON 1 but trying to remain calm in front of the kids, I unearth my diamond engagement ring from my desk drawer, underneath which I've placed a business card from my former Harlem downstairs neighbor, Michael, who buys and sells precious stones. "Bring it over," he says, when I call him and tell him I'm ready to sell. Later that day, he holds it up to the light and tells me he can give me around $1,800 for it, give or take, if he can match me with a buyer.

"What?" Surely he's mistaken about its worth, I tell him. My ex bought it wholesale for around $3,000 back in 1992 when we got engaged. "How can a diamond have depreciated by nearly half over the course of two decades?"

"That's the thing about diamonds," says Michael. "They're like cars. Once you drive them off the lot, they lose a big chunk of their value."

I did not know this, I tell him. I actually bought into the whole "diamonds are forever" marketing, assuming my $3,000 wholesale diamond was more like real estate: an appreciating asset I could one day sell if, say, a $6 bag of farm stand apples were ever out of my price range.

"No," says Michael. He tells me I have to take the stone to get it appraised before he'll consider anything. So a few days after my twenty-first wedding anniversary—I am, after all, still officially married—I put my ring into a plastic pillbox and head down to Fifth Avenue in midtown Manhattan, where a Hasidic woman checks the stone for flaws and gives me the two important numbers I need to sell it: It's worth $2,700 if I sell it to a dealer, she writes on the appraisal, but it will cost $7,100 to replace it.

The delta between those two numbers astounds me. "Why do we even bother with diamonds then?"

Irene Zisblatt, née Zegelstein, survived Auschwitz and its aftermath while periodically swallowing (and fishing out of her own feces) the four diamonds her mother sewed into her hem. I wonder how many of the ultra-orthodox women in this room, in fact, owe not only their careers to diamonds but perhaps even their lives. When did diamonds go from life-saving stones a doomed Jewish mother sews into her daughter's hem as a genocide survival tool of last resort to practically worthless?

"That's just the way it is," says the woman with a shrug. When I ask which store on 47th Street has the most honest reputation, she says, "I'm not allowed to tell you that. We have to be impartial." Then, a few seconds later, she whispers, "Some people have better luck with those online places."

Online places? I google "online sell engagement ring" and find I Do Now I Don't, a mix between eBay and a dating site for ring buyers and sellers. Cool. Still, I'm curious what I can get for the ring by just walking in off the street, so with my appraisal in hand, I choose the most bustling store on 47th Street. "How much would you give me for this?" I ask the older gentleman in a yarmulke, round-faced and portly.

"$1,800," he says dismissively, without looking at the appraisal.

"But it was appraised at $2,700," I say.

He shrugs. I walk out.

Back home, I set up a dating profile for my ring—something I have not yet done for myself—and I compose a little story about its origins. Stories sell rings, the website advises its users, and storytelling is the one fixed asset I still have. I list it for $3,900, hoping to get around $3,500, which would be half of its retail value and $500 more than my ex paid for it. Within hours, I start fielding a bunch of inquiries from random strangers until finally these opening lines hit my inbox, from a man named Aidan:

Hello, I am writing to see if you would accept an offer of $3,500 on the engagement ring you listed on the site. We are a young couple, very much in love, starting out and trying to save for our future . . .

Why does this one speak to me above the others? Because it's polite, to the point, the number is good, and I liked the part about saving for the future. I immediately write back:

Hi, Aidan, I've received many messages about the ring, but something about yours spoke to me. So I'm gonna do something kind of weird. If you're trying to save for your future, how about this: let's lop off another $100, which you have to promise me you'll place in a college fund for your future kids. I wish I'd done that instead of saddling my poor children with loan debts. Meaning, you can have the ring for $3400 with the caveat that you take that extra hundred you would have spent on my ring and not touch it until your first kid goes to college, deal? If those terms are acceptable to you, you have a deal.

Aidan lives near enough to me that we decide to simply meet in person to exchange the ring and its appraisal for his cash. He shows up at my door practically shaking, as if we're about to conduct a drug deal instead of an exchange of U.S. dollars for an engagement ring. But then I sit him down with my kids at our dining room table, and he relaxes enough to tell us his love story, wearing his heart on his sleeve so vulnerably and nakedly, both my seventeen-year-old daughter and I have tears in our eyes after he finishes.

Love moves us when we see it up close. It's not about the ring. It's never been about the ring. It has always been about hope. For what is a marriage other than two people throwing their lots in together without any proof that it will work out other than a gut feeling that it might? Empires have been built on far less.

When Aidan leaves, I head out to the store and buy some apples.

Money

In August, I receive both good news and bad. The good news is that I have an interview for a job as an editor for a new website called *Cafe*, a position I'd found on a job board. The bad news is that I've been rejected from the three-month holiday greeter job at The Container Store. "At this time," they write, "we are moving forward with other candidates for this position."

I burst out laughing when I first read this. Then I immediately start to cry. I've been holding it in for months now, all this fear and anxiety, the sadness and shame raging through me. The nightly sweats. The heart palpitations. The multiple faintings and feelings of hopelessness. Applying for that Christmas-rush position at The Container Store, which had been advertised with benefits, had been what I thought would be a rational solution to a critical problem, plus it would buy me another three months to find a full-time job. A no-brainer, I thought: the thing you do when you're unemployed with no other job prospects on the horizon.

The interview with *Cafe*, however, goes well. Really well. I meet with CEO Vinit Bharara, the brother of Preet Bharara, the then–United States Attorney for the Southern District of New York. Vinit has become wealthy, having sold his business Diapers.com to Amazon for $545 million. He will be self-funding *Cafe* at first, he tells me during our interview, before seeking investors, because he believes in good writing and wants to put more of it out into the world. That's his impetus, he says, above and beyond turning a profit, which of course he would eventually like to do but the writing should come first. (What a change, I think to myself, from my former job, where the writing was always an afterthought.)

Vinit comes off as kind, smart, and sincere in his literary goals, and the other three editors he's hired, who are also interviewing me at the same time, are similarly engaging. There's Peter, a warm and funny TV writer who weirdly happens to know my sister Jen well enough that he's been in my mother's house; Melissa, a big-hearted editor who tells me she's been a longtime fan of *Shutterbabe*; and Bill, a former U.S. Army captain and foreign correspondent, whose calm demeanor immediately puts me at ease.

I leave the interview elated. I've nailed it. I'm sure of it. Plus I love the team already in place. A flurry of phone calls and emails follow, during which start dates and terms are broached. I have breakfast with Bill the next week. Lunch with Melissa and Peter a few days later. The official offer, I'm told, will be arriving any day. Then an email from Bill lands in my inbox in mid-September: They love me, they love my work, but they've decided not to hire a new full-time editor at this point. "I want to emphasize the 'at this point,' part of that sentence," Bill writes. "I know you are probably going to have all kinds of other opportunities, but if circumstances allow we'd certainly like to stay in touch. For one thing, we expect to reevaluate after our initial launch in a few months, and I can envision several scenarios in which we might love to have you."

I cry again. Of course I cry again. Big, sloppy tears, a runny nose, the whole red-cheeked, face-melt mess. I don't have a few months to wait. I need a job *today*. "All kinds of other opportunities?" No, Bill. Only one. And it's a long shot.

A few weeks earlier, at the end of the summer, I'd flown to Los Angeles on my last remaining airline points for a bunch of TV pitch meetings set up by (let's call him, after the "Jewish Giant" in that famous Diane Arbus photo) Eddie. Standing six foot seven, Eddie was a photography nut, *Shutterbabe* fan, and TV showrunner who'd reached out via Facebook a few years earlier, the day after I'd first joined the social media platform in the summer of 2008. He was one of my first "friends," added only because we shared another friend in common and because he'd written an effusive message about my book, wondering whether the rights were available.

Back then, the option to adapt the book into a film had been passed from Darren Star and Dreamworks to Likely Story to Sundance to Participant Media. Now the option was once again up for grabs, and Eddie wanted to partner on pitching it as a TV series with ourselves as the showrunners, and this all happened so fast—two days from my "Yes, and . . ." reply to seven meetings scheduled starting the following morning—that I'd had to leave my eight-year-old alone with my seventeen-year-old. "The fridge is full, here are the numbers to call in case of emergency, I'll be back before the first day of school," I'd told them, handing my daughter a $100 bill from my engagement ring proceeds, praying no one would get hurt in my absence, and sprinting out the door up the two blocks to Broadway to take the A train two and a half hours to the airport, because the cost of a forty-five-minute taxi was out of the question.

They say money doesn't buy happiness. That depends on how you define happiness. It sure does buy time, convenience, childcare, breast scans, and professional opportunity, all of which can lead to greater happiness. So I'd like to amend that saying, if I may: An *excess* of money doesn't buy happiness, but having enough money does, and not having any money whatsoever buys nothing but fear, anxiety, and life-threatening heart palpitations.

I hated leaving my kids alone, but friends who might have watched my son were on vacation, as it was the week before Labor Day. It's hard for me to describe this period of need, shame, and instability without hyperventilating. It hasn't been easy on my heart either.

And yet I know how fortunate I am as well. I have three sisters, each of whom collectively answered my pleas for help after the engagement ring money ran out after my trip to L.A., and I still hadn't found a job. Together, they pitched in to cover my rent and utilities for one month each, which will get me through the end of November. Had I been evicted from my apartment after that money ran out, my friends the

Sylvesters said they had an empty guest room waiting for me and my kids at the top of their stairs on West 88th Street, should it come to that. It would have been tight, what with all three of us in one bedroom, and four of us during Thanksgiving and Christmas, or maybe my three kids could have shared bedrooms with their four kids during the holiday breaks—we never really dug into the exact logistics of this plan—but just knowing I'd have a roof over our heads that winter, if I lost my apartment, made all the difference.

Most people would rather talk about sexual kink than about money, which is odd because money—having it, not having it, earning it, losing it—affects the quality and stability of our lives more than just about anything else aside from love and health and sometimes more than those combined. I know I'm privileged to have been born white in a first world country with a solid roof over my head. I knew this even before I spent years visiting refugee camps abroad or shooting true poverty, drug addiction, gang life, and racism up close as a photojournalist.

The first roof over my infant head, back in March of 1966, was a one-bedroom apartment in Cambridge, Massachusetts, in which I'd slept in my parents' room for six months until we moved to a two-bedroom rental in Adelphi, Maryland. My father, twenty-four, was still in law school at the time, selling hand-drawn cartoon greeting cards for extra cash. My mother, twenty-three, had been a substitute teacher while getting her masters in education. Neither of my parents came from money. Both were second-generation Americans born of Eastern European Jewish immigrants whose parents had all fled persecution at the beginning of the twentieth century: Lithuania and Ukraine on my dad's side, Austria and Poland on my mom's. Dad had received a full scholarship to attend college. Mom had enrolled in a small, in-state college near her parents' home and then, after she'd met and married my dad, she transferred to be near him.

The year prior to my birth, the newlyweds were so busy with school and their side hustles that they barely saw each other. The only way they would be able to spend time together, they realized, would be to take a vacation, but they had no money. "You're either going to have to rob a bank or go on a quiz show," my dad joked. So my mother went on *Password* and won. The show teamed her up with comedy duo Marty Allen and Steve Rossi, and she took home $350 in cash plus a World Book

Encyclopedia, which she sold for $150, bringing her earnings up to $500. Their trip to Bermuda that June of 1965, including airfare, cost $550. Nine months later, on March 11, 1966, I was born. (Thank you, Allen Ludden.)

My sister Jen was born two years later, and in 1971 our family of four—soon to be a family of six after my identical twin sisters, Julie and Laura, came along in 1972—moved to Potomac, Maryland, a growing middle-class suburb of D.C. My parents had scrimped and saved to put down the deposit and get a mortgage on our $52,000 home in a planned, Levittown-type community where all the houses have the same late '60s/ early '70s look and feel: *Brady Bunch* split level, if I had to name the style. I shared a bedroom with my younger sister; the twins shared the bedroom next to ours. An addition was built on when I was a teenager, giving us each our own bedroom and my father a home office and art studio. My mother still lives in that house.

I remember the day in 1979 when Dad came home from work, beaming with pride. "Well, I just crossed into six figures!" he said. I had no idea what he was talking about until he explained it. We toasted his new salary with apple juice. One hundred thousand dollars? An un-thinkable sum. For all of us, including my father.

"Can I get a pair of Sasson jeans now?" I said, seeing a sudden chink in the armor of what had thus far been a fruitless debate. I'd just turned thirteen. The raging egocentrism of adolescence—this sudden, over-whelming need to fit in with my peer group—was in full bloom. Amer-ica, too, was on the verge of a crucial transition, from a thirty-year postwar tide lifting all boats to a trickle-down monsoon wrecking giant holes in every hull except those on yachts, while offering up luxury labels and gold lamé in recompense. If you couldn't *be* a rich person, dancing the night away with Andy, Liza, and Cher at Studio 54, you could at least dress like one. "The Me Decade," Tom Wolfe dubbed it, a name that seems quaint and premature in retrospect.

I could divine none of this nor could I place a pair of designer jeans in historical context. I just knew that many of the girls in Cabin John Junior High School were suddenly wearing Sassons, and I wanted to be like them. But at $24 a pair, the jeans were twice the cost of the Levi's I'd been perfectly happy to wear until that Sasson label began popping up on nearly every butt in the school hallways except mine.

"No," I was told. Our family had much more pressing needs than designer jeans, for heaven's sake! Furniture, for one. A new car to replace the decade-old rusted Gran Torino. A tiny house nearby for my widowed grandmother to live out the rest of her years. Four college tuitions in the not-so-distant future. If I wanted a pair of designer jeans, I'd have to pay the difference out of my own Levi's pocket. Twelve hours of $1-an-hour babysitting later, the Sassons were mine. But the acquisition, after a minor surge of elation, felt hollow. And I felt ridiculous for having spent my hard-earned money on manufactured hype. They were just . . . jeans. With a label signifying a level of expendable income that was not mine to signal.

My parents' astute refusal to pay twice the cost of a wardrobe staple became my first awakening, however absurd, into the subtle differences between middle- and upper-middle-class finances. I'd seen poverty up close for the first time when I was nine, during our trip to Puerto Rico and Culebra for my dad's work. "They don't have . . . pants?" I said, crying, when I saw children running around various slums, barefoot and half-clothed. But nearly every single one of my friends from Potomac was the child of a doctor, lawyer, government worker, or architect father and a homemaker mother. And more than half of them, or so it seemed, were white and Jewish. It didn't even occur to me that being Jewish put me in a tiny minority in the U.S. until after I arrived at college.

To help pay for my first year of college, Dad sold one of his paintings: a large canvas he'd splashed with multicolored acrylics. His lawyer salary covered our expenses, but Harvard was $16,000 a year at the time, meaning he made too much money for me to get a scholarship but not enough to have an extra $16,000 a year in the family budget, nor had he been able to save for his daughters' tuitions. (As is often the case with even upper-middle-class families.) Once ensconced back in Cambridge, Massachusetts, the city of my birth, my eyes were finally opened to the vast stratification of U.S. society, but this was back in 1984, when the delta between rich, middle class, and poor was less extreme.

I met kids who came from either nothing or next to nothing; students who'd studied at elite boarding schools such as Exeter, Andover, and St. Paul's; other public school suburbanites like me; and the children of foreign dignitaries and American royalty. Robert Kennedy's son Max, who'd gone to Andover, was my classmate. Samir Rifai, who would go on to become prime minister of Jordan in 2009, was the son of the 1984 prime minister of Jordan as well as a graduate of the then all-boys' prep school, Deerfield. Harvard had placed him and his security detail in my freshman dorm with a Jew who'd attended Andover and an Irish Catholic who'd attended Milton, like the joke about the Muslim, Jew, and Catholic who walk into a bar, but they're all wearing bluchers.

I'd heard of none of these prep schools before arriving in Cambridge. Or bluchers. And I'd certainly never noticed or understood the not-so-secret signposts of having matriculated from one: those L.L.Bean "blucher" moccasins, falling apart at the seams; the games of hacky sack; the Norwegian sweaters covered in tiny white dots, worn several sizes too large; the intricate wall tapestries from Nepal and makeup-free faces and pirated stacks of Grateful Dead tapes and slightly frayed navy pea coats and air-dried blond hair, even in winter, and what I can only describe as an unobtainable insouciance I've yet to master. Boarding school, to my mind, had always been where kids were sent after they either failed out of their public schools or set them on fire.

Not that I would ever admit this to any of my new classmates. No, instead of owning and embracing my solid, middle-class, public-school upbringing, I bought a Norwegian sweater at a Cambridge thrift shop and hid under it.

When people would ask where I grew up, I'd say D.C. instead of Potomac. When someone brought up the Social Register,[*] I feigned knowledge of its existence. When they inquired about my schooling, I'd evade. When they wondered where I summered, I'd pretend to understand what that meant. "On the Cape," I'd say vaguely, referring to our two weeks of family vacation in a tiny rental cottage in West Harwich, not to the whole summers many of my classmates spent in the Hamptons or on Nantucket or Newport in grand homes with ocean views filled with gently used furniture passed down through multiple brand-name generations.

---

[*] A list, first compiled in 1887, of the members of American high society—the descendants of robber barons, presidents, and other trust fund WASPs—published semiannually from then on. Joseph Pulitzer was the only Jew on that first list. By 1984, when I first heard of the Social Register, there were a few more Jews sprinkled here and therein, but the list was in its last gasp of social importance. Celebrity would take over as the U.S. societal sorting mechanism by the last decade of the twentieth century.

When my first college friend, Cordelia—descendant of Cornelius Roosevelt, the grandfather of President Theodore Roosevelt—invited me as her guest to the thirtieth International Debutante Ball at the Waldorf Astoria in New York that winter of 1984, I had no idea what a debutante ball was or how to dress for the occasion or that only the girls "coming out" ("Coming out from *where?*" I'd asked) were allowed to wear white. So I showed up in my all-white high school prom dress: a garish, sequin-covered number in polyester and Lycra that had seemed like a good idea when I bought it on sale at Montgomery Mall but suddenly, in that grand ballroom, singled me out as lacking whatever everyone else in that room had.

I remember standing there, feeling utterly exposed as a fraud as several female members of my college class, wearing puffy silk and satin white wedding dresses, minus the veils, were escorted into the ballroom by many of the male members of my class, all of whom were wearing white tie and tails: not that I even understood the semiotics of this particular garment either. Then—oh, god—I spotted Struan, the lovely and kind classmate I'd been dating that fall, having had no idea he was from this rarefied world of penguins and princesses.

We'd broken up, amicably if sadly, just after Thanksgiving of freshman year, when I told him I'd spent all of my high school years and even the summer before college in serious relationships, and I just wanted to be untethered for a bit, to see what that felt like. Struan is now the father of five and a kick-ass orthopedic surgeon who, when I tore my knee's meniscus during my third pregnancy, then waited twelve years to fix it for lack of time and resources, didn't lecture me about my stupidity but simply smiled his big Struan smile, scrubbed in, and fixed it.

"Deb!" he said, lifting me off the floor in a giant bear hug in the Waldorf ballroom. "What are you doing here?" Never before had my name sounded so idiotic. Deb! At the deb ball. In her totally wrong Deb dress. What *was* I doing there? But before I could answer this question, either to myself or to him, Struan was already being dragged by his new deb to the dance floor, where she and all the other girls in white dresses performed a choreographed courtship display dance with fans, like so many strutting flamingos in a National Geographic documentary. Afterward, the debutantes and their dates hopped into limousines and town cars heading north to various after-parties on Park Avenue, while I rode the subway downtown to my great aunt Ruth's place in Peter Cooper Village, a once-affordable housing complex built for World War II vets like my grandfather, who helped Ruth land her small one-bedroom two floors below. "How was it?" she asked.

"Fun!" I lied. How to tell the aging single woman with whom I watched every hour of Princess Diana's marriage to Prince Charles on TV that actually getting a chance to be Cinderella at the ball feels less like being welcomed into a world of prestige and glamour and more like walking through the hallways of your high school naked.

In other words, yes, I come from privilege. Immense privilege vis-à-vis most of the rest of the world and many others in the U.S. But it was not expendable-income safety net privilege. It was not trust fund privilege or here's-a-few-bucks-to-get-you-started privilege. It was solid middle-class privilege, which used to mean something to my parents' generation: an ability for a family to stay afloat comfortably enough, on one salary, from a four-decade career spent at the same firm, without tiring themselves out from too much treading.

But to my generation and those that followed, coming of age as the gap between rich and poor widened into a jagged chasm, being from a middle-class background has often meant that the minute we raise our heads above water, another sixty-foot wave appears: untenable childcare and housing costs; healthcare snafus, whether illness or loss of insurance; eldercare and sick parents; college tuitions that cost more than our yearly incomes; another round of layoffs without severance. This is particularly true if, having some vague notion of doing good in the world, we entered into less remunerative careers such as journalism, teaching, the arts, small business ownership, government, architecture, non-profits: all of which, in my parents' era, would have provided more than enough income to get by and then some. One of my dad's best friends, Jerry Landauer, was an award-winning investigative reporter for *The Wall Street Journal* who fled Nazi Germany with his parents in 1938 and was raised on modest means in Queens. On his journalist's salary, he and his partner, Roz, who was just starting out in her legal career, were able to buy a beautiful house in a leafy neighborhood in D.C. that would be utterly out of reach to any *Wall Street Journal* reporter today.

Visiting that house, in fact, when I was a young girl—seeing Jerry's light-infused home office, with its Persian rug and giant window, its messy desk stacked full with reporters' notebooks, files, receipts, newspapers, and books—that was the first time I thought: *That looks like a fun job*. I would eventually model my Harlem home office on the memory of his, down to the Persian rug my dog peed on.

When I left college at twenty-two to begin my life as a war photographer in Paris, I lived behind a particle board cupboard in the closet of a one-bedroom apartment I shared with three other friends from college, then on a pull-out couch in a colleague's living room for the rest of that first year. After I'd established myself professionally and could pay a little more rent—we're talking 2,000 francs a month, which back then was around $350—my first solo apartment was a *chambre de bonne* (a small room that used to be the maid's quarters) on the Rue Saint-Denis, a street famous for its prostitutes. My courtyard view out my one window looked straight into the apartment of an elderly *célibataire*, who cooked his dinner every night in the nude. My futon took up the entire floor space, such that I had to roll it up every morning to unfold a small table for breakfast. Sometimes, between assignments, I went hungry.

The man I met at twenty-four and would marry at twenty-seven had been orphaned as a young teen. He had neither income nor liquidity when we said "I do." In fact, he had student loan debts. I set aside one eighth of my monthly income as a TV news producer to help pay them off, just so we could start from zero instead of under water. We finally paid off his student loans in full after we'd had kids of our own, just when a new tsunami of housing and childcare expenses crashed down on us.

My three pregnancies set us back $9,000 each—$27,000!—for the deliveries and hospital stays, even though we had what was then considered good health insurance. My unpaid maternity leaves, when I was the primary wage earner, left us in debt. Then my husband, without informing me, invested all of our savings into an internet car-selling business that immediately went bust before losing his job in both the 2001 and the 2008 recessions. Suddenly, we were paying an extra $2,000 a month we didn't have in COBRA fees. My father was diagnosed with pancreatic cancer at the beginning of the recession of 2008, right after my husband was laid off.

A week after my father died, when I was still groundsunk with grief, my husband insisted—as much as I begged him to leave me alone to lick my wounds in peace—that I take the subway downtown to meet Dad's college roommate at his Midtown jewelry store to beg for a loan.

"No, I won't do that," I said. "Please stop." I was nearly done with a new book proposal. It would soon sell, in a two-book deal, and we would be back on our feet.

"We can't wait that long!" he said, growing frantic. Our landlord had just raised our rent another $1,000 a month. Our savings were gone. We were facing both eviction and loss of health insurance for COBRA non-payment by February.

It was mid-December 2008. Bell-ringing Santas stood on every corner of Fifth Avenue, soliciting dimes for the poor. I reflexively reached into my pockets to donate a few only to remember I'd already wrapped up all of our coins and lugged them to the bank to trade them for cash. Dripping with shame and fresh snow, I slipped into the silence of the store, the kind of place you need an appointment just to enter, worried that my slush-covered boots would stain the carpets. Inside that hushed interior, a thirtysomething blond in a full-length mink held the arm of a gray-haired older gentleman as they eyed an artfully illuminated case of necklaces encrusted with diamonds, emeralds, sapphires, and rubies. "That one," she said to their jewelry advisor, pointing to the largest necklace. No prices were listed, but by my estimate, the piece probably cost roughly the equivalent of a decent three-bedroom home.

Through a narrow hallway, I reached the inner sanctum where Dad's friend sat waiting. He'd hosted me in his Upper East Side brownstone during the summer of 1986, when I worked as a summer intern at a New York headhunting firm. He seemed appropriately stunned and confused by both my appearance in his office and by my request for a loan so soon—eight days!—after we'd shoveled dirt onto Dad, but he took pity on his former roommate's grieving daughter and sent us a check, two months later, for $25,000. (Yes, this, too, is privilege. Immense privilege.) We were supposed to pay it back, with interest, in three $8,333.33 installments over the next three years, and we were doing well on that front, after I'd landed the new two-book contract; and my husband found a new job with benefits; and we moved into the house in Harlem to halve our housing expenses. But then, after paying back the first installment, my husband got laid off from his new job. Corporate belt-tightening.

I still owe the last installment.

Yes, this is all humiliating to admit out loud, let alone in a book. I didn't want to. I still don't want to. But I must, because I'm hardly alone in my financial struggles, and shame shared by one, in my experience, becomes shame mitigated in others. Of all the motivations I have ever had to put pen to paper, this one sits near the top. If those of us in the non–one percent want anything to change, whether white collar or blue collar, we need to start screaming about income inequality, the ease with which we fire our workers, and the insanity of the costs of healthcare and housing in this country. That billionaires' wealth will rise by more than 25 percent, in the middle of a global pandemic, to $10.2 *trillion*, while eight million more Americans will slip into poverty, is both proof of our broken system as well as a *shanda*, as we Jews like to call a terrible thing that should never be allowed to happen because it's shameful, a disgrace.

"Billionaire wealth equates to a fortune almost impossible to spend over multiple lifetimes of absolute luxury," said Luke Hilyard, the executive director at a think tank that studies the societal effects of excessive pay. "Anyone accumulating riches on this scale could easily afford to raise the pay of the employees who generate their wealth, or contribute a great deal more in taxes to support vital public services, while remaining very well rewarded for whatever successes they've achieved."

Simply put? The reason Jeff Bezos is worth nearly $200 billion is because his warehouse workers earn $15 an hour. That's it. That's the whole tweet. Worse, he brags about these wages, as if he were being generous: "More than 40 million Americans—many making the federal minimum wage of $7.25 an hour—earn less than the lowest-paid Amazon associate," he'll write in his 2019 letter to shareholders, patting himself on the back.

On the one hand, okay, yes. Earning $15 an hour is quantifiably better than earning $7.25 an hour. On the other hand, dude, that still comes out to only $31,200 a year salary, which barely covers most Americans' necessities. In many cities, it will leave a family impoverished. Which raises the question: How many billions more than one does Jeff Bezos actually need?

Add a divorce into this broken system, if you're a woman, and the free fall is staggering, particularly for those mothers who, because our caregiving system is broken, and meetings are still called after 6 P.M., and men have yet to step up in any meaningful way, were forced to cut back on their hours or quit their jobs.

An American woman who files for divorce in her fifties—I was forty-seven when I got separated, fifty-two when my divorce was finalized, the financial disaster sweet spot for women—faces a loss of 41 percent of her household income after her marriage ends. And that's just her downward mobility if nothing else goes wrong; if she keeps her job; if her housing costs stay the same; and if she is receiving appropriate child support and/or alimony, neither of which I was receiving. Add on a hysterectomy, a rent hike, two college tuitions, a breast lump, a job loss, multiple extra hours of childcare, and $2,300 a month in COBRA fees, and those numbers go straight out the window, along with the woman's dignity, peace of mind, and hope for a better future.

In other words, when I lost my job at *Health Today*, I also lost whatever tenuous foothold I'd had on the middle-class ladder. The fall was steep. And (literally) heart-stopping.

Because of my Hail Mary trip to L.A., made possible through airline points and the kindness of my friend Julie, who let me crash at her house, Eddie and I were able to sell my *Shutterbabe* rights to Eva Longoria's company, UnbeliEVAble, for a nominal fee. Better yet, for a single mother in dire need of health insurance for herself and her family, I'd been hired to co-write the pilot. Eventually this will bring in $80,000 of income. The initial offer had been $38,000, but Eddie's agent had agreed to double my fee by lopping off a small chunk of his quote, which, because he'd been an executive producer on several '90s-era Must See TV shows, was significantly higher. This payment, in turn, will allow me to join the WGA (Writers Guild of America), the screenwriters union, which provides excellent, low-cost health insurance to its members, which will now include me and my family for the next two years plus each year after that, should I make $38,000 a year from then on as a screenwriter.

(I won't.)

The night I get the call from my agent alerting me to this life-altering news, I'm cooking the last of our pasta supply for dinner. I collapse on the black-and-white linoleum-tiled floor like a fallen rook, still gripping my wooden spoon. It's not like fainting. I don't feel the sound sucked out of my ears or the curtains falling over my eyes or that weird presyncope whiff of something resembling rubbing alcohol, if I had to name it, and I don't hit my head on the way down. It's more like having legs that can no longer support my body so they buckle. "How quickly does the health insurance kick in?" I ask. From my vantage point, sitting with my back up against the back wall of the galley kitchen, I spot one of the roach motels I've placed along the perimeter of the kitchen, teeming with new guests.

"The quarter after the quarter you're paid in full," I'm told, meaning I just need to stay alive in this chess game for six more months: to find health insurance as well as steady income until the script payment hits my bank account, which, my agent says, will take some time: Christmas, at the earliest, but probably later than that.

The next day, feeling emboldened, I call Bill at *Cafe* with a few follow-up questions. Had I done something wrong? No, he says. The company doesn't have the budget to hire someone full-time with my experience. The online job listing was premature. He's so sorry. There is no editor job anymore. And no, it's not as if the job has gone to someone else. They've just decided to wait until after they launch the website. He feels bad, he says, about wasting my time. I feel worse. But both his email and phone call have left the door open to future employment, and he seems bummed not to have an extra editor helping out with the launch, so I propose a plan: Why not hire me on a six-month contract basis? If I can prove my worth, we can renegotiate my contract at the end of it.

Sorry, he says. They just don't have the budget to cover my salary, even for six months.

What if I were just starting out? I ask, knowing that my TV-writing check will be hitting my bank account within six months to a year. I just need an income and health insurance bridge to get there. "You must be hiring entry-level writers, yes?"

Well, yes, he says, but you're hardly an entry-level writer.

I could be, I say. I can be anything you want me to be for health insurance.

Darren Star, of *Sex and the City* fame, has just started shooting a new TV show, *Younger*, based on the book by Pamela Redmond Satran, about nearly this exact scenario: a middle-aged mother, Liza, played by Sutton Foster, finds herself completely broke after separating from her husband, who lost all the family savings to gambling. Unable to land a job to suit her qualifications and experience, and viewed, by employers, as over-the-hill, she pretends to be twenty-seven years old and lands an entry-level job in publishing instead. I tell Bill I won't pretend to be twenty-seven, but if I'm hired to write for the website in any capacity, I can land an interview with Star on set as one of my first stories as a staff writer, as he's a good friend.

Darren and I met back in 2001, when he bought the film rights to *Shutterbabe* for Dreamworks. A few months later, the studio sent us to Paris together for research. The trip was supposed to have been a week-long, work-intensive, fact-finding mission, to help Darren write his script. And though we did work hard—meeting with all of the characters of my life as an expat; visiting every location where I'd once lived, loved, or worked in Paris—it didn't feel like a business trip. At all. "Our Big Fat Gay Honeymoon" I jokingly referred to it from then on.

Bill and I go back and forth a few more times until I finally come clean about my desperation for health insurance. Obamacare has now been passed, but because COBRA canceled my coverage more than thirty days beyond the required window for switching, I'm now in health insurance no-woman's-land until the next quarter. The ACA website won't even recognize my situation: It's not in the pull-down menu. Bill, hearing this, speaks to Vinit and comes up with a plan: a six-month staff-

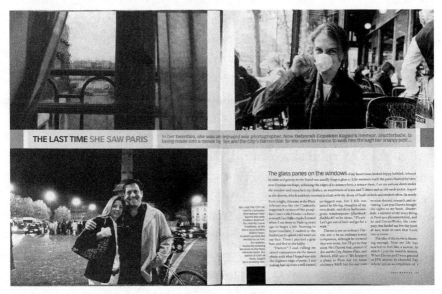

O, The Oprah Magazine, "The Last Time She Saw Paris,"
August 2002, © Deborah Copaken

writer contract—with that holy grail, benefits—at the equivalent of a $39,000-a-year starting writer salary. Meaning I will be earning $19,500 over the course of the next six months, with the caveat that I must produce a minimum of four stories a week. Plus edit as many as needed, plus recruit freelancers.

My starting salary at ABC News in 1992, nearly twenty-three years earlier, was $38,000 a year. My most recent executive editor salary, at *Health Today*, was $160,000 a year. I counter Bill's offer, since it does not cover my basic living expenses, never mind my son's college tuition, but the offer is firm, he says, and I have neither counteroffers nor financial runway to stretch out the negotiation. I need this job yesterday. I can freelance on the side, Bill says, to fill in the rest, no problem, as long as it's not an online publication. Print magazines are fine. Books, too. It can be a semi-nonexclusive contract.

"Deal!" I say, because this is what you do when you can't even land a job as a holiday greeter at The Container Store. You'll not only do anything just to keep your family afloat, including taking a job at a fraction of your worth, you're actually grateful for the opportunity: *Thank you, sir! May I have another?*

Note: This makes me officially employed in the eyes of the U.S. labor statistics, even though I'm not earning enough at this job to survive. Which, in turn, makes me officially a member of the working poor. According to one study during this era, *working poor* is defined as "full-time workers below 200 percent of poverty." Why look at 200 percent of poverty instead of just the poverty line itself when defining working poor? Because the poverty line is considered too low to account for metropolitan areas like mine, and it does not take into account how porous that poverty line can be: Millions of families fall in and out of poverty each year in the U.S., and all are at risk of poverty through job loss, medical emergency, or both.

By this measure, the year I am hired at *Cafe* at $39,000 a year, an average U.S. family of four considered to be "working poor" has a yearly income of $47,000 or less. And New York City falls far outside that average in terms of the cost of living.

Luckily, my son's new school, located in a low-income neighborhood with an average annual income of $22,776 a year, has free aftercare until 6 P.M.—let's place a *hallelujah* right here where it belongs—so I won't need to hire a babysitter. This is the rainbow's-end lifesaver for a working parent. With an hour commute to my new office, I'll just have to make sure to leave by 5 P.M. every day. And now that we live three blocks from his school, there won't be another half hour commute on top of that. We can just walk: *hallelujah* number two.

I immediately call Sloan Kettering and schedule my follow-up breast MRI for the week after my health insurance kicks in.

SEVENTEEN

At the Still Point
of the Turning World

OCTOBER–NOVEMBER 2014

The minute I sign my starting papers at *Cafe*, my heart starts to relax. Yes, I'm still worried about how I'll make up the extra income, and I still faint periodically or feel the PVCs rumbling when I check my bank statement or receive a new pile of old medical bills, but knowing I'll soon have health insurance and the breast MRI has magically given me back my health. I can sit and breathe through the episodes.

Step by step, I remind myself, as I walk the dog through Inwood forest every morning, watching the sun rise over its ridge. (*Hi, Dad. It's been hard since you've been gone, but I think things are getting better now.*) Step by step by step by step.

Now that my heart feels calmer, I turn my immediate attention toward its other pressing need, love. It's been a full year since my separation. Santi and I still see each other periodically on an as-needed basis, but I'm hoping, before I kick the bucket, to find something deeper, more meaningful, and less mutually exploitative than occasional sex with a willing partner.

What does it even mean, I wonder, to give and receive love from a mature and loving partner who sees you for *you*, who respects and adores you, who puts your needs ahead of his while you return all those favors in kind? I know such a thing exists. I've seen it up close in some of my friends' marriages, watching it deepen over decades. Tad and Amanda, Martha and Adam, Nora and Nick, Margot and Jamie, Marco and Abigail, Meg and Richard, Ayelet and Michael: These are just some of the names I roll call so often that my kids, still reeling from their parents' rupture, now end their antimarriage screeds with ". . . and don't tell me about Ayelet and Michael or any of the others. They are *outliers*, okay?"

My children are not wrong. Though I know plenty of marriages now entering their third decades, many of them are loveless or sexless or infidelity-plagued or filled with contempt, anger, lack of respect, financial shenanigans, lying, chronic sadness, or some other combination of these. I know this not only because I see some of the detritus of their broken vows and hearts up close and in person, but also because when you leave your own untenable marriage, you suddenly become the repository for the secrets from everyone else's.

This one, with the kind but aloof husband, has been seeking out emotional sustenance from another man for years. That one rolls her eyes so often in her spouse's presence, you wonder what their home life is like when no one's around. A woman I meet at a party confides that she is made to feel like a prisoner in her own home. "He controls everything," she whispers. One friend started counting the weeks between sex, then the months, then the years, now the decades. There's the woman who looks at her husband and feels nothing, another who feels only rage. The man who feels his wife slipping away but can't be bothered to try to win her back. The new empty-nesters who were fine-ish when the kids lived at home, but now find time alone together unbearable.

Friends and acquaintances ask my advice. They want me to tell them whether what they have is fixable, as if I've somehow become the expert on where the magical line exists between salvageable and not. I urge them toward therapy. Divorce is hard, I say. Avoid it at all costs. Or I quote Nora to them: "Marriages come and go, but divorce is forever." But I also know, when you're in the thick of a bad marriage, the impossibility of seeing the path ahead with any clarity. At a certain point in the cost benefit analysis, I tell them, if nothing changes in a struggling marriage, you're essentially choosing between two sadnesses: the sadness of staying and the sadness of leaving. Which sad is less sad? That's your sad.

I try going to more parties and work events, in the hopes of meeting someone, but all the men at the middle-aged gatherings to which I'm invited are married, plus many of the dinner invitations I used to receive when I was part of a couple have suddenly dried up. Note to readers: Your divorcing friends don't care if they're the odd woman out at a dinner party or the third wheel on your Saturday night dates, and they're not trying to steal your husbands. They are simply aching for a few hours of adult conversation during which they don't have to wash dishes or pretend to love Minecraft or sit alone on their bed, endlessly scrolling through other people's family vacations.

I ask my friends to set me up, and . . . crickets. I'm too ugly, I think. Too short, too big-nosed, too needy, too poor, too damaged, too loud, too *much*. "Is it . . . me?" I ask. No, they say. They just don't know any single men in our age bracket. They do, however, know this great woman who's also getting divorced, and though they don't actually say this, you know (because you know) that they're tired of hearing about her horrific custody battle or her controlling ex, so they pawn her off on you. This happens so often now that I throw my own dinner party for this new and growing group of once-married but now-single new friends, whose custody battles and court dates and copious tears I not only freely embrace, I welcome. There's strength in numbers. Power in group hugs. "Women Warriors," we dub ourselves, for together we feel like an army, less alone and fragile, proactive instead of reactive. I urge them each to bring someone new and equally broken to mix things up at the table. Yes, men are allowed to this gathering, definitely, bring them! We end up with twelve single hetero women, two gay men, and two straight men, both of whom are currently in relationships.

All the cool kids in my level three improv class, where we are learning a type of improv called the Harold,[*] are suddenly signing up for a new app called Tinder, but they tell me it's just for hook-ups. I ask one of them, the handsome and funny Shakespearean actor a decade younger—we'll call him Hamlet—if he wants to come see the Baldwins,

---

[*] A Harold is a structure of improv in which the characters and themes in the first act must recur throughout the rest of the acts as a series of connected scenes. This is really, really hard to do on the fly, without a script. Most Harolds fail in some fundamental way, but still can be quite funny to watch. A good Harold, however? A good Harold is a thing of genius, beauty, and awe.

an improv troupe at the PIT, with my son and me on Saturday night. Our weekly homework for improv is to see a professional show at least once every week, which is free if we see it at the PIT, plus our beloved level two teacher Meg is in the Baldwins. I'm the only one in the class with a kid who has to be at school early the next morning with a home-made sandwich and julienned vegetables, so seeing shows midweek with the rest of the class, followed by drinks and carousing, is difficult to impossible.

Hamlet, too, is reeling from a recent breakup with a long-term girl-friend. We also bond over the premature deaths of our parents: His mother died during his adolescence, also of cancer. The three of us — my son, Hamlet, and me, each broken in our own ways by parental loss and absence — fall into an easy Saturday night ritual, grabbing a cheap dinner before the show, cracking up during it, encouraging my son to call out the trigger word. The Baldwins know my eight-year-old will be in the audience every Saturday night, so they often call on him by name, because he gives good kid words like *cheese* and *zombies*. (Adults are more prone to shouting out words such as *penis* and *boobs*, which pro-duce less funny improv.)

After the show, we grab beers for us and a ginger ale for my son at the PIT bar and walk back to the subway together, giggling. My son lights up from Hamlet's presence and attention, as do I. Our Saturday night im-prov dates start to feel, for lack of a better word, like family. So familial that I now have feelings for Hamlet that go beyond friendship. To admit or not to admit? That is the question.

One night after a show, when my son is at a birthday party sleepover, and it's just Hamlet and me walking back to the subway together, I spend the whole twenty minutes working up the courage to say something, certain he's on the same wavelength but perhaps too shy to admit it. When I invite him to come back to my place, at the top of the subway stairs, he looks at me with a combination of horror and pity before grow-ing visibly upset. He thought I understood, from having shared so many of our private thoughts and feelings, that the kind of love he was seeking from this relationship was fraternal, not carnal. Friendship, not court-ship.

Ah. Got it. There will be no "You had me at hello." No swelling of music. No sharing of sweat or saliva. Yes, of course, I know, I'm over the hill and post-reproductive, while this man is still in the prime of his life. I wasn't imagining the two of us sailing off into the sunset or anything, just a couple of quick dips in the ocean before swimming off in different directions. Did I simply dream the electric charge between us or have I been out of the game so long, I can't even read the signals?

The A train takes an excruciatingly long time to arrive, during which Hamlet and I are forced to sit across from each other on our respective platforms for twenty minutes. He's heading downtown to Brooklyn. I'm heading uptown to Inwood. I feel like hiding under a rock. Instead, wholly exposed, I perform the modern-day equivalent of hiding under a rock: pretending to be deeply engrossed in my phone. I absentmindedly scroll through my various social media feeds, watching the endless stream of human faces and words rising up up up into oblivion.

What a strange race, the human race. Our desperation for connection is matched only by our ineptitude at connecting.

Derailed but not defeated, I sign up for Match.com. But after a week, I can't keep up with the psychopaths flooding my inbox, some of whom turn cyber-abusive if you don't respond. ("You think you're too good for me, huh? Well, die cunt!") I make a second attempt at signing up for eharmony, but there are still too many questions. I can't get through them. *What sports do you like? How much do you drink? What do you earn? Are you a smoker?* No, I click, for the last one, wishing for a third box to check for, "No, but I did for several years and boy do I regret that," because I would definitely date someone who filled in that box. *Are you willing to date someone with kids, yes or no?* Willing? Where's the box for "I'd rather"? *How would you describe yourself?* Right now? Um, sad, frightened, lonely, on the brink of homelessness, occasionally suicidal, and trying my best to ignore a near-constant arrhythmia. I click the boxes for happy, well-balanced, fulfilled, positive-minded, and at peace. *What's your idea of a perfect date?* Anything involving food, kindness, and sex, is there a box for that? *Do you believe in love?* Oh, for fuck's sake, yes, or I wouldn't be answering these annoying questions.

Yes, yes, self-love, self-partnership, you don't need a significant other to live a healthy and fulfilling life: I've heard and read all the arguments, political, feminist, celebrity, and otherwise, for trading love, marriage, and partnership for solo-living and self-reliance. But while I'm thrilled to be living in an era when this is a perfectly valid choice, when we women can have our own credit cards without needing a husband to sign off on them—I mean, let's all take a moment here to remember how recent that fuckery was—I'm also highly attuned to my own particular, individual needs.

These needs are both basic and embarrassingly mundane, but they are also strong and deep-seated and mine. I want someone to come home to; someone with whom to share dinner and stories of our days, to binge-watch the latest show everyone's talking about, to go out and see that new movie with the good review; someone to walk with me, hand in hand, as we unfold our vulnerable selves; someone to listen to me with the same attention and lack of judgment as I listen to them; someone to *see* me, fully, as I see them; someone to share the driving, to watch the leaves change, to catch me when I fall (literally, like when I faint, and figuratively, when things fall apart); to throw a dinner party together; to read books side by side and to trade off bringing each other coffee in bed; someone to share all those oxytocin-boosting, after-hours activities, such as lovemaking and storytelling and giggling and whispering and spooning and falling asleep in each other's arms.

"At the still point of the turning world," T.S. Eliot once wrote, "Neither flesh nor fleshless; / Neither from nor towards; at the still point, there the dance is." The poem is about time, but ever since I first read it in college, these words have, like a brain tic, always popped into my head whenever my body relaxes into the peaceful luxury of falling asleep in a lover's arms. "Except for the point, the still point, / There would be no dance, and there is only the dance." Time stops for me in a sleepy embrace. It is the most crystalline distillation of joy I know.

As much as feminist and political theory might want to throttle me for my basic-bitch needs, to tell me that engaging in or even wanting love and a traditional monogamous partnership requires subsuming the self and adhering to a patriarchal power imbalance it's my god-given duty, as a good feminist, to smash, raw science speaks otherwise. "Social isolation of otherwise healthy, well-functioning individuals eventually results in psychological and physical disintegration, and even death," sociologists Debra Umberson and Jennifer Karas Montez wrote in 2011, in the *Journal of Health and Social Behavior*. Meanwhile marriage, they say, influences "a range of health outcomes, including cardiovascular disease, chronic conditions, mobility limitations, self-rated health, and depressive symptoms."

Not that researchers are claiming all marriages are good for the body. Or for women, whose bodies fare worse in marriage than men's, particularly if the marriage is bad. A bad marriage, they remind us—as if I needed reminding—is as detrimental to one's health as a good marriage is beneficial. You'd actually be better off and less prone to illness alone. The key for reaping the benefits of a healthy relationship are the so-called "emotionally sustaining qualities of relationships": to feel loved, seen, and heard.

Knowing the effects of isolation, loneliness, and a lack of empathy on my own body, both while in a bad marriage and now not, I agree. I'm not talking about solitude. Solitude and I are good: We get along, we get things done, we walk, we play, we make stuff. In fact, I need my solitude as much as I need company, sometimes more so, and leaving a bad marriage has made me keenly aware of its benefits. But there's a difference between solitude and loneliness, a difference between the joy of having time alone with oneself to sit and think and the grief of having no one with whom to share your thoughts at the end of the day.

These days, songs like "All By Myself" send me spiraling. The loneliness, I cry to my sister Jen, is killing me.

So I download Tinder. And I start swiping, immediately horrified by the endless stream of human need and folly. If this is what "plenty of other fish in the sea" looks like, I choose land. Many of these metaphoric fish hoist literal fish, freshly caught, or guns or game or wait, is that a woman's hair he's tugging? Plus why are they all posing in front of their cars? Is that even his car, or did he go to a parking lot and flash his gang signs in front of the nearest Porsche? And what's with all the car selfies, bad spelling, group shots with other women, golf photos, and Ew! No! I don't want to see your hairy butt right now or ever. What does "Not looking for LTR" mean? I google "LTR": *long-term relationship*. Oh. Okay. Got it.

Some men list the many nonnegotiable conditions under which you might earn the chance to meet them: no gold diggers, no fat chicks, no bony asses, no drama, must be comfortable wearing stilettos, no heels, be tall, don't be taller than me, wear a dress now and then FFS (I look up "FFS": *for fuck's sake*), work hard, play hard, be relaxed, must be available to fly off anywhere at any time without a moment's notice, must have your own life, no games, no kids, be maternal, be sexy, and — my personal favorite, which appears so often I start to wonder who is the patient zero who started this — "If you're uglier than your pix, you're buying the drinks." I swipe left, left, left, left, left, wondering not only if these impossible-to-please men will ever find anyone matching their description of the perfect hard-working but always available, self-sufficient, childless, tall but not too tall, slim but not too slim, gorgeous madonna whore dominant submissive, but also what that poor woman's life will be like once ensnared.

My hopes that this part of leaving an LTR, FFS, might at least be a little bit fun and adventurous are quickly dashed. Finding love in middle age, I realize, will require just as much legwork, sweat equity, humility, patience, and compromise as finding a new job in middle age. You have to be single-minded, ruthless, open to new ideas, and willing to pick up and search under every moss-covered rock.

But not this rock. Three hours after downloading Tinder, I delete it.

My college-aged son sends me a link to a *New York Times* article about a relatively new dating app called Hinge. Unlike the others, at least at this particular juncture in the online-dating timeline, its algorithm depends on pairing you with partners with whom you share Facebook friends. That sounds like a more manageable, checks-and-balances, transitive property way to meet other humans, like going to a high school friend's college party. So I sign up. The first man to pop up on my screen is an artist — we'll call him Caravaggio, Gio for short — with whom I share thirteen Facebook friends, one of whom I call for a reference after swiping right and matching. She gives me her blessing.

I have never actually been on a blind date before. Or on an app date, as someone tells me they're now called when I apparently incorrectly tell her I'm about to go on a blind date with Gio. I didn't really "date" in my early twenties before meeting my husband at twenty-four. I met men in college, or on photo assignments, or through friends. Sometimes these men became boyfriends, and *then* we'd go out on an actual date, if we had money, or to a cheap Thai joint nearby where we could split a chicken curry. But these courtship rituals of my late teens and early twenties — "hooking up," as the kids call it these days — took place in the analog era, when I was either at school or off traveling the world, and now that world, in its digital entirety, fits in the palm of my hand. And three cheers for that, or I'd never meet any men who are vaguely in my age range. I just wouldn't. They're not at parties, they're not at work, and what am I going to do, spend $60 on babysitting just to go sit on a bar-stool with a paperback and hope?

Meaning I'm thrilled, heading into this first app date, not only to have matched with a seemingly handsome, interesting, intelligent man in my age range, but also to have done so relatively painlessly with some-one known to my friends. See? This is not so hard, I convince myself. Maybe this will even be fun. What am I looking for from this date and from him? Well . . . *love*, of course.

Which is my first rookie mistake.

No one on the apps is looking for love. Or if they are, they won't cop to it. "I'm just seeing what's out there" is the phrase I'll hear most often over the next three years of swiping. As if app dating were visiting a Brook-stone on a busy Saturday at the mall. Oh, look! A massage chair! Who knew? (You knew, that's who. That's why you wandered into the store.)

I'm shaking from nerves as I take the subway downtown from Inwood to meet Gio for lunch at the Upper West Side restaurant he's chosen, Peacefood Cafe, which, always looking for signs, I take as a good one. I like peace and food! Who doesn't like peace and food? Well, warriors, psychopaths, divorce lawyers, anorexics, and dictators, but most of us prefer peace and food, right? Maybe one day Gio or I will tell the story of how we met at the Peacefood Cafe and then found peace and emo-tional sustenance, together. Yes, okay, I realize it's premature, immature, and pathologically unrealistic to even imagine such a moment while I'm still hurtling underground through Harlem to meet him for the first time, but I can't help it. Being a hopeless romantic is a terrible burden. And yet between faith and cynicism, I will always choose faith. Love is my church, my mosque, my synagogue, my temple, and because I was lucky enough to be loved unconditionally by the first and primary man in my life—my father—my spiritual belief system is rooted not in magic or in an all-powerful being but in a tangible feeling I know exists be-cause I have felt it.

I wonder if I'll even recognize the man I'm about to meet from his one dating app photo, clearly a joke image—I like that it was a joke image, this already shows he doesn't take himself too seriously—in which he's smiling impishly next to a giant breast constructed out of sugar: part of an installation by artist Kara Walker that was built in the former Domino Sugar factory and that, for several months during the spring and summer of 2014, was on the ne plus ultra circuit of trendy art. ("I put a giant ten-foot vagina in the world," said Walker, "and people respond to giant ten-foot vaginas in the way that they do.")

I didn't visit the sugar lady. I didn't even realize her sugar boobs and ten-foot sugar vagina were out there for public consumption until they were gone, which shows you how trendy I am. I'm also dressed untrendy. Or rather I'm dressed in what might have once been considered trendy in the '90s, the only era during which my personal aesthetics matched society's: five-year-old Doc Martens, faded jeans, a peasant blouse, a long, gray wool shawl cardigan with a small hole in the right elbow, and no makeup. I want this stranger to understand that this is me, unadorned, in the clothes and face I normally wear out into the world. That I will always favor comfortable, unadorned, and slightly frayed over sexpot in lipstick and heels. I'm not here for his, your, or anyone else's porn-influenced viewing enjoyment. I'm here to take up space, to move freely through the world, and to be able to run from zombies quickly, should the need arise.

Our date, from the moment I sit down, goes well. So well that I can feel my heart trying to jump out of my chest as we dive into life's muck. His failed marriage, my failed marriage, his art, my books, addiction, love, sex, death, suicide, parenting, the nutritional value and cancer-fighting properties of butternut squash: No matter which turn our conversation takes, it opens yet another avenue of shared interests and stories spoken plainly, from the heart. He is, on this first date, the opposite of a man trying to show off. Rather, he seems unafraid to be vulnerable and real; to express confusion, ambiguity, raw emotion, faults, doubt; to listen and respond empathically. At one point, I'm telling him the story of my father's final hours, and his eyes mist over. I can literally feel the mirror neurons firing between us: something I have never felt being married to a man on the spectrum. I am equally consumed by Gio's dark, chiseled beauty, by his lofty ambitions, by his shyness and secrets, by the way he sometimes gasps for air between sentences, as if he has to remind himself to breathe.

Recycling, he says. He's really into recycling and reusing materials, whether it's mining junkyards for treasure or creating art out of old scraps. A show of his has just opened, he tells me, at a gallery in Chelsea: colorful sculptures made out of metal and blown glass. He shows me a photo of a wall he created out of beer cans. "Cool!" I say. Because "I love you," at this point, would seem both weird and premature.

Love at first sight: Does that even exist? As I walk away from the new object of my affections, I decide it must. I call my friend Ayelet before descending underground into the subway. "I just met the most amazing man," I say, heart waves rippling out of my chest with such intensity they feel like a forcefield. Turns out she knows and likes him, too, having met him at Yaddo, an artist colony, one summer. *Wow*, I think. *That Hinge algorithm* works! I make a mental note to try to interview its CEO for one of my first *Cafe* stories.

A week or so later, I invite Gio to a dinner party I'm throwing for Darren Star, who's just arrived in town to start shooting *Younger*. Gio shows up with an old friend of his from college. As I'm chatting away with this friend during dessert, Gio sneaks into my kitchen and washes all the dinner dishes by hand. A friend captures, in a photo, the growing electricity between Gio and me at the end of the night, as we play a duet on my kids' guitars. If thought bubbles were visible, mine would read, "I'm sunk."

Bad Judgment

OCTOBER–NOVEMBER 2014

I start my job at *Cafe* in mid-October, in a small office in the Flatiron Building with large windows and three long shared tables surrounded by Aeron chairs. I'm employee number nine, and these first six months of *Babes in Arms*–style "Hey, kids, let's put out a magazine!," where all of my colleagues are doing everything, including, in my case, shooting the photos, will remain one of my favorite employment experiences to date, despite not being able to make ends meet with my salary. On the days when my son doesn't have school but I have work, I bring him into the office. I don't earn enough to pay for childcare. I rely solely on his school's free aftercare. When he gets sick, I use up my own sick days to take care of him.

My first story out of the gate, "How I Got Rejected From a Job at the Container Store," originally published during the last week in October 2014 (but now sadly erased from the company's servers), goes wacko viral. "For years," I wrote, "we Americans have been fed the convenient lie: study hard, work hard in your chosen field, work hard at your marriage, save money, organize your flour, salt, and sugar into labeled bins and you will be in control of your life and your destiny. But control is an illusion during the best of times." Within twenty-four hours, the *New*

York Times op-ed section has linked to it on its homepage, recommending it to readers. *Forbes* asks to reprint it. TV comes calling. Radio, too.

The story—which is not really about not getting a job at The Container Store, but rather about the illusion of control—has struck a chord with American readers, many of whom are just waking up to the fact that they, too, are "just a single job loss, a single medical diagnosis, a single broken marriage removed from a swirling, chaotic, wholly uncontained abyss." It has also suddenly put the previously unknown *Cafe* on the map, digital and otherwise, which has, in turn, become a problem for our CEO: The journalists who are now interviewing me have logically started digging into my current income, asking me, point blank, if I'm finally earning a living wage.

"What should I tell them?" I say to my new boss, not wanting to lie but also not wanting to bite the hand that's not feeding me. $39,000 a year in the New York Metropolitan area is not a living wage for a family of four. In fact, according to MIT's living wage calculator, the minimum living wage where I live, in a household containing one working parent and three children—and that's not assuming that parent is also currently paying her eldest's college tuition, room, and board—is $112,816 per year.

"Tell them yes, you are earning a living wage," he says, immediately upping my salary from $39,000 a year to, well, not an official New York City living wage for a single mother of three, but to $80,000 a year, which is just under the living wage threshold for someone like me in Chicago. Six months from now, I will learn that my male colleague has, during this same period, been earning $200,000 a year.

My social media timeline and various inboxes have become choked with either the story itself or with queries from strangers about the story. One of those queries comes from Ken Kurson, editor-in-chief of the Jared Kushner–owned *New York Observer*. Kurson sends me a message through Facebook messenger. "We don't know each other," he writes, "but man, I loved your story so much. Please consider pitching *The New York Observer*." I explain I've signed a six-month contract with *Cafe* but tell him to feel free to reach out to me in five months or so. In return, he sends me a photo of him interviewing our CEO's brother, Preet. Which is weird, but whatever. A legitimate editor at a legacy media publication has reached out to me out of the blue to ask me to write for him. I can barely contain my glee. *One way or another*, I think, *I will crawl my way out of this fucking hole.*

We'll get back to Ken. He becomes a key character in my life's unraveling six months later.

After the Container Store story hits, I spend the weekend managing the influx of interview requests. Monday is taken up with speaking to reporters in various TV and radio stations around the city.

Then, Monday night, I'm doing my usual hour of cold-water dishwashing by hand, feeling nonetheless elated: I wrote something I was proud to have put out there; I got a raise during my first week of work; I've finally broken it off with Santi and have another date scheduled with Gio; my kids are adjusting well to our new home, despite the frequent cold showers and wearing hats to bed when the boiler breaks; the roach situation seems to be temporarily under control; the editor of the *Observer* likes my writing; I have an interview scheduled with Justin McLeod, the CEO of Hinge, and a *Younger* set visit and interview scheduled with Darren Star; I'll be getting my first paycheck in six months this Friday; I have a health-insurance approved MRI scheduled at the end of the month; my heart palpitations, for now, are under control.

I want to freeze this moment in time, when my heart, health, kids, work, and emotional well-being finally feel in alignment. When, for the first time in decades, I have the first stirrings of romantic love as well as hope for a less stressful future. When I can start to see the vaguest outline of what a meaningful path forward might look like.

Which, of course, is the exact moment when life says, "Oh, yeah? Watch this."

A notification pops up on my phone: Judith, my new colleague, has sent me an email. "A response to the piece is also now in Motherlode," she writes, with a link to the parenting blog* in *The New York Times*.

I lay my pink rubber gloves on the peeling Formica, sit down at the kitchen table, and have the out-of-body experience of reading a hit piece about my life in the paper of record, written by the *Times*'s parenting columnist, who has not called me either for comment or to fact-check. Rather, her story is an error-riddled reaction to the fact that her social

---

* The name of this blog, Motherlode, was rightfully deemed offensive enough that it was changed two years later to Well: Family, as the former name left out half of the population who should be shouldering the parenting load.

media feed, too, has been clogged with my story, and she and her Facebook friends have a lot to say about this.

"It's easy to imagine the few chunks of bad luck combined with *poor judgment* [emphasis added] that could land many of us in her shoes. But there was another reaction, about equally prevalent in my feed." Some of her Facebook friends, she wrote, were calling me "entitled, whiny, and worse." Then, conjecturing about the state of my mind and finances—again, without calling me to ask for a comment or even to spell-check my name—she continued, "One might even think that Ms. Kopaken [*sic*] did not actually want a job at The Container Store." Some of her other Facebook friends, she wrote, "saw *bad judgment* [emphasis added again], a lack of savings and a sense of entitlement—and in some cases added that they suspected that her New York-apartment-dwelling, sold-a-television-pilot self might be feeling stretched, but couldn't really feel the desperation she was laying claim to."

The kitchen light, which has been wonky of late, shuts off again. I've sent several texts to the super and three emails to the landlord about this, to no avail. I wiggle the ancient light switch to try to get it to turn back on and feel a jolt of electricity surge through my fingers and into my body. It flattens me, cartoonlike. This, too, has happened multiple times. "Oh, for fuck's sake," I say out loud, peeling myself up off the floor. With the light back on, a roach who was feeling cocky in the interim scurries anxiously up the kitchen wall back to safety. I start to cry. Again. Deeply but quietly, so as not to upset my kids who are doing homework in the other room.

I recognize this kind of woman-on-woman judgment journalism. I've been here before.

Like the journalist from *Talk* who, while interviewing me a few months before *Shutterbabe*'s publication, asked if I was worried others would call me a slut, then published her question and my horrified answer, thus appearing neutral over the issue of whether or not I am a slut while actually putting it out there—next to my smiling mug and a cleavage-revealing tank top chosen by the magazine's editors—that I could, in fact, be a slut.

Or the journalist from *Salon*, who wrote in a review of *Shutterbabe*, a book about the pitfalls of being a woman in the nearly all-male field of photojournalism, "The oddest part of her book is the absence of women

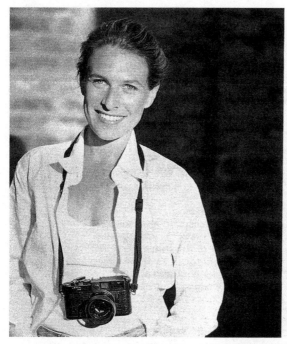

Kogan and I are to meet, but instead I find a tiny five-foot-two-inch woman, more handsome than pretty, wearing faded blue jeans and demure diamond studs and laughing the kind of laugh that immediately makes the people around her feel a little better about themselves. I ask if she's worried that her frankness will get her labeled a slut.

"I don't even like the word," she answers, looking pained. "How come there are no boy sluts? Why is it that Philip Roth and Norman Mailer can sleep around as much as they want and write about it but nobody calls them a slut?" As she

Talk magazine, January 2001 issue, photo of Deborah, © Oliviero Toscani

in almost any context. . . . So what happened? 'Maybe no one liked her,' a friend of mine suggests."

I have countless other examples, neatly collated into a scrapbook of tear sheets ripped from the pages of pre-digital magazines. These are not, I want to emphasize, bad reviews. Bad reviews I accept and can take, and they are an expected and necessary pitfall of putting a book out into the world. Rather, these are baseless character assassinations, often within the context of an otherwise good review, and misogyny hidden within rhetorical query. Like the review of *Shutterbabe* in Wellesley's feminist publication, *Women's Review of Books*, in which the female journalist praises the book while simultaneously insinuating, in the form of a rhetorical question, that I may be to blame for the unusual number of times I've been mugged and raped because that never happened to her as an undergrad: "Could there possibly be something about [Copaken] that invites these abuses?"

Or the journalist from *Talk* who blamed my rape on, you guessed it, "poor judgment": the kind a guidance counselor might point out, not her. She would never call me a slut with poor judgment in a national

Shooting star

by Deborah Solomon

Shutterbabe: Adventures in Love and War

by Deborah Copaken Kogan. New York:
Villard Books, 2000, 320 pp.,
$24.95 hardcover.

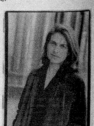

Deborah Copaken Kogan

Based on hearsay, I was fully pre-pared to have fun making light of this book. I was wrong. The book *was* fun to read, but too interesting (on several levels) to be simply dismissed.

Shutterbabe is really three books in one. The first is a memoir of Deborah Kogan's "glamorous" but brief career as a globe-trotting photojournalist—a career that lasted from 1988, when she graduated from Harvard, to 1992, when she traded the profession's flash and instability for the relative peace of the Upper West Side. The second is a pulp fiction-style rendering of Kogan's sexual adventures and misadventures with self-absorbed and often abusive men ("I circled Pascal's hairless chest with my finger. 'What about you? Why do you want to cover wars?' I asked him.") The third—really a combination of the first two—is the story of an ambitious and talented young woman coming of age during the tricky transition years (still going on) between the rise of feminist theory and its absorption into the mainstream.

As a vicarious adventurer, a former TV reporter—and as a woman—I was immediately sucked in by the opening sequence.

> There's a war going on and I'm bleeding... I'm squished in the back of an old army truck with a band of Afghani freedom fighters, who, to avoid being bombed by the Soviet planes circling above, have decided to drive without headlights through the Hindu Kush Mountains over unpaved icy roads laced with land mines... I

mean, what am I supposed to do? Ask the driver to pull over for a sec so I can squat behind the nearest snow bank to change my tampon?

She didn't... but me... wadded up toilet pa... return to "civilization... burned her bloody, gr...

Other insights int... woman abroad in Afg... wear a *burka* in order... subjects (she finally t... impeded not only her... ment but her view); an... she actually encoun... sojourn with the rebel...

of their days cleaning their Kalashnikovs) occurred when a land mine blew off the leg of the *mujahid* assigned to escort her away from the group so she could relieve herself in private. Yes, women on the road do have to play by different rules, physiologically as well as culturally.

The book includes some 35 of Kogan's photos, positioned to accompany the places and events she describes. They are technically adept and sometimes powerful, but since this is a memoir the focal point is not the pictures but the words, which Kogan can deploy as deftly as she wields a camera. Consider this vivid description of downtown Peshawar:

> Pedestrians, a variegated mix of clean-shaven Pakistanis, bearded Afghanis in their *shalwar* chemises—many of whom were amputees on crutches—as well as the random flock of Afghan women, walking in tight burka bouquets like boxes of crayons sprung to life, shared the bustling sidewalks with street vendors selling warm nan and various kebabs, whose steamy smoke mixed with the smell of burning trash and car exhaust to give Peshawar its distinct aroma: polluted mesquite, if I had to pin it down. (p. 32)

And consider, too, this blow-by-blow account of the professional at work—in this case, photographing an addict preparing his fix:

> I briefly contemplate using a flash, but decide to try to use the ambient light—a mixture of daylight and tungsten—instead. The

Kogan is also an acute observer of the arcana of her chosen profession, defining the importance to one's image of having the right kind of camera—a Nikon F2, F3, or FM2, preferably battered. And she can be mordantly funny. When she breaks off with a sometime lover, "[h]e reacted... like a true Frenchman, that is to say sadly but stoically, with a lengthy philosophical monologue concerning the meaninglessness of love in a life whose inevitable end is always death, followed by an invitation to spend the night in his room."

But this book, in addition to being interesting, is troubling. For starters, there's the unfortunate title, taken from Kogan's leitmotif: "With a couple of cameras hung around my neck, I was no longer the tiny mild-mannered homecoming queen from suburban Potomac. I was a superhero, a leaper of small land mines in a single bound; invincible. I was, now don't laugh—*Shutterbabe.*" I didn't laugh; I winced (or was it a shudder?).

I also winced at Kogan's six chapter headings: Pascal (he of the hairless chest), Pierre, Julian, Doru, Paul and Jacob. Yes, Kogan organizes her experience in terms of the sequence of men in her life (the last two being her husband and son). Whether or not this tits-and-ass orientation was urged on Kogan by a market-savvy editor, it seems a fair representation of her MO. Having lost her burdensome virginity at sixteen to a sweet defensive tackle on the high school football team, she "jumped from bed to bed with the glee of a frog in a lily pond, gently deflowering boy after gangly teenage boy." By the time she leaves college and heads for France she has

What's going on here? Am I hopelessly out of touch? Has the world changed so much since my own college years (characterized by an occasional flasher in the subway and tender consensual relations with sensitive undergraduates)? And should I fear for my preteen daughter? Or, as Kogan herself wonders, could there possibly be something about herself that invites these abuses?

Consider her choice of the most dangerous and depraved subjects—the

Talk magazine,
January 2001 issue

the Formica—she moves on to Cambridge, where she breaks a few hearts, gets date-

raped after she shows what a guidance counselor might call "poor judgment," magazine with a circulation of 670,000, thereby turning me into a person from whom hundreds of thousands of potential readers might think twice about buying a book. Thereby—and here's the real crime of sexism and misogyny—depriving me of potential income. It's a mythical *guidance counselor* who might deem my judgment poor for getting raped, not her.

Philosopher Kate Manne calls misogyny sexism's "law enforcement branch." Or, as she writes, "Sexism wears a lab coat; misogyny goes on witch hunts." One of the main hallmarks of these specific kinds of punitive witch hunts is using the opinion of others—groupthink—as a plausible deniability stand-in for the journalist's own unconscious biases: to punish "bad" women and reward "good" ones.

This new public flogging—which, like all public floggings these days, will live on long past my last breath—ends with a similar set of rhetorical questions, although now that we're in the Digital Age these are not so much disingenuous Socratic flourishes as they are prompts to readers meant to sway the jury and garner multiple responses and pageviews to attract advertisers: "How about you? When you read Ms. Copaken's story, or even the little I've shared here, do you identify with her or dismiss her—and more interestingly, why?"

My heart keeps snagging on this closing query—"do you identify with her or dismiss her"—which, I suddenly realize, contains within it the history of feminism. Not to mention the history of the labor movement. Women's health. Slavery and racism. Age discrimination. Rape culture. Politics. War. As if identification with a person or situation beyond your own individual experience must result in an either/or corollary construct. If you identify with her, then her story, a priori, is therefore worthy of recitation. The corollary being that *if you do not identify with her,* because you—like the journalist, I note—have health insurance, a wage-earning lawyer husband, no potentially lethal diagnoses requiring expensive tests and procedures (for now . . . eventually we all die of something), ample savings, and zero need to seek emergency employment outside the home, either in the service industry or anywhere else that might have you, then you must dismiss this woman's too-bad-to-be-true story outright. Identify or dismiss, those are your options.

The responses in *The New York Times* comments section, today's

Roman Colosseum, pour in almost immediately, each cruel reply another stab to my heart.

I call my friend Ayelet again, less than two weeks after calling to tell her about my successful first app date. I'm crying so hard at this point I'm unable to catch my breath. "Fuck her," she says. "Kicking another woman when she's down. It's bad journalism, and it's bad feminism." Over the next three minutes, she simply listens to me as I sob, emitting an "It's okay" or an "I love you" or "I know" during inhalation breaks in my lamentations.

Ayelet has had her fair share of factually inaccurate, unwarranted takedowns, too, like the time she wrote a Modern Love essay about loving her husband more than her kids. It was meant to be provocative: to define the difference between romantic love and maternal love; to say to her fellow mothers, who are so often shamed into trying to achieve the unachievable goal of maternal and feminine perfection, that this unrealistic, sexist paradigm is hurting us, our kids, and our marriages.

"I . . . I . . . whyyyyy?" I say, when I'm finally able to speak. "She even spelled my name wrong!"

"And," says Ayelet, "she referred to being diagnosed with breast cancer as 'possibly preventable-but-who-can-plan-for-everything.' If I ever get breast cancer, I'm going to insist on the preventable kind."

I burst out laughing. "I love you," I say.

"I love you, too," she says. "Just promise me you won't read the comments." Ayelet and I have half joked that when all the men are dead and gone, we'll move into adjoining houses in one of those tiny-house colonies together.

"I'll try," I say, but of course I fail. I can't help myself. I've never been good at leaving scabs alone either. "The problem with Ms. Copaken's story," reads one comment, "is her tone . . . It [*sic*] so whiny and smug and that you wind up rooting against her."

Tone. I slam my computer shut. There's that fucking word again. Tech CEO Kieran Snyder became interested in the idea of tone, specifically of the gender bias in the critical language used to describe the way women communicate. She reached out to colleagues in her industry and collected 248 of their predominantly positive performance reviews (because those were the only reviews, she knew, people would be willing to share with her). The results of her study, "The abrasiveness trap: High-achieving men and women are described differently in reviews," were startling. Seventy-one out of ninety-four women were criticized in these otherwise positive reviews for their tone, while only two of the eighty-three men were taken to task for it. That's 76 percent of successful females versus 2 percent of successful males being told, *in positive performance reviews,* "Watch your tone."

Five years later, Emily Khazan, a graduate student at the University of Florida, will conduct a similar study on gender bias in evaluations of university TAs (teaching assistants). Posing online as a female TA for half the class and a male TA for the other half of an asynchronous online course—meaning, some students saw a photo of their female TA, the others saw a photo of a male, but they never met the TA in person—Khazan performed her normal TA duties the same for both groups: grading papers, answering emails, etc. By the end of the semester, the "male" TA received much higher evaluations than the "female" TA. More critically, the "female" TA received *five times as many negative reviews* as the male, who received . . . none. Even though the "male" TA and the "female" TA were the same person: Emily.

I finish the dishes, put my little one to bed, fold the laundry, walk the dog, take out the trash, help my daughter edit her college essay, kill some roaches, answer several work emails seeking immediate answers, and crawl into bed, which feels emptier and colder than usual tonight, like being the lone penguin on a dark ice floe. I don a wool cap and a sweatshirt, pull out my laptop and read the takedown once more, hoping for some different interpretation, but no. It's just heartless and hateful.

But then, as I'm wiping new tears, a miracle occurs, in real time, as I refresh my browser. The ratio of cruel comments to kind ones flips: compassion, for once, is winning out. "The Wicked Stepmomster" from Philadelphia writes, "Are we really vilifying a person who tried to get a job? This recession has taken more than our money if that's the case." Amon from Texas writes, "When I read the piece, I rooted for her. As I hope others would for me." Another writes, "What happened to this author could literally happen to any one of us who is not in the hallowed 1%. Be smug at your own risk." And Anon from New York writes, "If we find fault in her, her fault explains the problem, and we can free ourselves from having to contemplate the very real possibility that this could be any of us."

I try to find compassion, both for the blogger and for her projection. Clearly something about my story must have personally triggered her, and I bet I know what it is. One of the dirty little secrets of human nature is that, while on the surface most of us are charitable or at least consider ourselves to be, subconsciously we judge or in some cases abhor misfortune's victims. This is a form of psychic protection against the very real possibility of our own downward spiral: Blame the person falling off the ladder, not the system that sent them plunging.

I find the blogger on Facebook and block her.

Unrequited

NOVEMBER–DECEMBER 2014

The rest of my first month at *Cafe*, including the Friday after Thanksgiving, I write, shoot, and report one story a day after another, often struggling to make it to after-school pickup by 6 P.M. I also take on freelance work after hours, during lunch, and on the weekends to make ends meet. I shoot CEO and author headshots and bar mitzvahs, dragging my son along to the shoots. ("So boring," he deems them, but he knows this is what we have to do if we want to eat.) I write book reviews and moonlight articles for other magazines. Nevertheless, I am elated with my *Cafe* job itself, despite its daily trials. *"I love my job!"* I tell everyone who asks, because I do, even though my heart's PVCs are back in full force and small red dots called petechiae have started to appear all over my legs and torso, which doctors originally diagnose as leukemia—those are a fun three days—until they finally decide no, the burst blood vessels beneath my skin must be stress- and/or cardiovascular-related, because there's no other medically viable reason for the thin tubes carrying my blood to be bursting and leaking.

After confirming (via a skin biopsy of one of the larger groups of spots on my thigh, which leaves a permanent scar) that I am not suffering from any other form of known disease, I choose to ignore the bleeding

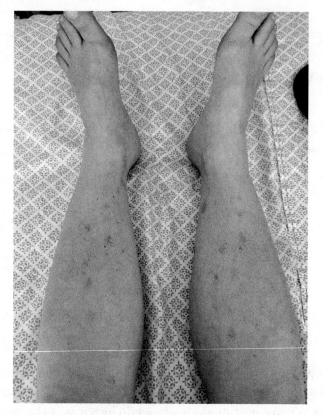

Petechiae, © Deborah Copaken

vessels and soldier on because rent is due, and my spots are more ugly than bothersome. So I visit the set of *Younger* and interview Darren before rushing back to the office to tap out my story. I interview Justin McLeod, the CEO of Hinge, the dating app I used to meet Gio, and I ask him what I consider to be a throwaway question: "Have you ever been in love?" His moving and surprising response will stretch far into the future for both of us, but not yet. I write a story about the role of art in healing pain and about my cousin Jeremy's avoidable death from undiagnosed diabetes and about Bruce Jenner's transition to Caitlyn.

Mostly I've been tasked with writing personal stories, so I write about wearing the black Zara sweater Nora gave me as a protective shield against the sadness of facing my first Thanksgiving, her favorite holiday, as a solo parent. I create a series called A Day in the Life of My Instagram Feed, which is essentially an examination of the differences between the public face we show the world and our private selves. I write about not being able to zip my own up-the-back zipper on the day I'm supposed to meet my ex-husband on neutral ground, to talk about tackling our divorce. I write about the comfort of holding hands in a church with Dan, an old friend from college, at a Roches Christmas concert, both of us reeling from heartache, and what it feels like to be a Jew on Christmas. I write about selling my engagement ring and postmarital app dating and being invisible as a middle-aged woman and having a spouse on the spectrum. I pour all of my pain and shame into my writing, and this daily reckoning with the catastrophe of my life along with my morning walks in Inwood Hill forest saves me. It also, apparently, has begun to save others: "Thank you," strangers write. "I thought I was the only one dealing with ____."

In a few years, *Cafe* will transition into a political site, and nearly every single one of these essays will be erased from the company's servers. This will not pain me as much as I thought it might. I think of it as my sand mandala, blown away with a gust of wind. Writing my way through this period while having adequate health insurance is the point. That it temporarily feeds me and others is the gravy.

Meanwhile Eddie, my *Shutterbabe* pilot co-writer, has been flying in and out of Manhattan for four-day weekends, so we can write the pilot together in the same city. He leaves his wife and son behind in Los Angeles and rents a room at the Standard hotel, with stunning views of downtown Manhattan, to use as our office, and I take off personal days and vacation days from work—I can't afford to go anywhere on vacation anyway—to give us four consecutive days of writing. We work long hours at the desk in his room, with the L-shaped bench around it, then I go home and feed my kids. Mostly my seventeen-year-old daughter takes care of her eight-year-old brother during the daytime hours on these weekends, but when it's college application crunch time for her, my friends Meg and Richard volunteer to watch him at their place.

"This room must be a huge expense every time you come out here," I say to Eddie. It's a nice room. We haven't been paid yet. He's investing a lot of his own money in this project, including round-trip business class tickets. He literally cannot fit his six-foot, seven-inch frame into a coach seat.

Eddie shrugs. Because he was a showrunner on many of the most popular TV shows, which still generate millions in residuals, he doesn't think about the cost of the hotel or expensive meals or really any price of anything for that matter. "I couldn't spend all of my money if I tried," he tells me one day, which feels like an unbridgeable disconnect between us.

I like Eddie. He's slightly arrogant, in the way that many of the boy nerds who landed in Hollywood in the late '80s and early '90s and hit it big in TV comedy tend to be, but he's funny and adept at script structure. Plus he loves photography, so we'll often visit one of the nearby Chelsea galleries on our way back from lunch. Sometimes I get the middle school Spidey-Sense that Eddie *likes* me likes me. That maybe he's telling me about all the money he has and reached out over social media six years earlier not just because he was interested in acquiring the rights to my book but because he was interested in acquiring the rights to me, and now that I'm spouseless, my option's up for renewal.

One day, during our lunch break, he admits that his marriage has been in the toilet for years. I make it clear that I'm in love with Gio, to draw a strict boundary, and though this is a factually correct statement on my end, it is not on Gio's. In fact, my love for the artist has become increasingly unhealthy and one-sided. Unrequited, one might even call it, which is ironically the name of a book that Ron Charles, the editor of the *Washington Post* book section, sends me to review at the darkest moment of my self-abasement. With this new man, I write in the review, I am turning into a woman I no longer recognize. "She was needy, this new version of me, and overbearing. She sent epic texts and indulged in unearned sentiments. This wasn't healthy. For either of us. And at 48, I'm old enough to know better."

Though I have forgiven the needy embarrassment of a woman I became during this moment of scarcity with regard to all things, including love, my romantic obsession with Gio remains, to this day, a nearly bottomless source of self-loathing and shame. But at the time in question it is also fair to say that he kept giving me enough crumbs of hope to keep my heart pining and in a near-perpetual state of arousal.

What happened was this: Our nascent relationship turned physical quickly, but it was nearly impossible to find the time, space, or babysitting dollars to keep it going. Plus Gio has a second home out west, where he often retreats to make his art; a third home out east, where he spends time with his teenage daughter; a fourth home in his new art studio in Brooklyn, and a fifth home in his head, where he feels safest, having been tormented as a child by his father. Any hours we do spend together have to be squeezed out of the tiny sliver of overlap between his time in New York and out of his head, and my time not at the office or taking care of children: in other words, hardly ever.

In fact, the first time I'm able to spend the whole night at his place, instead of rushing home to my son, will turn out to be our last. My breast MRI is scheduled for early the next morning, and Gio's apartment is near the hospital, while mine is more than an hour away by subway and crosstown bus. Moreover, the scan is scheduled for a Saturday morning, and my teenage daughter will be away that weekend visiting colleges, so she can't watch my son.

In my memory, Gio reached out and invited me to stay at his place the night before the MRI, but in retrospect I'm nearly certain I asked, and he conceded. It's also a testament to how desperately I wanted the former to have been true that I can no longer recall the details of the latter.

A grown-up sleepover date on a Friday night, when you have a young son, an old dog, and neither car nor taxi fare, requires the strategic planning and foresight of a requisitions officer. First, I take my hour-long subway commute home from work and pick up my son at aftercare before walking him home and feeding him. After doing the dishes and packing first my son's overnight bag, then my overnight bag, then a bag with the dog's food, I shove the dog himself into a fourth bag, a dog carrier (because all New York City dogs must be contained in a bag on the subway), bundle up my child against the cold, and then crazy bag lady with her four big bags and small boy take the train downtown to my friend Rebecca's, who has agreed to watch the dog. Then my son and I hop back on the subway with our two remaining bags and head farther south to my friend Ariel's, who read my Container Store story and answered my not-meant-to-be-serious closing plea for someone to please babysit my child on the Saturday morning of my MRI with a "Bring him here! I insist!"

I leave my kid with Ariel and her two daughters, none of whom he's ever met but thank goodness for the blithe amenability of third children, and Gio meets me outside in an Uber. I hop in his car, grateful for the ride, and we head farther downtown to his place, a five-story brick building in the countinghouse style.

His interior renovation of this historic landmark, much like his renovation of his historic self, is a whimsical, Willy Wonka–esque marvel of recycled materials mixed with mad scientist genius, with old couches reupholstered in silver, a punching bag that magically descends from the ceiling, and a fireplace that he's constructed out of vintage metal lockers. *This is a man,* I thought, when I first visited his home, *who takes thoughtful care.*

It's after 9 P.M. when we finally arrive at his place, four hours after I left work. I could have traveled to D.C. or Boston during the same time period it took me to first perform then absolve myself of my human and canine responsibilities. In moments like these, I'm jealous of my divorced and separated friends who co-parent with their ex-spouses or have their own parents nearby or money for an overnight sitter. Had I left my office at 5 P.M. and taken the subway straight here, I would have arrived by 5:20 P.M. That's three hours and forty minutes of extra time to relax and commune with an empathic and nice-smelling man. Meanwhile, over on Facebook, photos of my ex-husband's new girlfriend have started to appear in my feed. He's moved into her apartment and is renting out his on Airbnb. They seem to go camping a lot.

Gio places a bunch of soft pillows on the floor in front of the locker fireplace, throws some logs inside its cavity, and starts a fire, in front of which he holds me from behind with my arms tucked inside his, the way I used to swaddle my infants to calm them. "Thank you," I say, still tense from the logistics of getting here but finally melting into the embrace.

"Breathe," he reminds me.

Later, he digs up some dried sage from the vintage apothecary cabinet he's turned into a bedroom storage unit, lights it on fire, then blows out the flames. As the dried leaves start to smoke, he waves the billowing herbs around my body like a conductor with an orchestra of one. It's a protective shield, he claims—half seriously, half tongue-in-cheek—against a breast lump recurrence.

"There," he says, smiling, after a few soothing minutes of my being the sole object of another human's attention. "Now you're safe." He's referring to the alleged protective properties of the sage, but I feel it more on the level of this act of care than as anything having to do with magic herbs. Our more intimate acts that night are equally tender, and as I fall asleep, cradled in his warmth, I once again allow myself to imagine what it might be like to be held like this forever.

The next morning he brings me coffee in bed, and we stand up on tippy toes to gaze out through the window in the eaves, watching the streaks of red and pink fan out behind the Brooklyn Bridge. Then, to calm my nerves before the MRI, I do a little yoga by the bedside.

Gio drinks his second cup of coffee in bed and, smiling, watches my middle-aged skin jello as I attempt to place my right foot against my left knee into a tree pose. I feel no shame over my naked body—I forgot to pack workout clothes—nor over its lack of grace while it struggles to find balance, which is one of the few boons of losing your marriage, your home, your mentor, your industry, your father, your job, your uterus, your calling, your money, your health, your freedom, your friends, and your health insurance all at once: I, you realize whenever you catch your reflection in a storefront window, still exist.

The silly things I once found shameful about my body, beginning in my early teens and stretching onward into adulthood, are all just part of the scaffolding holding up my brain, in which the real me resides. In fact, once I find my balance in the pose, I feel more rooted in the earth than I've felt in decades. I feel seen. Adored. At peace. That pesky organ in the middle of my chest, which has so often been rumbling trainlike with PVCs for the past year, waits instead at a level crossing, calm for once, to the point where I'm not even aware of its pumping nutrients and oxygen to the rest of my body.

"Are you okay going to the hospital by yourself?" says Gio. He mumbles something about a client he's supposed to meet.

"Sure," I say, losing the pose. "Of course." The sturdy tree reverts to flesh and skeleton, feeling the sudden need for a fig leaf. I grab one of Gio's towels. Wrap it around me. Throughout my mercifully short breast lump odyssey, I have always gone to every appointment and needle biopsy and scan and clip placement on my own, so it's not that. It's that he'd previously offered to come with me, and I'd gone ahead and allowed myself to believe in magic. I ask him where I might find the closest 6 train.

"You're not taking the subway to your MRI," he says, ordering me an Uber from his phone. As the car whisks me off to my scan, I choke back tears I find distasteful and weak. I concentrate hard on trying to make them stop. You're strong, I remind myself. You can do this and everything else alone, just like you always have. Why should you even care that Gio doesn't want to do them with you?

Because I do. I care. I care more about this than I can even admit to myself at this moment. Why is it so hard for me to say, "Please, come with me to the hospital. I would really appreciate it," instead of thanking him profusely for the generosity of the Uber and pretending my heart doesn't hurt? Why am I so afraid to admit that, though I *can* do everything on my own, I don't want to? The tears won't stop, hard as I try to force them.

Both the clouds in the sky and those in my head suddenly clear as the car speeds up the FDR Drive: Last night's paradisiacal union, I realize, will be our last. My heart rebels: *No, no, no, you're perfect for each other. He has work. Responsibilities! Cut him some slack. He just needs time to process this burgeoning love and give himself fully to it and you.*

"What are you doing for Christmas?" I'll text him a week later, after trading brief texts over the results of my MRI, which showed that the lump was still gone. First he tells me he's headed to his house out west, then he seems to get annoyed, but I'm not sure, because tone in texts is impossible to decipher.

We're not in the same emotional place right now, he explains digitally, his preferred mode of communication, so I can never gauge the direction, force, or pique of the air behind the floating text bubbles or the depth of the space between our emailed lines. Christmas together? No. This is not what he wants. He needs time to be single after a big breakup with his last long-term girlfriend. He went from a long-term marriage straight into another long-term relationship then into another, without a break between any of them, and he doesn't know who he is anymore by himself.

Fair enough, I think. I understand the need to hit the reset button alone.

He also needs time, he says, to bond with his daughter. He could potentially see the two of us getting back together romantically in a little while, after he's had time to heal from the last rupture, or after his daughter leaves for college in two years, but right now he's not ready for love, just casual dating: something he's never tried but wants to pursue.

I do not want to date casually. I don't even know what that means at our age other than lying to Peter to play with Paul, so for the next few months, though we continue to text now and then and meet up once for breakfast, during which he repeats his desire to date others before maybe getting back together in the distant future, I mourn the loss, hop back on the dating app train, and move on.

The Church for Wayward Hearts

FEBRUARY–MAY 2015

Valentine's Day evening, 2015, I arrive home from a slice of pizza date with my kids to a giant bouquet of magnolias outside my front door. And I mean giant: three feet wide, two feet high, arranged into the shape of a small tree, with a card containing a hand-drawn heart but nothing else. My kids are as perplexed as I. "Maybe Dad sent them?" says my daughter. I text my ex-husband: *Did you send the kids and me flowers?* An immediate text bubble appears with three dots followed by a long pause and then: *No, should I have?* I text my college boyfriend, the one from senior year who never married or had kids. We'd fallen into bed two weeks earlier for old time's sake, both of us quickly regretting it after. Of course. They must be from him: a way of acknowledging the sweet time warp we shared while at the same time accepting we can never be. How kind. The flowers are not from him either, he writes back, but he wishes he'd thought of it, and oh, happy Valentine's Day. Then I notice a clue on the envelope: the phone number of the florist. I call the number and ask if they'd mistakenly forgotten to include another card with actual words on it instead of just a heart. No, says the florist, and, sorry, no, she's not at liberty to divulge the identity of my secret admirer. He's asked to remain anonymous.

I'd redownloaded Tinder and had been on two other app dates: a lovely one with a younger shrink, who lived far away in Kentucky, so oh, well; another with an alleged designer of T-shirts who claimed to be fifty-three on his dating profile, but who, when I arrived at the appointed meeting place at the appointed time, looked to be in his early seventies: my parents' generation, not mine. "You're disappointed, aren't you?" were the first slurred words out of his mouth, after I finally located him nursing what must have been his third or fourth martini.

"Well, yeah," I said. "Because you lied. So that doesn't really start us off on a good footing, now does it?" I didn't take off my coat or sit down. I'd already prepared the perfect escape, in case the date was a bust, in the form of a large industry party to which I'd been invited. Our date was officially over before it even began because of his lie, I told him, but if he still wanted to come to the party as planned, that was fine with me. Maybe he could meet someone more age appropriate there. Still trying to argue the case for why he had to lie—"You wouldn't have swiped right on me!" (*Yes, precisely.*); "I deserve love!" (*We all do, dude, but we also all deserve honesty.*)—he followed me around the corner to the party, and I lost him in the crowd.

When he finally reemerged, an hour or so later, he seemed concerned. "What time are we leaving?" he said.

"We are not going anywhere together," I said. "I told you. There's free booze and food, though, so please, enjoy yourself."

"But I have no place to stay!" he said, grabbing my arm. On his profile, he'd claimed to live in Brooklyn, so I was confused. He explained he'd driven all the way down from his home in Vermont for our date. His son lives in Brooklyn, but his son was mad at him for whatever reason (*Like maybe because you're a pathological liar?*) so now he couldn't stay with his son, as planned, so he was hoping he could stay with me.

Suddenly realizing I was dealing with more of a sociopath than a bad date, I made an excuse to leave the party early and headed for the subway. The man offered to escort me, saying he was heading uptown anyway to try to sleep at an old girlfriend's. "That's okay, I can make it home myself," I said. He followed six steps behind me. "Please stop following me," I snapped. When he later tried to stick his tongue down my throat on the crowded subway car, I ended up shouting to the other passengers, "This man was my Tinder date. I've been trying to get away from him all night, but he has followed me onto this subway and just kissed me against my will. I'm going to get off at the next stop to get away from him, so please make sure he stays on this train and does not follow me again." Thankfully, two men obliged, holding him back as I gave him the slip. I have no idea what happened to him next, but could he have sent the Valentine's flowers? That would mean he somehow figured out my home address. Fuck.

I do a reverse search using the phone number of the florist, click on the Google Maps link next to the name that pops up, and suddenly, with a sigh of relief and a snag in my throat, I understand: They're from Gio. The flower shop is around the corner from his apartment.

I start to tear up, my heart bursting outward like a time-lapse magnolia into blossom. He's back, I think. He's seen the light. He has come to his senses and realized how good we were together. He's not only sent me a heart—his heart—he's filled my home with flowers. So what if he didn't write a card? He's an artist. He uses symbols to communicate.

As a preteen in the mid-1970s, I tore through Nancy Drew mysteries faster than my parents could replenish them. Everything, to Nancy, was a possible clue, like that time she found a witch tree symbol that eventually led her to Pennsylvania Dutch country to hunt down a thief. Or that time she went to the Loire Valley to figure out the mystery of the ninety-nine steps.

Putting on my Nancy Drew hat, I google "magnolia symbolism." I read: "Magnolias symbolized dignity and nobility. In ancient China, magnolias were thought to be the perfect symbols of womanly beauty and gentleness. In the American South, white magnolias are commonly seen in bridal bouquets because the flowers are thought to reflect and emphasize the bride's purity and nobility."

Oh.

I text Gio, thank him for the flowers. He responds with a single red heart emoji. We're back, I think. And it only took a few months of patient waiting. "Do you want to come to a Valentine's party with me tonight?" I text back.

My friend Dan, a professional artist I met in our college photography class, was born on February 14 and has been having a party every year on this date in the scruffy but lovably punk home his friend Jimmy has dubbed "The Church for Wayward Hearts." It's a birthday party, first and foremost, but it's also a refuge for anyone who finds themselves alone on Valentine's Day or just hating it or maybe not in the mood to be bilked by all the candlelit restaurants that jack up their prices every year because they can, simply by stringing up some paper hearts on the walls.

Dan's walls are a graffitied work in progress. If you feel like drawing on them, you can. Gio, I think, will love it.

Gio can't come to the party, he says. He's home sick with a cold. I offer to bring him some chicken soup on my way down to Brooklyn. I make this offer *after* buying the chicken soup, which is a mistake. He doesn't want me to drop by with soup. He's about to go to sleep. If I ring his bell in a half hour, he'll have to get out of bed to answer the door. Ah, right, of course, I think, clutching the still-warm container on the subway.

If you are smarter than I and have already figured out the plot twist to this particular Nancy Drew mystery, yes, another woman is there with him, though it will take me another four months to figure this out on my own. The clue? A radio interview he'll do with her that spring to promote their short-lived design company. When asked to explain their company logo, she'll say to Gio, with a coy giggle, "Okay, this is going to be embarrassing, though . . . I saved a Valentine's card. It was a Valentine's card I gave to you." To which he'll respond flirtatiously, as I cry, "You stole my card back?"

"Chicken soup? Cool!" says Dan, when I bring the container to him instead. I explain its origins: The Mystery Magnolias, Caravaggio's Cold. (Two totally decent, alliterative titles for Nancy Drew books, in retrospect.) Dan says, hmm, that seems a little odd. He's protective of me. Of all of his friends, really. No, I say. He's just sick. No biggie. Dan smiles and gives me a hug. "Welcome to the Church for Wayward Hearts! Wait, I want you to take a photo of Megan and me on the moon." Megan is the winsome, loving actress to whom he's committed himself since the sad Roches Christmas concert when we both bawled. She plays an FBI agent on a network TV show and will give birth to Dan's child a year later, which is the thing he's wanted more than anything since I've known him: to be a father.

She's sitting on the edge of a giant cardboard moon he's set up and illuminated in his otherwise pitch-black photo studio. He sits down on the moon and melts into her. Watching them interact, I suddenly feel

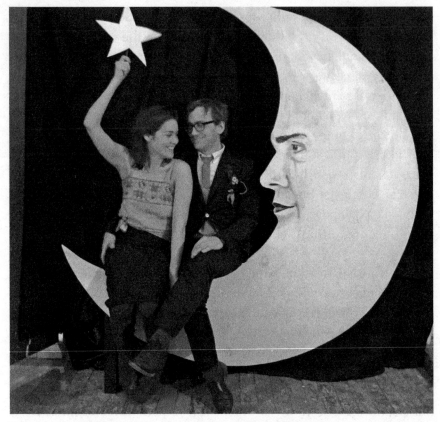

Megan and Dan, February 14, 2015, © Deborah Copaken

like I'm shooting a musical. Or a dream. She's stunning. They're stunning together. It's impossible to take a bad photo of these two, with all the love ricocheting between them. Dan's heart, now full, seems suddenly out of place at his own Church for Wayward Hearts. Soon, he will tear down the whole house to the studs and rebuild his punk playground into a family home.

"You two give me hope," I say, hugging them.

My heart, on the other hand, still feels wayward, on both the health and love fronts. I've been put on a beta-blocker to calm my panic attacks, but by lowering my already low blood pressure, the medication turns me into a fainting machine. Once I stop taking it, the blackouts decrease, but then the palpitations come back. Sometimes they get so intense, I feel as if I'm having a heart attack. As for Gio, I'm . . . confused. A single hand-drawn heart tells me nothing. Magnolias tell me nothing. The Nancy Drew in me is stumped and fresh out of clues.

Does he love me? I ask the Magic 8-Ball I buy for my son in the toy aisle of our local drugstore, but really the ball's for me. $10 to know the future? A bargain. "Ask again later," the ball responds. *Have I reverted to a fifth grader?* "It is decidedly so."

Post magnolias, Gio and I step gingerly back into each other's lives. That is to say we write novela-long emails, argue about inane things as stand-ins for bigger issues, make up, and share a meal now and then. But my assumption of the flowers as lover's olive branch is wrong. "Friends first," he says, drawing a strict boundary, which in his mind means still holding hands when we go out for dinner, spooning in front of his fireplace, fêting me on my birthday with our kids, and giving me both epic foot rubs and the kind of generous gifts you'd give a lover, but the rest, he says, is off the table for now. Which seems like an odd line to draw in the sand with my bare foot in his hands or my back cradled up against the warmth of his stomach, all of which feel equally if not in some ways more intimate to me than the clinical definition of sexual intimacy.

I finally lose it in an email, utterly baffled, after hearing the radio interview with the other woman. Why did he send me those Valentine's flowers if he was with her that night?

He insists he and the other woman are just friends. His plumber and his mom also sent him Valentines, if that helps. Once again, I'm just reading into things and making false assumptions. He sends me a link to a new Emmylou Harris and Rodney Crowell song, "The Traveling Kind," and I comb through its lyrics in search of new clues. *We were born to brave this tilted world, with our hearts laid on the line* . . . Well, yes. That's the only way that love happens. Through vulnerability. Ripping one's chest open. Exposing the contents. For the next week, I listen to the song on autorepeat, mining it for hidden meaning like a moony twelve-year-old. A few weeks later, he sends me a link to "The Lion's Roar," by First Aid Kit, and once again I put on my Nancy Drew hat and sift it for clues: *And I'm a goddamn fool, but then again so are you, and the lion's roar, the lion's roar has me seeking out and searching for you* . . .

"I'm right here!" I shout, when I hear the song for the third time. "You don't need to search!"

Meanwhile, the cockroach situation in my apartment becomes so untenable, I finally go against building rules and call an outside exterminator to deal with the infestation. That night, my son and I walk into a massacre, with thousands of exoskeleton husks crunching underfoot, and a noxious odor so intense, it's impossible to stay inside the apartment. My son screams at the sight of cockroach Antietam. Then he starts to cry. "We can't stay here tonight!" he says. He's right. Even the dog is hovering in the corner of the living room, shaking. It's 6:30 P.M. I can't afford a hotel room. I can't cook us dinner in a kitchen littered with dead roaches on every surface. And I don't have the mental capacity, after a day at work, to deal with this right now.

Gio, whom my son adores, offers to feed and house us when I text him a photo of the stomach-churning husks. He fixes up his guest room for the two of us, and we take the hour-long subway ride downtown to his apartment. "I like it here," my son says, looking around at the whimsical yet cozy bedroom, as I read him a bedtime story. "Does he have roaches?"

"No," I say. "No roaches. Maybe a few mice. But he's getting two cats to deal with that."

"Good," he says. "I like cats." This was spoken as if they might one day be his cats, too. He has asked me, several times, if Gio and I are getting married. Gio's daughter is a sophomore in high school, and he worships her. He has let it be known that he would be open to having her as a stepsister.

I love this young woman as well. One day, after I shoot her portrait, she tells me she's interested in writing, so I suggest she write an essay for me to edit, and I'll see if *The Mid* (the rebranded name for *Cafe*) wants to publish it. Within a few days, she produces a story that does so well on our site, it gets republished by PBS.

Soon thereafter, author, psychotherapist, editor, and fellow single mother Lori Gottlieb reaches out over Facebook to offer me an assignment in Paris during my son's spring break in April. "You up for being my photo assistant . . . in Paris??!!!" I say to my son.

"Oh my god, yes!" he says. Croissants and crepes? His favorite food group.

Gio and his daughter will be in Paris over spring break as well, in a hotel across the Seine from my son and me. We are staying with my friend Marion at her apartment in the tenth, but she works during the day, so Gio and his daughter volunteer to babysit my son on the afternoon I'm scheduled to shoot the Musée de l'érotisme: not the best place to take an eight-year-old, with its six-foot-tall wooden dildos sprouting up from a planter, and vintage porn.

The four of us meet up for lunch at Le Meurice, Alain Ducasse's Versailles-modeled restaurant on the Rue de Rivoli: the kind of place that gives women menus without prices on them, which we all find appalling, but the butter is molded into the shape of a nipple and tastes—oh my god—like heaven, so we suck it down along with our righteous indignation. Plus Gio has insisted on paying, and he'd rather we not know the prices anyway. After the meal, I stand up to take a souvenir photo before heading off to shoot the sex museum, and the three of them suddenly burst out laughing. Apparently, my fly is open. And they have noticed this simultaneously. The stuffy French waiters are none too pleased with our loud American peals of mirth, but the resulting shot of the three of them is as joyful as any family photo I've ever taken.

I am aching, as much as my son, for the family in this photo to be real enough to frame.

Later that spring, I help Caravaggio plant a green roof atop his art studio in a Brooklyn neighborhood that was once designated a Superfund site until cleanup began in 2013, sparking a near total transformation. They even have a Whole Foods now. A gourmet pie shop. Restaurants. Coffee shops. "Beautiful!" he says, when I finish wrapping fairy lights around a discarded toilet I've transformed into a marigold planter. "I love it."

"I love you," I blurt out, looking down at the glowing toilet, my dirt-caked nails, the oasis we've created out of old trash and new blooms.

"Love you, too," he says, after a too-long pause, giving me a platonic squeeze.

It's easy now, in retrospect, as I sit here and catalogue the non-trajectory of this non-relationship, to be ashamed of my part in my own debasement. Not only did I not run, I was the one leading the charge, begging for crumbs. And that's on me. Time spent on Planet Caravaggio felt so magical and hypercharged, my heart kept shushing my brain.

Eventually, however, the truth becomes unavoidable. Even to me, who takes twice as long as most to see it. The public parade of the various other women on his dance card starts to scroll by on social media, that wretched picture book without context, speaking louder than any of Gio's frequent silences between texts. Nearly all of these other women start following me, one by one, on social media, seemingly out of the blue, until I see Gio show up in their feeds and think, oh. Got it. Another one.

As each subsequent photo of him and a new her scrolls by, my chest starts to feel more and more like the hay-filled target in my childhood archery class, after our instructor had shot all six arrows into its center. "You have to ease them out slowly, between two fingers," he said. "Otherwise, the face will tear." It will be years before I manage to slowly yank out all of Gio's arrows from my own hay, and not without significant tearing.

At one point, mid-yank, I notice Gio has started liking all of the photos posted by Maya, my ex-brother-in-law's ex-partner: my former sister-in-law, in other words, with whom I'd shared six years of holidays, family meals, and weekend sleepovers. "How do you know him?" I ask Maya.

She went out on a blind date with him, she says.

"Same," I say, and Maya gasps. *What?!*

"I had no idea, Deb," she says, when we meet up at a lecture at Columbia University a week later, for the paperback launch of Rebecca Solnit's *Men Explain Things to Me.*

"Don't worry! Neither did I." The lights in the lecture hall dim. "Clearly," I whisper, "at least one man explains nothing to any of us." My ex-husband and Maya's ex-partner are identical twins. Neither of us can stop laughing.

Lunch with Ken

JUNE 2015

en Kurson—the editor of the *Observer* who'd originally contacted me in the wake of my viral Container Store story—reaches out at the end of my contract at *Cafe*, as promised, and invites me to lunch to discuss jumping ship and coming to work for him. My basic expenses are still greater than my income, so I'm anxious to hear what terms of employment he has to offer.

At this point, *Cafe* has become *The Mid* (a site specifically geared toward middle-aged women), before purchasing *Scary Mommy*, which already has a large, readymade audience of middle-aged female eyeballs. I'm now on staff at *The Mid* with an at will contract. "At will" means you can be fired at any time, without cause or severance. This is both a uniquely American idiosyncrasy of labor law as well as a highly controversial one. With roots stretching back to an 1884 Tennessee Supreme Court doctrine, "at will" employment puts all of the eggs of the employer/employee relationship into the employer's basket. "The assumption is that the employee is only a supplier of labor who has no legal interest or stake in the enterprise other than the right to be paid for labor performed," writes labor lawyer Clyde W. Summers. "The law, by giving total dominance to the employer, endows the employer with the divine right to rule the working lives of its subject employees."

Conservative American scholars love at will employment. It allows corporations to expand and grow unimpeded by financial responsibility to their employees, which creates more value for shareholders. Legal scholars and economists more sympathetic to human rights and to the dignity of workers, however, see at will contracts exactly for the power imbalance they are: codified modern monarchical masochism, with the corporation as king/sadist and the worker as serf/masochist. "It is employment at will and its fundamental assumption which is the major barrier to establishing a system of collective bargaining," writes Summers. "In American labor law, the monarchy still survives."

Vinit Bharara, the CEO who hired me at *Cafe*, installs Scary Mommy as editor, and the axes begin to fall. First Peter is fired. Then Michelle, our new editor. Both of them have been doing excellent work and did not deserve to be fired, but at will contracts are indifferent to good work.

Scary Mommy makes clear from the moment we meet that she does not like me. Or my writing about the pains, pleasures, and humiliations of both dating and solo motherhood after a long marriage.

I try ingratiating myself with her in the company of some of our co-workers, after all of us ordered boxed lunches from a nearby food truck in Madison Square Park. "I love the Brussels sprouts here!" I say.

"Of course you do," she says with an eye roll.

One day, as I'm biking home from the office, Scary Mommy calls my cellphone, and into my earbuds, as I'm huffing and puffing, delivers the following message: "You know, Deb, everyone here seems to love you, and I'm sure if we got to know one another I would, too, but I have to say: Every time I read one of your stories, I just want to dumb it down and make it shorter. And that doesn't seem like a good place for us to start if we're going to work together."

I want to hop off the bike and have this conversation on the side of the road, but I'm already late to pick up my son at aftercare, so I continue to pedal the rest of the thirteen miles home, panting from both the effort and from mortal fear of losing yet another job. I remind her that nearly all of my online stories have gone viral. And that one of them, "The ABCs of Adulthood," has just sold as a three-book deal to a publisher. Vinit has been happy with my work, I tell her, increasing my salary twice in six months. She reminds me that she's the boss now, and what she says goes: shorter, dumber, or I'm out. Most of her mommy bloggers on *Scary Mommy* write for free anyway. I should feel grateful I'm getting paid at all.

"Get off your bike!" my agent, Lisa, yells at me, when I call her next. "Just sit on a bench and breathe." I'm crying so hard at this point, I can barely see straight.

"I can't!" I yell back, hyperventilating. If anything, I have to pedal twice as fast to get to my son's school by 6.

I choke back the tears and splash my face with the dregs of my office water bottle before I pick up my son. My entire goal and ethos as a parent has always been to be the Not-Scary Mommy. And that means holding it together, as best I can, when I'm falling apart. Not that I always live up to these ambitions—far from it—but I try.

A few days later, I meet Ken Kurson for lunch on an unusual scorcher of a late-spring day, so I'm wearing a sundress to cope with the heat. I squeeze into a crowded banquette. He takes the chair opposite me inside Mercato, a small, cozy Italian joint around the corner from the *Observer*. Almost immediately, our conversation takes a turn for the cringey. "So," he says, "how's the breast? Were you able to finally get that MRI? Is the cancer still gone?" He stares straight at my chest.

This line of questioning is illegal in a job interview, but never mind. The story of mine that prompted this lunch was about the combination of having a breast lump and no health insurance, so I decide to give him a pass. It's understandable, if unfortunate.

I tell him I'm fine and give him the vaguest denouement details of my stage 0 breast lump story, trying to steer the conversation away from my former illness and toward the present job offer, his eyes away from my chest and toward my face.

"Wow," he says, "it's so weird—here we are talking about your story about your breast cancer while I'm staring at your breasts." He cracks himself up, inappropriately.

Every woman has a creepy man meter in the basement of her soul. The questions we ask ourselves, when its dial zooms past ten to trigger the alarm, must be answered both instantaneously and calmly. *Am I in danger?* (No.) *Am I alone with him?* (No, we are surrounded by other diners on either side.) *Is he married?* (Check, wedding ring on the left hand. Not always a good indicator of safety, but sometimes.) *Is he a psychopath or just awkward?* (Just awkward, I think?) *Is the harm he's inflicting with his words or actions intentional or unintentional?* (Unintentional? Again, it's unclear.) *Is this a job interview, a date, or a conversation with a stranger who suddenly appears out of nowhere?* (Job interview.) *Should I remain stonily composed or throw my iced tea in his face?* (It's a toss-up.)

I take a sip of my tea, ignore his new comment, and ask, once again, about his job offer.

After talking about his close relationships with both the *Observer's* owner, Jared Kushner, and their mutual best bud Rudy Giuliani, he asks about Vinit; about the funding for the website; about Vinit's brother, Preet, the U.S. Attorney for the Southern District of New York; about proprietary information about the company I don't feel comfortable sharing because not only do I not know enough to speak with any authority on any of this, it's not relevant to our discussion. So I tell him instead about Scary Mommy's comment about dumbing down my writing and making it shorter, about the Brussels sprouts eye roll, about how she doesn't seem to like me no matter how hard I try. That's why I agreed to meet with him today, I remind him: to talk seriously about his job offer.

"Is she fat?" he says. He grew up fat, he says, so he knows all about what it's like to hate thin people, so it could just be that: Of course a thin person would love Brussels sprouts. Or maybe she actually has a shitty marriage, he says, and the fact that I escaped mine could feel like an affront to her. People in bad marriages have to hate those who escape their own. It's practically a rule. He wants to know what it's really like dating after a long marriage, not just the stuff I write about. His wife hates him right now and has told him she wants a divorce, but he doesn't want a divorce, so they're trying to work it out, you know, although he thinks the whole postmarital dating thing might be fun, is it?

I don't want to answer any of these inappropriate questions or talk about deeply personal stuff with my potential new boss, so I once again try to steer the conversation toward the reason we're here: his job offer.

Oh, right, he says, he can offer me $65,000 a year to jump ship and join the *Observer*. I tell him I'm earning more than this at my current job, and he says, yeah, but that place might fold any day, and I'm offering you a permanent job at a legacy publication. I tell him I'd like to think about the numbers and get back to him.

A week later, Vinit calls me into his office: Scary Mommy isn't happy with my writing. It's nothing personal. She just wants me to—

"Dumb it down and make it shorter," I say, cutting him off. "I know, she told me."

Vinit looks as pained to have to impart this information to me as I feel pained to hear it, so I admit I'm being courted by the *Observer*, and he looks relieved not to have to fire me. Just give me a week or so to figure out the details, I tell him, and I'll leave of my own accord.

I send Ken an email saying I would like to accept his job offer at $65,000 a year, which is $27,000 less than I'm earning now, but at least it's better than my original $39,000 a year offer at *Cafe*, which was $73,816 less than what MIT's economists determined is a living wage for a solo mother of three in New York. And it's not zero, which is where I'm heading if I don't land a new job. Next time a smiling, over-pancaked newscaster waxes rhapsodic over robust employment numbers, please think about the delta between a living wage and the working poor, and remember everyone's lying. Employment numbers tell us nothing. Being employed in the U.S. rarely translates into being able to pay one's bills.

Ken responds immediately to my email. I'm relieved by this alacrity until I open his message. "I'm not even sure there IS an offer!" he writes back. Uh-oh. "I am a slow mover. I have never edited you and I don't know how you'd fit in here yet. I know you can write like a bastard, and I can see that your work ethic is positively amish [*sic*]. But I would need to know you better before making an offer. That said, somewhere in the 62,5 range and if I changed Pizza Tuesday to Alpo Tuesday, maybe 65. Benefits are good though."

I read the email several times. "Know you better"? How is this relevant to my work? Isn't that why he reached out: my work? I write back to remind him that he did, in fact, offer me $65,000 a year over lunch, after writing me six months earlier to say he loved my writing and wanted me to work for him.

Ken sends another confusing email back which says, "I'd have to work with you a bit first—edit a story or two and discuss story ideas."

I stand up from my desk and head toward the office kitchen in search of a glass of water, but my heart is doing its beat-skipping thing again as I stand up, and the oxygen can't reach my brain, and suddenly the curtains fall over my eyes and the chatter of my co-workers slides into a silent echo and my fall is broken by the edge of the kitchen table as it smacks against my forehead. Bill, the angel editor who fought to hire me, rushes over with ice. Embarrassed, I explain it's no big deal, I'm just a fainter, I'll be fine. I rashly insist on riding my bike home, instead of leaving it locked up outside the office, and I faint again ten blocks later while waiting at a red light, so now the bike's on top of me, I'm bleeding profusely, and I'm blocking traffic.

I stand up, brush myself off, lock my bike to the nearest pole, hobble down the subway stairs, and ride north in an actual subway seat because when the other passengers see me boarding the crowded car, they gasp and clear a path. A good Samaritan hands me tissues and a wet wipe for my bleeding forehead and bloody knee and urges me to go immediately to the emergency room.

"I will," I lie. "I promise." I'm not in the mood to explain anything about my broken life right now.

It will take another two years and dozens more fainting spells for me to finally seek out a diagnosis for my "beat-skipping thing." The cardiologist will diagnose premature ventricular contractions (PVCs)—so that's what they're called, huh?—as well as orthostatic hypotension after I faint during a tilt-table test within the first thirty seconds of being tilted. Orthostatic hypotension is defined as a rapid decrease in either systolic or diastolic blood pressure within three minutes of standing up from a sitting or supine position. When I stand up too fast, I faint. If my body's reacting to extreme stress, I faint. The cardiologist will put me on a Holter monitor for a month, to gauge the percentage of skipped heartbeats to regular ones. I'll have to wear the complicated contraption 24/7 except when I shower, which is totally fun when you're a middle-aged woman on the app dating circuit. When one of my Tinder correspondents sends me a naked selfie, and he asks me for the same in response, I'll shrug, set up the self-timer, and send him this (see opposite page):

He'll never write back.

The human heart beats 100,000 times in a single day. According to the results of my month-long Holter monitoring, my PVCs are interfering with approximately 16,000 of those heartbeats, which is on the cusp of too high. At 20,000 PVCs a day, the heart is at risk of damage and failure. My cardiologist will warn me that if we can't get my extra heart-

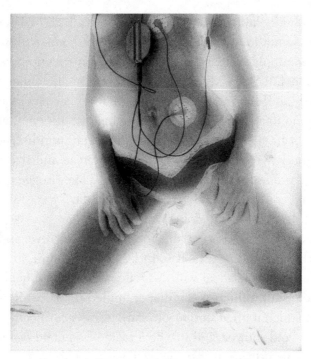

Self-portrait with Holter monitor, © Deborah Copaken

beats under control, a pacemaker might have to be installed. We try a
bunch of drugs to get my heart to comply. None of them work. A couple
of them make me feel worse than taking no drugs, plus they mess with
my ability to concentrate at work, which subsequently increases my
stress and the frequency of the PVCs. You know what finally makes my
PVCs disappear? A livable wage plus reciprocal love, both of which are
still far off in the future.

I go back to Vinit with my tail between my petechiae-spotted, bandaged legs. Please, I say. I'll write shorter and dumber. I'll do anything to
keep my job. But Scary Mommy, he says, is firm. This is her team now,
she doesn't want me on it, and he has to allow her the independence to
make her own choices as the newly installed editor. And no, he's sorry,
as per my at will contract, I will not be getting severance.

"But I put us on the map!" I'm now ugly begging on top of ugly crying. "Please! Just give me a little time to search for a new job."

The two of us are sitting in one of the two rooms with doors that shut
in the open-plan office, but this closed conference room also has a giant

windowed wall looking out over the rest of the staff, all of whom are trying to pretend not to watch a grown woman cry. Vinit, with whom I've had nothing but pleasant and even meaningful interactions, seems visibly upset, too, but Scary Mommy has fired most of the old guard at this point already, and I'm one of the last of the original soldiers still standing. Seven months! That's how long we've been at this euphoric experiment in utopian, anything-goes publishing: seven months. And we did well. Gloriously well, in fact. Our stories were read and shared widely, without paid promotion. They made headlines. They forged friendships. They sparked community, conversation. Every day I went to work, I felt good about showing up and doing my job.

"I'm so sorry," says Vinit, unable to look me in the eye, and all I can think, uncharitably, is that he'll soon be heading home to an already cooked, well-balanced meal with his wife and private-school-educated kids, in their multimillion-dollar diaper-funded home, while I'm heading home to uncontained shit: roaches, mold, geysers of bathtub sludge, live wires, a cold shower, and maybe a plate of rice and beans the kids and I will share, if I can muster the energy to cook it.

Oh, but wait. Doh. I forgot. My daughter is going out. And I have a date tonight. And a sitter, whom I can no longer afford now that I'm no longer employed, is already on her way to my apartment to watch my son until 9:00 P.M. I check my watch. I'm already running late. Red-eyed and trying to hold it together, I leave the conference room and grab my computer. Place it in my bag.

Whelp. I guess that's it. We had a good run here, my trusty old MacBook and me.

One of the advantages of working in an open-plan office is that you haven't had your own desk in which to shove and store random shit as the months accumulate, so when you get fired, you have no desk to clean out. Leaving means simply walking out the door, with your water bottle, computer, and whatever shreds of dignity you still have left intact. On the far wall, by the exit, Abraham Lincoln speaks his quiet wisdom in hand-painted letters, under which I'd set up and shot *Cafe's* first self-timer group photo just six months earlier.

"The written word may be man's greatest invention," it says. "It allows us to converse with the dead, the absent, and the unborn." Yes, Abe, I think. You're right. Thank you for reminding me from the grave. I

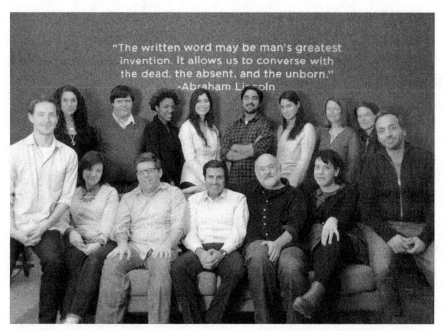

"The written word may be man's greatest invention. It allows us to converse with the dead, the absent, and the unborn."
-Abraham Lincoln

The original staff of *Cafe,* 2014, © Deborah Copaken

wonder, with a quick chuckle-turned-sigh, how Scary Mommy might edit this down for optimal SEO traffic. *The written word rocks! Yay, language! The top three reasons why writing will make you immortal!*

Melissa, my editor, friend, and ally, who will soon leave *The Mid* to run *Lifehacker* before landing as a Culture and Lifestyle editor at *The New York Times,* follows me out beyond honest Abe's words and stops me in the hallway between the office and the elevator. "What can I do?" she says, giving me one of her signature warm hugs.

"Nothing," I say. "I'll be fine."

Melissa had encouraged me to set up a GoFundMe on my forty-ninth birthday several months earlier, after noticing, with horror, my still-spotted legs. "There's no shame in holding out a hand," she'd said. "You need to pay Sloan Kettering. You need to pay your son's bursar. And you're not earning enough money here to do that. Meanwhile, there are millions of people out there reading and sharing your words, many of whom are entertained enough to write in *every day.* That's *worth* something, Deb. Words have value, even if no one wants to pay us for them. Phrase it that way when you write up the GoFundMe, like, 'Hey, guys, thanks for reading and sharing all of my stories of postmarital insanity on social media, really appreciate it, but for my birthday this year I'm going to ask you to chip in for reading them.' Go full Amanda Palmer. People will understand." (In two years, a new company called Substack, a subscription-based newsletter platform, will make this their business model for journalists seeking actual payment for their work instead of pennies: "We believe that journalistic content has intrinsic value," they'll write in their mission statement, "and that it doesn't have to be given away for free.")

Melissa had been both right and wrong. Many of my friends had understood and donated what they could. One of them—Ariel, who'd also watched my little one during the night I spent at Gio's before my MRI—showed up at my office on my birthday with a cupcake, a lit candle, and a small box containing several crisp one-hundred-dollar bills. "Do not pay me back, ever," she said, handing them to me. Abby, always my champion, kicked in a typically generous gift as well after throwing me a surprise birthday lunch. Nicole, an old friend from high school, offered not only financial help but a place to stay in Evanston whenever I wanted to visit my son at college. A stranger, Tony—one of the then-coaches of the UC Berkeley football team, who'd bought a copy of *Shutterbabe* for each of his three daughters and had friended me on Facebook—had sent a check to my apartment for $1,000, along with a letter of praise and empathy, saying others had been kind to him when he was down on his luck, and now it was his turn to pay it forward.

Others would be less generous. A journalist I'd met once at a party wrote a story for *The New York Times* mocking my GoFundMe and others' over her "sneaking suspicion that someone of considerable (or at least ample) means and/or connections is asking for help." When she messaged me for a quote, I begged her to keep me out of her story—why not write about the underlying economic conditions creating this surge in tin cups held out by white-collar workers and single mothers in America rather than shaming the cup-shakers?—but she wrote about me and my cup anyway, albeit without attribution.

Another woman stopped my literary agent after their $36-a-pop Soul-Cycle class to lend her opinion. "Now that Deb has a book deal," she said, "maybe she should take down her GoFundMe." That book deal, for *The ABCs of Adulthood*—a thin graduation gift book with photographs—was worth $20,000, which then had to be split evenly between my co-creator and me before being divided further by Uncle Sam, who'd take 30 percent, and my agent, who'd take 15 percent. In other words, I would net around $5,000 (or the equivalent of 138 SoulCycle classes) for that book, give or take. The woman who said this—and many of our mutual friends, she insisted—thought holding out my hand was unseemly and wrong, which a large shame-filled part of me obviously thought, too, but I also felt cornered into choosing between two wrongs: 1) Don't ask for help/don't pay MRI co-pays, medical bills, and my son's college tuition; or 2) Do ask for help/do pay the medical bills and my son's college tuition. Worse, this warning had come from a woman whom I considered to be a good friend. I'd even blurbed her last book.

I'd actually loved this woman's book, unequivocally, and wanted to give it whatever boost I could. Short and sweet, it was sad, hopeful, and inspirational in equal measure, but also funny and charming about the indignities of a failed marriage, after which she quickly got divorced, found a new spouse, and lived happily ever after: a real-life divorce fairy tale. The sad irony is that her words in that book had given me hope, back when I was still in the throes of figuring out how to leave my own marriage, that I, too, could have a second shot at life and love. And that all of the struggles in between might be madcap and slapstick, but the time period would be short, and the logistics would be manageable.

This does not feel short. Or manageable. It's been nearly two years since my separation, with no denouement or divorce papers in sight. And though I try to laugh and put on a good face for my kids and friends, mostly I feel lonely, scared, and stressed-out all the time.

"What about the job at the *Observer*?" says Melissa. "Your lunch with Ken Kurson."

"It's complicated," I say. "There was a job. Then suddenly there wasn't a job." I press the elevator button. "Sorry, I gotta run. Unfortunately, I planned a blind date for tonight."

"Oh, no! Of all nights."

"Oh, yes." I laugh. "How bad do I look?"

"You look fine."

"I look like I have pink eye."

"No," she says, holding my shoulders, looking me straight in my swollen eyes. "You look beautiful and strong. You've got this."

She's lying, I know, but I appreciate her conviction. "I'm going to miss you," I say, hugging her once more, almost clinging to her generous embrace. "Oh, god." I pull away. "What should I tell my date when he asks what I do for a living? 'Well, Jonathan, up until about thirty minutes ago, I used to converse with the dead, the absent, and the unborn. Now I do fuck all. You?'"

Melissa cracks up. I crack up. A full-throttled, almost crazy belly laugh. It feels good to laugh, even if there's still a plaintive wail underneath.

I wave goodbye to the woman with whom I've spent nearly every hour of my waking life these past seven months. "I love you!" I shout as the elevator doors shut. My heart skips several beats—ba boom, ba ba boom, boom, boom-ba-boom—my laughter reverts to tears, and I descend.

PART V

CERVIX

2015–2017

TWENTY-TWO

Kind of a Tinder Date
and Kind of Not

JUNE 2015

Sorry I'm late," I say. "I think I just got fired."

My blind date with Jonathan, the Hollywood screenwriter, is off to a smashing start. Picture a sweaty woman with humidity-frizzed hair who's just walked the twenty-four blocks between the Flatiron office she loved, but will never see again, to the appointed East Village restaurant, Prune, which, post-cry, is what her face looks like. She walked, even though Google Maps said this would make her eleven minutes late, both to save the subway fare, now that she suddenly no longer has an income, and to clear her head. Her red polka-dotted skirt has a small stain on it from her last app date, but only if you look closely. She'd considered canceling at the last minute, after catching a glimpse of her swollen eyes in a clothing shop window, but her date was already at the restaurant, the babysitter had already arrived at her apartment, and it would have been rude to cancel on both of them five minutes after the appointed time.

"You *think* you got fired . . . or you got fired?" He's thin and compact, my date, with a downturned mouth, dark eyes, unremarkable features, and gray, curly hair. Yet somehow when it's all put together, it works well, like a room in an Ikea catalogue.

I try to explain, but it sounds insane, so I deflect and ask him about him. He tells me about the films he's written. I'm both impressed—they are well-known, top-grossing films—and unable to respond graciously, as I've seen none of them and don't want to lie and pretend I have. "Cool," I say, followed by a long, uncomfortable pause where appropriate praise should have been.

Our date is kind of a Tinder date and kind of not. I've been set up by Jonathan's friend, with whom I matched on Tinder but have never met because the friend lives in L.A., and he happened to match with me during the few hours during which the app's location services pegged him in New York. If you think this is a crazy basis for meeting a decent single man in my age range—the friend of a Tinder match you've never met— you are not nor have you ever been a lonely middle-aged woman, relegated by society to invisibility.

We are not, suffice it to say, invisible. We are flesh, and we have needs. In fact, I believe it's crucial to talk openly and honestly about both the joys and horrors of casual sex in middle age, in the same way I once felt it was important to talk about both the joys and horrors of casual sex in the lives of twentysomethings and war correspondents. The subtitle of my first book was "Adventures in Love and War," and I meant it. At the same time, I have a strong and I hope understandable desire not to be publicly slut-shamed again. And yet to tell an honest human story without admitting the messy truths of who we are behind closed doors feels both false and willfully evasive.

Eros and Thanatos—love and aggression—are the two opposing forces that drive all of our narrative arcs, but one cannot write openly about the former, as a woman, without triggering the knives of the latter. These slut-shaming knives are wielded, I was both surprised and also not surprised to learn, not by men but rather by other women, many of whom self-identify as feminists.

Why? It's a question I've often asked myself, over the course of these post-adolescent decades, and the obvious answer I've been able to come up with is this: One of the more destructive by-products of sexism is that, given the impossible choice between madonna and whore, some women will reject the absurdity of this binary duality by projecting their anger over it onto other women and subconsciously judging them by the same patriarchal standards.

In other words, your basic garden-variety internalized oppression.

But there seemed to be more at play—and social science now backs me up—with the vitriol levied at women by other women. "Women's participation in slut shaming," writes sociologist Elizabeth Armstrong, "is often viewed as internalized oppression: they apply disadvantageous sexual double standards established by men. This perspective grants women little agency and neglects their simultaneous location in other social structures." Specifically, Amstrong and her co-authors argue, they are "unconvinced that women would engage so enthusiastically in slut discourse with nothing to gain."

So what *does* a woman have to gain by slut-shaming another woman? According to their study, two things: class advantage and status. "High-status women employ slut discourse to assert class advantage, defining their styles of femininity and approaches to sexuality as classy rather than trashy."

I apply this sociological theory to the slut-shaming I've both witnessed and experienced over the course of my life, and, yep. Fits like a dainty white glove.

My conversation with Jonathan, after its rough start, begins to flow with ease. We realize we know people in common. He's recently relocated to New York after decades in L.A. and waxes rhapsodic over what it means to be able to walk everywhere instead of getting into a car each time you want to visit a friend, the grocery store, a movie theater. I listen to the story of his divorce, which he recites without rancor. This is an unusual and welcome break from the men who mercilessly savage their ex-wives, like the man who also disparaged, over the course of our one hour together, a hotel I'd just said I liked (*Third-rate*); the last man I'd dated (*Poofter*); and the restaurant in which I thought we were enjoying a delicious meal (*Terrible service*).

Jonathan also reveals that he had a postdivorce relationship that just broke up a couple of weeks prior, and he's still quite raw from it. He speaks glowingly of his kids. He's courteous to the server. He listens well and doesn't interrupt.

After coffee and dessert, he asks where I'm heading. The D train stop at Broadway–Lafayette, I tell him. That's right near his apartment, he says. We should walk there together.

This is the part of the date I always find the most confusing, even at—no, *especially* at—my age. Is he asking me up to his apartment? Or is he just being polite and offering to walk me to the subway? Do I want to have sex with him, if he asks me upstairs? The answer to this question often depends on my attraction to the man as well as to how many months it's been since I've been touched by anyone. More than three months? Sure, why not? Less than a month, I'm a little pickier.

My most recent app date had been with a tiny but dazzling Italian musician, whom I met on a Friday night at a bar around the corner from my apartment at 10 P.M., an hour when I often do my grocery shopping after my son falls asleep. I'd recently called the local precinct, to ask if it was legal to leave a sleeping eight-year-old in his room while I went out around the corner to buy milk and eggs, and the officer who answered the phone said, "Look, I was raised by a single mother. You do what you gotta do in the hours you gotta do it. Kids these days have cellphones. And he'll get pissed if he doesn't have milk in his cereal tomorrow morning."

After a quick beer, the musician and I made our way to a bench in Inwood Hill Park, across the street from my apartment, where we engaged in what my mother's generation would call "heavy petting." Apt, because I have fully become a 1950s teenager, only without the local drive-in, lookout point, or Thunderbird for privacy. Butting up against the limits of public decency, we took the equally teenage risk of tiptoeing into my apartment, sneaking into my room, and making out for another hour behind a locked door before I made him tiptoe back out into the night around midnight, because, to paraphrase the nice cop, Mama's gotta do what she's gotta do in the hours she's gotta do it.

The next night, as I was heating up spaghetti sauce for dinner while my son was busy doing his homework at the kitchen table, the musician's first name followed by "From Tinder" where his last name should have been flashed across the screen of my iPhone.

"From Tinder" has become a growing family name in my contact list, not to be confused with "From Bumble" or "From Hinge," like the way Europeans often have last names with a *de* followed by their region of origin.

I put down my spoon and picked up the phone. The Italian thanked me for a wonderful time. "What are you doing right now?" he said. His accent was thick.

"Stirring tomato sauce and boiling pasta."

"In honor of me?"

No, in honor of the gods of Whatever's in the Pantry. "Sure." I laughed. "In honor of you."

"So . . ." He paused. "I have an important question of you." *Of you.* I love it when foreigners insert their own grammatical peculiarities into English.

I turned the heat down to simmer, gave the pasta a quick stir. "Okay, shoot. What's the question?"

He got right to the point. "Are you into threesomes?"

I froze. I was not about to talk dirty while preparing dinner in front of my kid, but I was also curious: I'd never had a threesome. Maybe that would be fun? But how to make my response to his question G-rated and anodyne? "That depends," I said. "Will the team you're trying to build for this particular project consist of two men and a woman or two women and a man? The former would probably be the better way to achieve your objectives and goals."

"Two women and a man?" he said, but in the next breath he was giving me the task of finding us the other woman. "How quickly do you think you can find her? By next week?" Suffice it to say, nothing is less sexy to a mother than being asked to add one more line item to her to-do list: Order more laundry detergent, answer work emails, sign the permission slip, locate succulent for son's school project, run the bath, walk the dog, take out trash, straighten the toys, *and* find a willing and sexually available woman for a threesome with the man I just met last night on Tinder? No. No, thank you. I'll take a pass. Unless she can show up with Tide pods and a cactus.

"Sorry," I said, "I'm a little too busy right now to take on a new project." I hung up.

"Who was that?" said my son.

"Just this guy I know who needed an extra person on his team."

"You didn't want to be on his team?"

"Nah. I would have had to do all the work."

His new school was really into group projects. He knew all about what it was like to have to pull the weight for the others. "I hate when that happens."

A few days later, I was sent a reminder text, also while I was cooking dinner: "Before the end of the universe I would love another time in my life to have the privilege to share a bed with two smart and sexually vibrant women. ☺ I know it's a lot to ask to the world. Just sharing with a smart woman. Hope you are doing well."

Once again, I politely declined his offer to help find another woman for a threesome. He was not asking it *to* the world. He was asking it *of* me. I still get the occasional mass email about his performances, but otherwise that was our final communication.

Several celibate weeks passed. How many? Let's see: There were buds on the trees in the park where the Italian and I made out, so it was early spring. Now, as we approach the screenwriter's building, it's hot, nearly summer. Meaning it's been at least a month or two since anyone but my mirror has seen me unclothed, so I'm leaning toward going upstairs, if it's offered. Even though this hasn't exactly been a love connection. But there are other issues to consider. The screenwriter seems deeply sad from his recent breakup. I'm both sad and panicked from my job loss. So the timing of this otherwise semi-promising date is completely off. It's also late, and I'm tired. My ex is still living in California, and sex after work can add on another $40–$60 to my babysitting costs, plus I can never sleep over, so then the question becomes truly mercenary: Is this man's touch tonight worth an extra $40 in babysitting or should I save it for lightbulbs?

Yes, lightbulbs. The wiring in my apartment is so old and jerry-rigged, that my lightbulbs—particularly those in the two kitchen ceiling fixtures, the ones with the live wires that frequently shock me—burn out faster than I can replace them. Even the new LED ones, which are supposed to last forever, burn out after only a few weeks. I'm nearly always standing on a ladder after work, replacing at least one of them, or ordering a steady supply of replacements online.

"I'd invite you up, but my daughter's in the apartment," says Jonathan.

"Of course, no worries. I have to get home and let the sitter go anyway."

"Oh, god," he says with a sympathetic eye roll. "I remember those days." His children are around the same ages as my older two. "Must be hard trying to date with such a young one." (Translation: *I'm not sure I'm up for dating a woman with such a young kid.*)

"Yeah," I say, but only because the truth is too complicated to explain. Yes, my postmarital dating life would be much easier and less expensive if I hadn't had a third child nine and eleven years after his siblings. No question. But the everyday exigencies of caring for my little boy; of coming home from work to his guileless hugs, his moon cheeks and stories; of watching him sleep as an antidote to hopelessness: This is my life raft. *Our* life raft. We may not be able to see the shore, but we bob along together, buoyed by love.

Anyway, that's that. I don't have to choose between sex and lightbulbs tonight after all. Maybe sex wasn't even on the table, who knows? Maybe he took my distracted lack of presence during the date as a lack of interest in general. Maybe he's physically repulsed by me or simply not attracted. Maybe he believes there must be something wrong with me if I got fired. Maybe my young kid is a nonstarter. It's so hard to read between the lines when it's been a quarter century since you've had to deconstruct them. I seem to always live in the dark these days, both literally and figuratively.

"Thanks for dinner," I say. "It was nice talking to a grown-up." Ugh, what a weird thing to say! *It was nice talking to a grown-up?* I talk to grown-ups every day at work. Or rather . . . I did. As of two hours ago. Now what? Jonathan and I will make a few halfhearted attempts to get together again, but the timing will never work out.

"How do you do it?" my friends ask. "How do you keep going on these dates that go nowhere, week after week, without losing your mind?"

"Easy," I say. "With zero expectations that any of them will go anywhere." In fact, I explain, to keep my sanity, I've begun to treat every date like a journalism assignment. Though my first app date with Gio went unusually well, I've since learned that going into any app date hoping love will blossom is like taking a pickaxe to pyrite and expecting gold. The trick is not only to anticipate the fool's gold but to appreciate the luster and heft of each nugget. Then each date becomes an opportunity to bear witness both to the refraction of someone else's light and to the weight of their burdens.

How do they weave their own particular narrative? What do they emphasize, and what do they leave out? Are they as forthcoming with their own missteps and failures as they are with their successes, or is every defeat the fault of another? So much can be learned from asking the simplest questions: Where did you grow up? What was your relationship with your parents like and how is it now? Do you have siblings? Are you close to them? If you could snap your fingers right now and do anything else or be living anywhere else, what and where would that be? What's keeping you from making that change and why?

My married friends like to help me swipe, which is fine by me, as I find that part of dating as tedious and soul-sucking as they find it titillating, but otherwise I refuse to swipe in public. It feels like a private act, meant for bathroom breaks or while spacing out on the couch after a child's bedtime. One time, bored, I started swiping while in line for coffee, but when I happened to catch the eyes of the woman behind me, staring at my screen, it felt akin to having been caught masturbating in public.

I think of my hour or so of nightly swiping before falling asleep as a job but with different goals: love, not money; companionship, not collegiality; relaxation, not industriousness. Swipe! I pretend I'm a casting agent, searching the slush pile. Swipe! A college admissions officer, filling a class. Swipe! An overpaid TV host, deciding who gets the golden buzzer. Swipe, swipe, swipe, swipe! Love's in there, somewhere, I think, watching the dominoes falling off the screen one by one.

I'm not looking for nor do I believe in the concept of a *bashert*, which is the word Jews use to describe that one perfect soul mate, out there in the ether, just waiting for me to find him and only him. But I do believe in the ability of dating apps to facilitate the search for a decent romantic partner who can one day grow into a mate for my soul, and I believe in the existence of multiple decent romantic partners for each of us seeking co-pilots, which is what I want: a best friend who smells good, has acceptable hygiene, makes my heart thump when I look at him, likes to have sex, loves me with the same combination of ferocity and gentleness as I love him, and treats me, as I treat him, with reverence, kindness, and empathy.

Rare, I know, and perhaps a MacGuffin in the still-unfolding narrative of my life, but I have to keep believing romantic love is possible. That this millstone of loneliness might one day be lifted. Even my ridiculously long computer password, during this period, bears the deadweight of my conditional tense concerns followed by my age: "WhatifLovewerereal?49."

An American "epidemic of loneliness," it's being called, in research papers, the press, even on an official U.S. government website. Two in five Americans are unhappy with the relationships they do have. One in five Americans feels lonely and socially isolated. Loneliness, these researchers warn, is as lethal as smoking fifteen cigarettes a day; can lead to suicide, Alzheimer's disease, and other dementias; messes with our immune and cardiovascular systems, and more. Loneliness, in other words, is killing us.

So every night, like a bedtime prayer, I open my apps and swipe.

TWENTY-THREE

Durkheim

JUNE–OCTOBER 2015

One night, I swipe right on (let's call him) Durkheim, a ruggedly handsome, fifty-something sociology professor from coastal New Hampshire who's a dead ringer for Steve McQueen. "It's a match!" the screen tells me as the covalent bond of our encircled faces draws together. I feel that dopamine rush familiar to every retiree feeding quarters into a Vegas slot machine who suddenly sees a row of three sevens and hears the crash of metal below. I text a photo of Durkheim to my friend Soman, who's gay, for his expert opinion. "Hot," he writes back, although he's a little concerned that my potential paramour has a close-up of himself surfing, which means he had to go to the trouble to make this photo happen, so like how does that work and what does that say about him? I ignore Soman's misgivings. If I had a face and body like that and could surf, I'd probably go to the trouble of attaching a GoPro to my surfboard, too.

I start a chat with Durkheim. He's in New York helping his mother take care of his stepfather, who's being treated for cancer at Sloan Kettering. "No way," says Soman. "An actual good Samaritan?"

"Way," I say.

"Okay, okay, go for it. What do I know?"

Our first date goes well: a 7 A.M. Sunday stroll through Inwood forest with my dog followed by takeout coffee and blueberry muffins on a park bench overlooking C Rock: the Bronx high cliff onto which Columbia students have painted a giant C, and off of which adolescents jump into the Harlem River and adulthood. We discuss his failed marriage. His regret over not having kids. The sociology of suicide, his lifelong area of interest. Because my son always sleeps late on the weekends, and I always take the dog on a long walk before he wakes up, I can relax into this conversation and really listen.

"I'm grateful you were game to get up so early," I say.

"I figured I'd try to make it as easy on you as possible. Must be hard dating as a single mother."

I laugh. "What, you mean other women on Tinder aren't inviting you to 7 A.M. dog walks?"

He laughs. "What are you doing tomorrow night?" he asks, which never happens at the end of a first date. The unwritten Tinder rule seems to be, in my limited experience, to play it cool and make your date wait a few days for a follow-up text.

I tell him I'm sorry, but I can't go out with him the following night, as I'm scheduled to perform live storytelling. He asks if he can get an extra ticket to the show. Sure! I say, I can even get him a comp, and he can join us for the dinner I've planned prior, with friends who will also be coming to the show: my new pal Justin, the CEO of the dating app Hinge, whom I interviewed for *Cafe*; and Kate, his long-lost girlfriend with whom he'd recently reunited. "Just keep it on the down-low that we met on Tinder instead of Hinge," I laugh.

"Promise," says Durkheim.

Justin had flown across the Atlantic to declare his love for Kate after I'd urged him, during our interview for *Cafe*, to do so. Or rather, I'd asked him that throwaway question at the end of our interview—"Have you ever been in love?"—and this turned into an off-the-record, tearful truth session. For both of us. I recounted my missed connection with the man I thought had stood me up in Paris but hadn't; he told me about losing Kate to his youthful addictions and immaturity. I urged him to act, before it was too late.

Justin, like the star of his own real life rom-com, had arrived in Switzerland to declare his love for Kate one month before she would have married another man. Now Justin and Kate were living together. And Ken Kurson—the *Observer* editor who'd reneged on his full-time job offer but had given me, as a consolation, a $600-a-pop freelance column—was sending me emails and calling me on the phone to say if I could write a feature story about the dating app CEO who found love the old-fashioned way, he'd splash those lovebirds across the front page. "And hire me full-time, like you said?" I said.

"Sure, maybe."

Fuck his *maybe*, I thought.

With my lease on the roach-infested apartment now up for renewal, I've been toying with the idea of moving to the surrounding suburbs or even exurbs, but the rents there are just as onerous if not more so than mine, and the added commute, if I move far enough away to make a difference in my monthly nut, would mean I'll never see my child, never mind the added babysitting costs and new costs: gas and car payments. Plus my son loves his school and hates upheaval. But the real issue is that Freedom Debt Relief—one of those money-grubbing debt consolidation companies—has destroyed my credit, so no one will sell or lease me a car or a home anyway, not that I even have a down payment for either.

The Freedom Debt Relief flyer had arrived in my mailbox, promising a step-by-step path out of debt with their friendly support staff and help. Stupidly, I was a sucker for this pitch and believed them. In three years, Freedom Debt Relief will be sued by the Consumer Financial Protection Bureau (CFPB) for illegally charging people in advance for debt-relief services; for charging debtors without actually settling our debts; for hiding the fact that many of the leading banks have a standing policy of never working with a debt-settlement company; and for instructing desperate consumers like me to "expressly mislead" creditors when asked if I was enrolled in a debt-settlement program.

Freedom Debt Relief will not admit guilt for any of these illegal and immoral acts. Rather, they will reach a settlement with the CFPB and several affected consumers, not including me, because I will not hear about this lawsuit until well after it has been settled. Instead, for the next six years, $600 will get auto-deducted from my account every month and deposited straight into Freedom Debt Relief's pockets, while my marital credit card debt—whose burden I took on, as a stipulation of our divorce—will balloon from $38,000 to more than $45,000 while it sits there, unsettled and unpaid.

"What do you mean, 'Maybe?'" I said to Kurson. "Haven't I proven my worth already?" My essays for him have done well. He's told me this himself multiple times, and I can see their mushroom proliferation on social media with my own eyes.

"I mean, if you get me the Hinge CEO story, I'll think about it."

I hang up the phone, infuriated. I don't want to hand over a potentially great love story to an editor who promised a job then yanked it away. What kind of mind games is he playing? I'm happy to write the occasional *Observer* column for him, as poorly as it pays, to keep giving my middle-aged voice a professional platform, which could lead to the promised job, but Justin and Kate's story deserves a better publication. Or at least a publication whose editor isn't sending me weird threatening emails if I don't write it for him.

"I consider this the *Observer*'s story," Ken writes in an email on July 1, 2015, "and you know I come from a grudge-holding desert people." Then he adds, peculiarly, "Have a great 4th. Don't go to any touristy terror targets."

"Wait why re: terror spots?" I email back. "What's your insider info?"

He writes back: "On Monday, I emailed Jared [Kushner] to tell him I was hearing chatter from Rudy [Giuliani] friends about how AL Queda [*sic*] and Isis never really cared about American symbolic dates. But homegrown lone wolf sympathizers will." The email goes on and on with his theories, his proof, his paranoia, and his doubts that his intelligence is even true, but, he adds, "All I'm saying is I wouldn't be choosing this weekend to visit, say, the observatory at Empire State Building."

After my first column was published, I'd answered Ken's invitation to visit him at his office to get a hard copy of the paper for free. Not wanting to be alone with him, after his comment during lunch about my breasts, I brought my little one along as a buffer. "Who's this guy we're meeting?" said my son, as we walked into the *Observer* lobby. I'd bribed him with the promise of pizza afterward.

"My new boss," I'd said. "Sort of."

"Why sort of?"

"Because he said he'd hire me full-time and then didn't."

"That's mean!" said my son.

"Yeah," I said. "It wasn't nice." But maybe if he sees you, I think—an actual child who needs to eat—he'll reconsider.

Ken had a turntable in his office, and he kept putting on records to test my nine-year-old's knowledge of 1970s rock. Seeing my son growing more and more uncomfortable, I was trying to figure out a way to signal Ken to stop, without further embarrassing my son, when, with a sigh, Ken told us that he'd once been the lead singer in two punk bands, neither of which I'd ever heard. This explains a lot, I thought: a man trapped in a spinning record of regret over his unlived rock stardom. I remembered him telling me over lunch that he'd been bullied as a kid for being fat. I felt a sudden surge of empathy for this man trying to rewrite the wrongs of his past, along with annoyance and discomfort, but not enough to keep us trapped in that room indefinitely. I suggested he give us a tour of the rest of the office. "We have dinner plans," I said. "I don't want to be late." Not exactly a lie, but also it wasn't like we had reservations for two slices of pizza. As a parting welcome-to-the-*Observer*-but-not-really gift, he handed me an *Observer* T-shirt, suggesting I take a photo of myself in it and send it to him. A joke? I wasn't sure. Clearly this man has boundary issues, but he also has cash and column inches to give me.

And yet.

And yet. Those boundary issues often rose to the level of disturbing. In response to an email I wrote after my first column was published, asking him where to send an invoice and thanking him for giving my voice a new platform, he sent me instructions for invoicing the paper along with this: "Thank YOU. I'm so glad we met. In another life, I'd be Mr. Copaken." In response to an email I sent asking him if he'd received the story I'd written, at his behest, on the vagaries of dating after a marital rupture, he wrote, "Yep. That and the other one are in hand. I love your sloppy seconds!" When we were trying to come up with a name for my column, and he wrote, "What should we call your column? I was thinking 'All the Single Ladies'," to which I responded, "But I don't want to tie it to being single. A) It's not really about being single; and B) I hope I don't stay single for much longer." His response? "Are you proposing marriage to me?"

The first weekend in July 2015, Durkheim is able to visit from New Hampshire and actually stay over at my place, as all three of my kids are miraculously away at the same time. The next morning, before our hike in the woods, I give him both the *Observer* T-shirt and the story behind it. "I love it," he says. "Thank you." He thinks it's both fitting and funny for a sociology professor to have the word *Observer* splashed across his chest, which I hadn't even considered. I just wanted him to have the T-shirt. I take a photo of Durkheim wearing it in the woods and attach it to my response to Ken's email about Jared Kushner and Rudy Giuliani warning him of possible Fourth of July terror in New York City.

"I have my new beau visiting this weekend," I write. "We will probably stick close to home anyway." The boundary-drawing subtext being: No, I will not wear the T-shirt you gave me and send you a photo of my boobs in it.

The next day, Ken sends a response: "Becky's review: 'Oh. My. G-d. Can you ask her to see if he'd take a picture with his shirt off?'" Becky is his soon-to-be ex-wife. Did she really say this? I've never met her. Why did he show his wife the photo of my new boyfriend? Then there's his

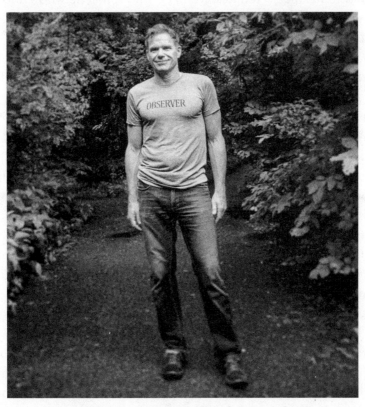

"Durkheim," July 4th weekend, 2015, © Deborah Copaken

spelling of god, G-d, which I recognize from my Hebrew school days. It's the way religious Jews spell *god*, in order to not write the full name in a place where it could get discarded in the trash or erased. I'd heard Ken was religious, but I did not realize to what extent.

Ken needn't have worried about either the word *god* or his email being erased. That email, among many others yet to come, will become part of his FBI file.

I spot Durkheim beaming in the audience as I perform onstage the next night, and a smile immediately spreads across my face. Our second date, and already he's shown up—literally—more than his predecessor. When Durkheim and Justin, the Hinge CEO, were busy talking during our preshow dinner, Kate had leaned over to me. "I like this one," she whispered. She'd liked Gio, too, since my meeting him on Hinge had led to my interview with Justin and then ultimately to Justin's flying across the Atlantic to declare his love, but she did not like seeing me suffer from reluctance. "You deserve to be with someone who wants to be with you," she said.

"Yeah," I laughed. "At a bare minimum."

By the end of the summer, after dating exclusively for three months, Durkheim and I begin to tiptoe around the pressing subject of our future once the school year begins. Because of his stepfather's cancer treatment, he's been spending most of the summer in New York, but now reality hits: We live in two different cities.

I leave my son in the care of friends and take the bus up to visit him in Portsmouth, New Hampshire, where he teaches me to surf. Standing up on the board, feeling that frictionless propulsion: I don't have the words to describe this euphoria. I could compare it to feeling like an air hockey puck gliding over a table, but that doesn't really do it justice or get at the joy of the movement through space, the heat of sun on wet skin, the smell of salt, the sound of surf, the rush of air, or that distinct and sudden feeling of being strong enough to tackle any whitecap life throws you. Get knocked over by a weird break in the wave? No problem. Lose your balance and fall down? No worries. There's always another swell on the horizon, so stand back up and try again. From my first successful ride, I instantaneously understand the lifelong hunt for the perfect wave that overcomes so many: There are worse ways to live out one's days, but I'm not sure there are too many better.

Afterward, we lie on the beach holding hands, and I stare out at the fairy dust sparkles on the water's surface, which fill my eyes with fresh tears. From their blinding brightness, yes, but also from my body feeling, on a cellular level, both the nourishing perfection of this sunny reprieve and its ephemerality. Like every wave, however seemingly perfect on the surface, our relationship will soon crash against reality's shores. Am I in love with this man in a forever way or am I just desperate for companionship? That I have to ask, I fear, already answers the question.

Or does it? This man is kind. He's smart. He's humble and easy on the eyes. He makes me feel at peace when I'm with him: shoulders dropped, pulse steady. Isn't that, on some level, love? Has love in my life been so historically interlaced with pain and self-denial that I cannot recognize or accept it when it arrives on a blindingly bright summer day? "WhatifLovewerereal?49," I type into my computer to open it, day after day, but perhaps the more salient question is this: Am I too broken by life, at forty-nine, to accept real love into it?

I also wonder if my hesitation to both accept and embrace this new love is more about logistical roadblocks than barriers of the heart. Durkheim has tenure and can't move to New York. His apartment is a bachelor's one-bedroom, with no room for a child. Yes, he could move, but he owns and loves his place and can afford it on his own. What if we were to move to a larger, more expensive home, share the costs, but then it doesn't work out between us? He also—though previously married— has never been a father. What will it mean for him to suddenly have to help raise another man's young child for the next decade? Moreover, I have no possibility of earning a decent enough living in the coastal tourist town he calls home to cover my older two children's education. What I really need to focus on at this crucial moment, now that I'm struggling to pay two college tuitions, is money. A lot of it. And fast.

Durkheim and I end things that fall. Or, rather, he starts his semester, and I resume my job hunt, and I take my son up to visit him one peak foliage weekend in October, just to see what that would be like, and when the three of us are together, it suddenly feels wrong. Not that he's not wonderful with my kid, because he is, knowing exactly when to stop for a chocolate crepe and where to find the best Legos in the toy store. But his living room couch makes an uncomfortable bed, says my son. And while he likes the professor, he sees the chalk on the blackboard and does not like where this is going. "I'm not moving here, if that's what you're thinking," he says, when we're alone. He loves New York. He loves his school and his friends. We just moved from Harlem to Inwood only a year ago, he reminds me, and he doesn't want to move again. His father is gone. The Commune is over. His sister just left for college. Isn't that enough upheaval for one nine-year-old for now? What he's asking for is both age appropriate and understandable: a moment of steadiness amidst the near-constant chaos of his childhood thus far.

Durkheim is heartbroken but understands. The grace and kindness with which he handles the breakup is the moment, ironically, I feel unequivocal love for him. I ask myself whether we could ever have a future later on, after my son's a bit older. After I've built a proper nest egg and ferried my big kids through college. But I cannot ask a man to put his life on hold while I sort out my own. That's exactly what Gio had been asking of me for over a year, and I wouldn't want to inflict that kind of noncommittal pain on anyone. In love, as in grief, timing is not just important: It's everything.

TWENTY-FOUR

Public Relations

OCTOBER–DECEMBER 2015

I will be a monk, I decide. I will forgo all love and sex and fun and friends and dedicate the next few years to my son's steadiness and to my older children's education: to paying off their tuitions; paying down debt; figuring out a way to get divorced. For this, I know, I must trade the work I love for a job that pays significantly more than journalism's increasingly meager, non-living wage while I wait for *Shutterbabe*, the TV show, to be greenlit for production.

Thanks to a tip from my friend Ariel, I've had several interviews with her friend's husband, Sharky, as well as with the rest of his team at a large and successful marketing and PR firm: all former journalists, all collateral damage of the internet era, all working for what I understand is a living wage in a new department called "synergic journalism."

Synergic journalism, as far as I understand it, after landing this job with its fancy-sounding title—Vice President and Deputy Editorial Director, Health—is a new way for companies and brands to tell their own stories. Or rather for those of us with actual journalism chops and boots-on-the-ground experience to tell those stories for them, only without professional skepticism or objectivity. Beyond this I know only that, at first glance, the team I'll be joining seems competent and maybe even fun?

Leslie used to work at a popular celebrity magazine and is now in charge of "Consumer," meaning well-known consumer brands you've definitely heard of. Steve used to work at *The Wall Street Journal* and is now in charge of our business vertical. Sharky used to work at *Fast Company* and has apparently become a marketing genius after his massive win, including a silver Clio—the Oscars of the advertising world—for one of his recent campaigns.

Sharky is confident, exceedingly tall—so Brobdingnagian that when one of our colleagues tries to take a photo of the two of us standing together, she has to move back several feet just to fit us in the same frame—GQ-handsome, floppy-haired, tattooed, and scrappy, with humble beginnings in the Deep South. He keeps a turntable on his desk and is a master at music trivia, only unlike Ken Kurson, he doesn't test nine-year-olds (or anyone) on the gaps in their music knowledge. He has a taste for the occasional finger of whiskey, and, like every male manager in PR, he comes to work each day dressed in head-to-toe black. On occasion, he mixes it up with fancy white sneakers or patterned shoes.

A former solo parent himself, Sharky understands the vagaries of my own particular brand of parenthood without my having to explain it. He even came right out and said, without prompting, "Look, I know there will be times when your kid has to go to the doctor or has a school performance in the middle of the day or some need you can't even conceive of right now, and I want you to know that I understand you are the only one holding up his world." Which made me tear up. He's offering a solid six-figure salary to join his team: $190,000 a year, more than I've ever earned annually in my entire life. It's still not enough, after taxes, debt, and basic living expenses, to finance two college tuitions out of pocket, even with financial aid—which, frankly, is ludicrous, can we fix this, please?—but it's more than twice my former salary, plus I'll be subsidizing it slightly with my *Observer* column, which Sharky says I can keep, as long as it doesn't interfere with my PR work.

"Welcome to the team," he says, showing me to my desk in the open-plan office, which is next to Leslie's and two seats down from Stefanie, who leads "Creative" on health. Creative? What does that mean? New terminology and acronyms fly at me like tennis balls from a machine, too fast for me to return every lob—KPIs, CPMs, owned media, paid media, ROIs, oh my!—but I love Stefanie from the moment she hugs me. In my experience of working with women, you can always trust the genuine huggers with your secrets and your life. The handshakers? Depends on the grip: the firm-grippers are usually trustworthy; the weak-grippers can be hit and miss.

Leslie's handshake is weak. Her snack of choice is carrots. When I offer her my snack of choice, peanut M&M's, she politely declines. She's a long-distance runner, wiry and taut. We become fast friends, but only at work. I invite her over for dinner three times, but each time she turns me down. Always good to know where the boundaries are.

I'll be leading our health vertical, which means once again creating content for the pharmaceutical industry, just like back in my *Health Today* days but with big budgets and only myself to lean on as the writer. Am I selling my writing skills and soul to Big Pharma so that my children can get a college education and health insurance? Yes. Yes, I am. Do I feel bad about this? Yes. Yes, I do. But I have sent out well over four hundred letters, emails, and résumés, hitting up literally every person of any journalistic influence in my Gmail contact list and then some, all to no avail. Those who take the time to write back keep repeating some version of the same story: *So sorry, Deb. Right now we're cutting jobs not adding them. Good luck out there. I know it's rough.*

After nearly a full week of watching mandatory corporate videos about sexual harassment, citizenship, and compliance, I get my first assignment to work with Stefanie in Creative on a brand manifesto for an estrogen-replacement product aimed at the menopausal market. "It says here that it's a treatment for vaginal atrophy?" she says. Both of us are reduced to giggling teenagers in a sex ed class. "You basically stick it up your twat and it remoistens you. Or something like that."

"Ah," I say, "the marvels of middle-aged womanhood." Thank goodness I'm not yet worrying about such things. It's no longer the Amazon rainforest down there, but we're a long way from the Sahara. Let's call it Switzerland: neutral, blue-skied, still skiable. At the same time, many of the single women in my middle-aged warrior women dinners are dealing not only with parched deserts but also with Grand Canyons. Though I can tell this is a painful issue for them to deal with in private, in public, many of them treat the whole ordeal with black humor and brutal honesty. "Honey, with enough lube," said a newly single friend of a friend, a successful business owner, "I could fit three dudes up there. And a couch."

"I know exactly the tone we need to take to appeal to women of our generation," I tell Stefanie.

"Go for it," she says.

First I quickly google "brand manifesto." What's a brand manifesto? Then I read the materials on the estrogen product, sit down at my computer, and bang it out: "Oh, the irony of menopause!" I type. "Just when you have time to really explore your mature, adventurous, sensual self, your vagina goes on strike . . ."*

There's a lot more. I'll spare you.

I print out the page and show it to Stefanie.

"Yes!" she says. "Oh my god, yes! I love this! And I'm betting the client will, too."

She's right. The client loves it. I'm thrilled. Sharky's thrilled. My first assignment, and I've hit it out of the ballpark.

Then I immediately erase the win with a massive if inadvertent error.

At the end of each week in the marketing and PR world, you have to account for each of your hours, just like a lawyer: a task which, every week, fills me with dread. Not just because the computer program the company's created for this weekly millstone is as counterintuitive as any I've ever used, and it doesn't automatically save your work, so you are constantly losing it. It's more that my brain doesn't neatly divide creative work into precise fifteen-minute intervals. Sometimes my best work is done in my head in the shower before I get to the office. Or while walking the dog. Or on the weekend, while thinking about something else entirely.

My first week on the job, I keep careful track of all of my hours and fill out my timesheet accordingly, allotting two of my fifty hours to writing the brand manifesto for the estrogen replacement company.

Big mistake.

"Two hours!!!???" Our money guy, who's in charge of all the budgets for Creative, is now yelling into my left ear. "We negotiated with the client for twenty!" Apparently, the client was so happy with my work, they'd called not only to gush over the work itself but also to thank us for doing it far under the expected budget.

---

* Fans of *Emily in Paris* will perhaps recognize this as the brand manifesto Emily creates for the fictional company, Vaja-Jeune. We'll get to that, I promise.

"But I did it in two," I say, utterly confused. What I don't yet under-stand—my colleagues have to explain this to me, after the money guy goes back to his desk—is that when I was assigned a twenty-hour project, this meant I was supposed to have *used* all twenty of those hours: no more, no less. In any other job I've ever worked, efficiency was an asset, not a liability.

In essence, it was beginner's luck. Brand manifestos don't usually come fully formed onto the page. You're supposed to spend time re-searching the market, understanding the customer, learning about the product, brainstorming at least three avenues of approach then choosing one. Alas for me, I *was* the customer. The research was already done, the understanding of the product implicit. And because I did the job in 10 percent of the time allotted, we got paid only 10 percent of our pro-jected budget.

My time, as a vice president in PR, is worth $300 an hour to my com-pany. In other words, in my first week on the job, I've already made a $5,400 error.

Another error like that, I could lose my job.

I saw what happened to the older gentleman on our team. He'd spent most of his life at the company, working in PR crisis management, which is what large corporations pay PR executives giant sums to do when they mess up on a grand scale: crashed planes, murderous medical devices, E. coli'd burgers, spilled oil. But crisis management had become a bru-tal business, requiring precision weaponry and a soul of ice to turn im-ages of ducks slicked in oil into a story about the fossil fuel industry's deep love for planet Earth, and the older gentleman was kind-hearted, avuncular. Old school PR, not new. So he'd been put out to pasture on our floor. He was vivacious, charming, and curious: the kind of man who would tell you in great detail about the doorstop biography he was read-ing or the off-Broadway production of *Orestes* he'd just seen the previous night. Everyone loved him. I loved him. But he was not billing enough hours. A few years shy of his retirement, he was coldly cast out with a paper plate of goodbye cake.

My days begin to feel like an Ionesco play, a theater of the absurd from which the only escape is sleep, and even then my sleep sometimes gets interrupted by late-night pings requiring immediate response: SLIDE 3 OF THE RFP IS MISSING! All caps with a red exclamation point. At 11:30 P.M. As if we were all doctors on call instead of tiny cogs in the giant wheel of the pharmaceutical industry. "It's PR, not brain surgery," goes the classic PR joke, but only because so many people in PR have to be reminded that a missing slide from an RFP—request for proposal—is not the same as a missing chunk of human skull.

One morning, I'm invited to help brainstorm some ideas for a new drug to combat OIC. "OIC?" I say, plopping down on a chair in the conference room after sprinting from another. "What's that?" My Google Calendar is packed with these back-to-back meetings. I often have no idea which pharmaceutical products I'll be helping to hype until minutes before I'm supposed to provide intelligent solutions to hyping them.

"Opioid induced constipation," my colleague says. OIC, she goes on to explain, is a common scourge among opioid addicts, only she doesn't call them addicts. She calls them "people living with chronic pain."

"So it's a drug to help addicts stay addicted to a different drug. Am I getting that right?"

"Constipation is painful!" she says.

"I know. Believe me, I know. But wouldn't it be better to try to get them off opioids?"

"That's not our job. Our job is to market this drug, and we need a journalist's perspective."

I'm not sure she wants my journalist's perspective on this one, actually. But my colleagues, I know, do not want to hear soapboxing. It is not our job to question or rail against the morality of the products we're paid to market. It is our job to market them.

"Cool," I say with a smile. "Let's help addicts poop!"

With this one sentence, I cross a Rubicon. Any fantasies I once held of how I could work in pharmaceutical marketing and avoid the pitfalls of moral relativism have just been shattered. My father's words rattle around in my brain, daily: *You have to know where the line is. If you earn your money off the suffering or deaths or exploitation of others, that's not a moral income. That's blood money.*

Meanwhile, the act of writing, which used to bring such joy, is now devoid of it when my words are wielded as weapons of mass manipulation instead of as pathways to shared connections with readers, which, when I stumble across them in my favorite books, feel like love.

One morning, seeking counterbalance, I open up my laptop on the subway to work and start writing the interwoven stories of Justin and Kate, Gio and me, and the long-lost love who I thought had stood me up in Paris back in 1989. My subway, the A train, gets packed during rush hour, and I'm always squished in an aisle between this one's backpack and that one's sweaty armpit on my way home from work, but my morning commute is different. I live at the end of the line, two blocks from the 207th Street stop, which means on my way to work every day, as crowded as the train gets, I usually get a seat. If I'm lucky enough to nab one of the chairs perpendicular to the window, at a slight remove from the crowds, I can put on my noise-canceling headphones, tune out the world, and write during the entirety of the fifty-minute ride: my daily act of quiet revolt.

I begin typing: "My interview with the baby-faced CEO was winding down when I tossed out one last question: 'Have you ever been in love?'" The story flows out of me not like blood from an artery but more like lava from a volcano. It spews! It smokes! It solidifies from liquid thought into hard word chunks on the way out. I feel, in this glorious, all-too-rare moment, like the story's amanuensis, not its creator. By the time the conductor calls out, "Next stop, Canal Street!" I have the first draft of . . . something.

I'd already published a Modern Love essay in *The New York Times* several years earlier, so I know the chances are slim of publishing a second, but I polish the threads of my story over the next few mornings, during my commute, and then I email it to Dan Jones, the Modern Love editor.

"Very nice!" he writes back, with two excellent suggestions for excavating it more deeply, agreeing to publish it if I do a quick rewrite with his edits, plus he wants me to add on another 150 words: a welcome change from "Dumb it down, and make it shorter."

On the day the story is published, under the title "When Cupid Is a Prying Journalist," I coincidentally have a lunch planned with a different editor at *The New York Times*, who I'm hoping can help yank me back into the journalist fold, prying or otherwise. I'm not sure how much longer I can handle the mental pretzeling required of my job. I was hoping the extra money to pay for my children's tuition would counteract feeling morally compromised every hour of every day, but it doesn't. In fact, "going over to the dark side," as it's often called whenever journalists make the transition to public relations, has taken such a toll on my mental health that I've started seeing a shrink again. "Why are you here?" he'd asked during our first session.

"I feel stuck," I said—I keep saying—"and I can't envision the pathway out." The words spill out of my mouth as fast as the snot leaks from my nose. I go through half a box of tissues before admitting that the only time I feel like myself these days is during my fifty-minute "writers retreat" on the A train to work.

The shrink remains silent, but his tilted chin and raised eyebrows say it all: *Then that's your pathway out.*

"No, no, you don't understand," I say, trying to clarify the writing-for-hire landscape for those who are not used to seeing it up close every day. "There are no jobs. The internet ate them. No one has the ad dollars to pay me to write stories for them anymore, hard as I've tried, because 70 percent of those dollars now go to Google or Facebook." It's not lost on me that I'm now helping to create digital marketing campaigns specifically tailored for Google SEO and Facebook virality. I'm now part of the problem. "I also wrote a feminist indictment of the literary world in *The Nation* back in 2012, and now I can't sell a new book to save . . . to save my . . ." my voice trails off, unable to finish the sentence.

"To save your life?" says the shrink.

"Yes," I say, "my life," before rushing back to a meeting to discuss marketing a new drug to treat Chronic Obstructive Pulmonary Disease (COPD), an illness whose primary risk factor, I learn, is smoking. At this meeting, it is decided that I'll do a "deep dive" into the disease, which means spending the next two weeks interviewing every pulmonologist and COPD patient on the pharmaceutical company's payroll: definitely not the way I've been trained to do reporting. Experts and patients who are paid to give their opinions are always swayed by the money.

The New York Times editor invites me to meet her at the same restaurant where I'd first had lunch with Ken Kurson: apt, since I'm still hoping to land a full-time job at the *Observer,* but he keeps stringing me along with vague *ifs* and *maybes*. On my Google Calendar, I have written, "Meeting with a potential client outside the office," to avoid having a meeting scheduled during my lunch. No one in my office writes "lunch" on their calendars. You can't charge for an hour you're not at your desk "working," even if working means shoving a sad desk salad down your throat while scrolling through Facebook and Zappos.

"Deb! Oh my god," the editor says, when we sit down at our table, several hours after my essay has gone live online, "your essay is going gangbusters! It's already on track to become one of the most popular Modern Loves we've ever published."

"Wow!" I say. "That's great." Before leaving my office for lunch, I'd checked Facebook and had noticed it was popping up all over my time-line, as well as all over my Twitter mentions. Most publications will not reveal to their freelancers how many clicks and shares their stories garner, even after they've clearly gone viral, so I'm glad to have this information, however vague and nonnumerical. It also makes me wonder: In exchange for the $250 I was paid for my 1,500 words—16 cents a word or 0.05 percent of my prior worth as a magazine writer—how many ad dollars did *The New York Times* earn? This is a serious question, not a David/Goliath indictment. I'm actually curious how many ad dollars a viral Modern Love brings into *The New York Times*. "What are the chances I can parlay that into a full-time job?" I say.

"Zero," says the editor, laughing. "All of us are holding on for dear life." In three years, this kind and brilliant woman will be the next victim of media budget cuts.

Private Relations

LATE FALL 2015–EARLY WINTER 2016

As promised, Ken Kurson has taken his "I come from a grudge-holding desert people" revenge on me for my publishing the essay about Justin and Kate in *The New York Times* instead of the *Observer* by ghosting me.

In the middle of the summer, he'd sent a reminder email with the following header: "When will you know if the Hinge story is a go? I love it . . . Would be good for you to start your new chapter with a cover story, too, and we lavishly illustrate." He wanted an "excellent draft" by July 13.

Justin and Kate, I told him—and kept telling him, even prior to his email giving me a deadline—did not want their story published in the *Observer*. This was true, even if I probably could have convinced them otherwise. But this was also my line in the sand: You promised me an actual full-time job, motherfucker, not some vague, barely remunerated "new chapter," and you reneged on that promise. So I'm under no obligation, as a freelancer without a contract, to give you or the *Observer* my best story. He'd also been sending me more odd and inappropriate emails throughout the summer, culminating with this one: "Can I ask you something private and personal, unrelated to this?" This was in response to an email I'd sent asking him to please correct my byline from

Deborah Copaken Kogan, which I had not used since my separation, to Deborah Copaken.

A quick side note: I did not change my last name to my husband's when I got married. Rather, I'd changed it in a pique of postpartum frustration and ire two years after my wedding, when a postal clerk refused to give me the baby present sent to my infant son because the last name on his package did not match mine. I'd waited for over an hour in line to retrieve it, my five-week-old strapped to my chest, wailing with hunger. When we finally got to the window, and I handed over the pink package slip and my drivers license—"Who are you?"; "His mother"; "Well, how am I supposed to know that?"; "Our address is the same, and he's attached to me?"—I was told I would need both his birth certificate and my marriage license every time I wanted to retrieve a package for him or for any future children I might conceivably have. This is not actual law but rather what Columbia law professor Elizabeth Emens called "desk-clerk law": rules about women's names that become normalized when a desk clerk or government official decides they are.

I walked the eight blocks home from the post office, breastfed my baby, changed his diaper, gathered my various IDs, my son's birth certificate, and my marriage license, and trudged back to the post office just in time for the lunchtime rush. This time I waited long enough that I had to whip out my boob again, right there in line, and change my baby's diaper on the post office floor. Finally in possession of the package, three and a half hours after having originally left the apartment to do so, I opened it up, shoved the gift—a tiny new onesie, all this for that—into the diaper bag, and took my new miniature human and all of my various forms of ID straight down to the Social Security Administration to change my last name to his, both of us cranky.

Had I known that two decades later I would need my ex-husband's signed and notarized permission to change my name back—more desk-clerk law, not real law—I might have thought twice about this seemingly rash but tactically rational act. But postpartum hormones are strong, and my imagination for the kind of further clerical barriers I might one day face down the line was weak. Being a woman in a country where only the men are created equal feels a lot like playing an RPG videogame in which every door between your avatar and the pot of gold has a lock, a chain, bricks, a desk, another door, several more doors, quicksand,

sharks, and a fire-breathing dragon lurking behind it, while the only barriers blocking the male avatars' doors are knobs.

One can hardly blame them for getting upset when their knobs get
stuck. "There is a chance," Ken's "private and personal" email began,
"—a small chance, thank G-d, but a bigger chance than there was before the summer—that my wife is going to dump me," he wrote, followed by much throat clearing and then by what journalists call the nut
graf, in which he wondered what his "chances" would be "on the open
market." His guy friends, he went on (and on and on and on), "all seem
to go through this embarrassing pussy chase," and he didn't want that.

Then his email took a turn for the wildly inappropriate, considering
I'd met him only once for a job interview and a second time to pick up
a copy of the paper from his office with my son. He wanted to know if it
was realistic for him, "given what you know about my finances, appearance, mental state . . ." (*Nothing! I know nothing about your finances or
mental state, why would I? Ugh!*) for someone with his "pilgrim soul" to
"find someone suitable (must be Jewish)" or did I consider him a "fat
and disgusting misanthrope" who needed to lower his expectations?

I felt nauseated over his word choices—*open market, pussy chase,
pilgrim soul*—but I nevertheless tried to answer vaguely, with both compassion for a man having trouble turning his knob on the door of life and
with the precaution of a giant moat around my own castle. It was not my
job, as a freelance writer he'd contacted via social media to write for his
paper, to pump up this man's ego and to tell him how wonderful he was
or how great a commodity he might be on the "open market." For one, I
hardly knew him. For another, he held the keys to one of my doors of life
with the pot of gold behind it.

"The short answer is you'll be fine," I wrote. "The longer answer is
don't get divorced if you can possibly avoid it." Then, because I couldn't
help myself, I addressed his use of the phrase *pussy chase*, which had
stuck in my craw. "The 'pussy chase' of which you speak is actually important dating," I wrote. "I know it's been a long time since you've been
single, so let me spell it out: Anyone who is unattached at our age—
whether having never married or going through a divorce—is damaged
in some way. Hurt. Angry. Struggling. Sad. And all those awful feelings
in between. So there's a lot of dating. It's part of the process."

For my own part, after breaking up with Durkheim and realizing

that, with my increased workload and unremitting parenting responsibilities, I was in no position to be a good partner to anyone, I made a
deliberate decision to stop looking for a forever love and to start looking
for love in the here and now. The conditional logic of this choice, once
made, seemed obvious enough: Given that we're all going to die, and we
don't know when; given that the chances of my finding a new partner at
my age were statistically slim and growing slimmer by the year; given
that I found celibacy untenable and pleasure pleasurable, I would therefore choose to enjoy, without apology, whatever stolen opportunities for
physical affection I had left. A sex life, to me, is nonnegotiable. My body
needs touch and release in the same way it needs air, water, sunlight,
food.

So that fall, after turning forty-nine, I decided to widen my opportunities for imbibing this particular elixir by lowering the age parameters
on my dating apps from a minimum of forty-five to a minimum of thirty.
I also rewrote my profile: "Two years separated from a long-term marriage. Open to whatever comes along. Still believe in love, despite everything." Once I'd opened up the playing field to "whatever comes along"
while leaving the door open for love, a team of players actually showed
up in my dating app messages, and I could suddenly be a lot pickier
about whom I'd choose to meet in person.

It turns out that many men in their thirties are either not ready for
committed relationships; or they're recovering from broken ones; or they
see an increasingly stagnant economy and lack of wage opportunities for
men of their generation as barriers to getting married and having kids, so
they feel stuck in an endless economic limbo. These younger men—
"All the Young Dudes," I would later dub them, in an *Observer* essay—
liked dating women in their late forties and early fifties in the same way
older war journalists, back in my war photographer years, had once provided comfort in foreign cities under siege to an adamantly single, twentysomething me. Our sexual needs aligned. The end.

Would I ever refer to my new dating protocol as a "cock chase"?
Jesus. No. Never. The male language of domination and conquest—of
notches in belts, subjugation, commodified acquisition—had nothing to
do with what these men and I shared together, with emphasis on the
word *shared*. In fact, once I stopped looking for a new forever partner
and accepted that I might never find one, I started to let go and to really

enjoy myself: to explore what I liked; to ask, in great detail, for what I needed; and to try new things with those patient enough to take their time.

Yes, yes, app dating still sucked, and for every successful date I endured ten bad ones. Or men who canceled at the last minute. Or ghosted me. Or became weirdly verbally abusive when I turned them down for sex: "I had friends in from out of town! I could have gone out with them tonight instead of trudging all the way up here to Inwood to have drinks with you!" yelled one sock entrepreneur, eight shots of tequila in. Or they sent unsolicited photos of their penises, butts, chests. Or they were pathological liars. Or had three weeks of dishes piled high in their sink. Or they would text "your cute" (*you're you're you're!* I'd want to text back—scream, really). Or in one case I was simply stood up on Manhattanhenge, on one of the most gorgeous spring nights of the year, and wound up weeping, alone, on a bench in Washington Square Park, from which I observed seemingly everyone else walking hand in hand with their partners into the perfectly grid-aligned sunset. And yet all of this bad behavior and bad grammar notwithstanding, I suddenly felt grateful to find myself single and game at the precise moment in history when seeking out the occasional partner for sex became as easy as ordering up a dish of pad thai.

Ken never responded to my answer to his "pussy chase" email. I sent him several new story pitches. No response. A new essay. No response. Another new essay. No response. Finally, Lorraine, my day-to-day editor, wrote to say that the paper could not take any more of my essays in 2015, even though Ken had asked me to produce a column every two weeks. They'd run out of budget for the year, she said. Also, from now on Ken and I would have to discuss the topic of my essay before publishing, which was not only not part of the deal we'd originally struck, it was an impossible protocol to follow, given that he'd stopped answering my emails.

I send Ken another email: "I don't actually have time to spend a week writing a story that doesn't get published. I was under the impression that you needed me to write a lot, not that we had to discuss and approve ideas prior to writing them. I need to understand the parameters here, thanks."

Twenty-six more days go by. No response.

Then, the week my Modern Love is published, Ken finally responds: "I can't believe a writer of your skill and elegance is insecure but this job has taught be [sic] that ALL writers are insecure when they don't hear back promptly." Once again, the email is long, rambling, and inappropriately personal. "You know I am not quite myself lately," he writes (*No. Why would I know that? I do not know you*), "as the emotional and financial blows are rained on me like Joe Frazier taking out Muhammad Ali in their first fight at the Garden . . . I'll be back to myself soon enough. I'm destroyed right now, but already glimpsing that better days are ahead."

His sadism, I finally realize, is both real and lacks subtlety. He publishes the two essays he claimed not to want to publish, but then says he can't pay me for them. He keeps dangling the possibility of a full-time job in front of my face—"You are such a nice writer," he writes in one email, "I wish I could afford you on a full-time basis"—but then in the next email, when I tell him I'm still interested in a full-time job with adequate pay, he yanks it away with a backhanded compliment—"If you were a tech writer with tons of sources, you'd be making $150k. But a brilliant essayist with a huge heart and silky prose? It's rough." He also keeps crossing boundaries. When I land a two-week gig in L.A. as a consultant in the writers' room for *Younger*, and Ken finds out, he sends an unsolicited email both to me and to the author of the book upon which the series is based, though she is not a writer on the show, and I never asked him to introduce us. "Pam, meet Debbie," reads the subject header, followed by: "You're both *Observer* contributors and both my friends, despite your weird refusal to fix me up with your hot single Jewish friends."

I tell Sharky, my boss at the PR firm, that I'll be taking my two weeks of vacation all at once, to work on *Younger*. Darren wants me for four weeks, but oh, well. Because I'm a new employee, two weeks is all I have.

TWENTY-SIX

On-ramp

MARCH 2016

By March, my ex has moved back to New York, so I can now actually travel for work again without organizing sleepovers for my son or paying for extra babysitting. I have Wednesday and Thursday nights to myself, to see friends or go on dates or take myself out to the movies. I have every other weekend alone now as well to work on other projects or to just sit and think and stare into space: the kind of lost, formless time that had wholly disappeared when my marriage ended.

"You're not leaving us, I hope," Sharky says, when I tell him I'm taking my two weeks of vacation to work on *Younger*, and I not only promise him that I'm not, I reiterate how grateful I am to have my job.

Then, in preparation for my trip to L.A. to work on *Younger*, I hit a roadblock: my lack of a credit card, due to my involvement with Freedom Debt Relief.

When I travel for the PR company, I use the company American Express, but because I haven't been able to afford a real vacation in four years, booking travel without a credit card had not previously reared its head as an issue. I end up having to call Darren to explain that I, a newly minted fifty-year-old, have neither the credit nor the cash to book my own travel.

Darren has been a Hollywood wunderkind since he arrived in L.A., struggling for only a short span of time, while living in an apartment complex that would later serve as the inspiration for *Melrose Place*. He created the smash hit *Beverly Hills, 90210* while still in his twenties. *90210* was based, in part, on the dynamics and subtle class differences in the large suburban public high school we both attended, albeit five years apart.[*] Darren's father was an orthodontist, his mother was a journalist— unusual, in that era and suburb, for a mother to work—and he grew up in Camotop (yes, that's Potomac spelled backward), which was the newer, wealthier side of town with the substantially larger houses. In *90210* parlance, Darren would have been the Jewish, gay Brandon Walsh while I would have been Andrea Zuckerman.

Darren always insists on paying for dinner whenever we go out, except that one time I argued that he can't always be the one to pay, and he let me pick up the tab. He understands I've been going through rough times, because he's my friend and because he reads what I write and publish, but it's one thing to have a vague understanding of a friend's struggles and quite another to be told, "Look, I just paid my ex's $12,000 tax bill, because we're still married, so it's suddenly and quite unexpectedly my tax bill, too. So now I have less than an $800 cushion in the bank and no credit cards, so I can't pay for my hotel, car, or meals with my ATM."

He seems both shocked at this state of affairs and also compassionate. "No problem," he says, he'll make it happen.

My shame over this runs deep, but it also echoes the financial struggles of Liza, the protagonist in *Younger* played by Sutton Foster, who finds out, after separating from her husband, that his gambling addiction has bankrupted their family. Which is one of the reasons she ends up moving into her artist friend Maggie's loft in Williamsburg, Brooklyn, in the first place and has to pretend to be a twenty-seven-year-old ingenue to land an entry-level job as an assistant to the head of marketing at a publishing house, after trying in vain to land a more senior job commensurate with her skill set as a former book editor.

Economist Sylvia Ann Hewlett has studied this phenomenon of the

[*] No, we did not know each other back then, though his younger brother and my cousin were classmates and friends, and therefore his mother and my aunt know each other as well.

brick wall middle-aged women hit after taking time off from the corporate world, which she calls off-ramping and on-ramping. Of those women who off-ramp from a full-time corporate job to care for ailing parents or children, only 74 percent of those who want to rejoin the workforce manage to on-ramp back into it. But that number is also deceiving, because of those 74 percent who manage to find jobs, only 40 percent find full-time, professional employment. The rest are relegated to permalance, freelance, part-time, or self-employment. "The implication is clear," Hewlett writes in the *Harvard Business Review*. "Off-ramps are around every curve in the road, but once a woman has taken one, on-ramps are few and far between—and extremely costly."

Before heading to L.A. to work on *Younger*, I'd been having frequent dinners with Darren in New York, now that he's bicoastal. He became fascinated with the twists and turns of my dating life. Of my refusal to give up at my age and throw in the towel. "You're like a gay man!" he said, proudly, as he mined me for material, and we dissected each paramour or almost-paramour as if we were Derrida deconstructing Heidegger.

There was the conceptual artist who told me, before heading off to live in a spinning wheel for several days, that he'd just ended a long relationship in Berlin and was still a little raw. "What was she like?" I said.

"They," he said. "I was the third in a throuple."

There was the widower who admitted that he wasn't all that upset to have lost his wife; the divorcé who wasn't actually divorced.

There was the twenty-seven-year-old who pretended to be forty, until I happened to mention that I'd covered the 1989 San Francisco earthquake, and he accidentally revealed his lie: "Awesome! I was born on that day!"

There was the miniatures artist who created intricate dioramas depicting his favorite movie scenes. It took me a Where's Waldo while to notice, in the photos he texted, the round hole cut out in the bottom of each one for his erect penis. Which he would dress up as one of the characters. "Wanna bring your camera over and come help me shoot my latest creation?" he texted. "I just have to find a miniature Princess Leia wig for the tip of my cock."

"Um . . . no, thanks!" I wrote back. "But good luck with that."

There was Juan, the Spanish banker from London, deep in the early throes of marital implosion, whom I met and befriended at the tail end of my friend Josh's fiftieth birthday. When Juan found out I'd written *The Red Book*, he smiled slyly and said, "You're not going to believe this, but I actually have that book on my nightstand right now." Which I thought was one of the lamest pick-up lines I'd ever heard and told him so. He insisted we walk a few blocks away to confirm it. Lo and behold, there was my novel, right there on his nightstand, at the top of the pile.

"No way," said Darren.

"Way!" I said, laughing.

"So what happened next?"

"We talked. About love. About marriage. About the end of love and the end of marriage. About my father's death. About death in general. About books. About art. About what it means to be a good human. He's really brilliant. And funny. And age appropriate. And handsome. And a *gifted* lover, good lord." I sighed. "I really liked him. A lot."

"So?"

"So that's it, the whole three-act arc in one night. And it's all it ever can or will be because of circumstance." Juan and I had each taken note of the alchemy in that room, spoken of it out loud in ways that sounded both absurd and like treacle, even to our own ears. And yet we both cried, too, both from the surprising joy of those eight hours and from our concomitant understanding, even while they were happening, of their loss. "The next morning, we went out for breakfast and coffee, I came back to my shithole in Inwood, he went back to his flat in London, and now I'm back to marketing pills to help opioid addicts poop. He sends me adorable emails with poems attached. Poems, Darren! Poems I actually like!"

"So what's the problem? I don't get it. Why not see him again?"

"He lives between London and Madrid with his kids. I live in Inwood with my kids. He's from a totally different world of wealth and privilege. His family were patrons of Gaudí, for fuck's sake. There's an entire park named after them in Barcelona. He's either Spanish aristocracy or royalty. I didn't ask. He didn't offer." In fact, he was deliberately vague about his upbringing. It was Danna, Josh's wife, who later filled me in on his family's storied background.

"So what's wrong with dating a prince?" said Darren.

I shrugged. "I don't want to be rescued." Also men like that, I added, attract gold diggers. I would always be looking over my shoulder.

One night, I introduced Darren to Zane, thirty-one, a natural blond, blue-eyed guitar player and singer in a band you've probably heard of. Although at the time we met on Tinder and planned a guitar lesson instead of a date, I had not. But when I asked my then nine-year-old if he'd heard of the band—which Zane had started with two of his college pals on a lark, and then suddenly there they were on Letterman and Conan, despite his plans to become a journalist—my son tween–rolled his eyes and said, "Duh, Mom. They wrote that song that the fifth graders sang at graduation last year."

A few months later, I introduced Darren to Finn, a young Texan entrepreneur who knew his way around both China and its many factories, having lived and worked there for several years, spoke fluent Chinese, and was game for any adventure and then some: naked yoga, shaman visits, forest bike rides, living room tango. "So handsome!" said Darren, when Finn left the table to find the bathroom.

"Too handsome," I said. Several times when we were out in the world, people had stopped Finn on the street to ask him to take a selfie with them, mistaking him for Bradley Cooper.

These latter two, both nineteen years my junior and each cognizant of the other's existence, are mature, empathic, thoughtful. They don't play games. They text back. They're open to anything. They arrive at the meeting place on time and prioritize female pleasure: a welcome change from the many men of my generation who were taught all about putting condoms on bananas but nothing about locating the spadix in a calla lily. Moreover, because there is zero preconception that these relationships are heading down any aisles or must conform to any traditional standards of monogamy, they have freed me to explore the idea of love for love's sake. Of being present. Of showing up. Of letting go. Of throwing out the standard rule book and writing a new one, with only one basic rule: live and let love.

It was during one of our date-dissecting dinners, in fact, when Darren admitted he enjoyed hearing about my love life not only because he loves me, but also because no one in the *Younger* writers' room was actually a middle-aged divorcée going through these same humiliations and joys. Seeing an opportunity—an on-ramp, let's call it—I grabbed it. Why don't I come out to L.A. and share my experiences with the room?

Younger

MARCH–APRIL 2016

Every single day in the *Younger* writers' room is more than just fun. It's the most fun I've ever had at a paid job either before or since. Work starts at the humane hour of 10 or 10:30 A.M., after which people drift into the writers' room: a sunlit, all-white, large but cozy space on the Paramount lot. We're each also given our own offices off a winding hallway, and when I walk into mine on my first day, I shut the door, open my window, and tear up. It has been two years since my rejection from the job at The Container Store. Three years since I contemplated throwing myself out my office window in Harlem. Four years since Nora died. My thumb hovers over her name in my iPhone, itching to call her. Or at least to text her a photo of my office and the Hollywood sign, which I can see from my window if I lean out really far: no, not the kind of leaning out born of a death wish. Now that I have this job, all I want to do is live.

From 10 A.M. until 1 P.M., with a giant pile of snacks between us, a dozen of us take turns telling real stories and pitching fictional ones around a conference table. At the end of the table, Joe, the writers' assistant, types every word spoken into a daily file and organizes it into narrative threads and themes, while Dottie, one of the showrunners, starts to build a board of index cards with the dramatic beats on them. "What if Liza goes on Tinder and gets stood up?" I say, or "What if Josh decides he wants to have kids?" or "Maybe they should stand there on the street, hand in hand, watching Manhattanhenge." After a generous break for lunch at 1 P.M., we come back around 2 P.M. and continue batting around ideas until 5 or 5:30 P.M. at the latest, but sometimes we break for the day as early as 4:30. When that happens, I take advantage of the extra hour to drive out to Venice Beach to watch the sun set behind the drum circle. And every morning, when I drive onto the Paramount lot and park my car in my appointed spot, I cannot believe how lucky I am to get paid to do this. There's real joy and camaraderie in that room: laughter, creativity, a feeling of teamwork and friendship. It's also fascinating, as someone who normally writes alone in her bed or on an Ikea Poäng chair in her living room, to engage those same areas of the brain as part of a larger community.

I'm told by the others that this level of everyday laughter, friendship, and mirth is unusual in a comedy writing room but not unheard of. For one, Darren's rooms have an equal number of men and women, whereas many half-hour comedies can be frat houses. For another, he picks his groups carefully, for optimum collaboration without too many egos stepping over one another.

Before I leave to head back to New York, I tell Darren that I would be totally open to taking a leave of absence from my PR job, relocating to L.A. with my son for twelve weeks, and joining the writing staff for season three, if he has any openings. "Let me see if I have anyone who leaves," he says, keeping the door open. But when the door actually does open several months later, and I ask Sharky if I can take a twelve-week unpaid leave, he'll say no. I'm too valuable to the team. Because my full-time job is too valuable to my kids, I'll accept his no, mourn the loss of opportunity, and keep my nose to the corporate grindstone, wishing I had the financial wherewithal to say yes to such a rare and possibly life-changing break.

What's so often left out of the bootstrap narrative in this country is privilege. White privilege and male privilege no doubt, but also sheer monetary privilege which, as the divide between rich and poor grows ever wider, becomes increasingly crucial. The summer after my sophomore year at college, I applied for and got accepted to an internship at

NBC that I ended up having to turn down, not having realized it was unpaid. The money I earned each summer during college was crucial to paying my living expenses during the rest of the year, so I wound up working at a headhunting firm instead, which bored me to tears but provided enough spending money for both semesters. (My job? To help run background checks, in those pre-digital years, on future CEOs of multinational corporations, which meant calling up their college registrars and former places of work. I won't say all of those men—they were all men—lied on their résumés, but close.) The next summer I was offered an unpaid internship at Magnum Photos, which I decided to take knowing I'd have to spend every night after work as a waitress as well. My days that summer felt endless: 9 A.M. until 4:30 P.M. at the photo agency; 5 P.M. until midnight at the New Fuji Sushi and Steak house; 1 A.M. until 7 A.M. for sleep. But the contacts I made at Magnum were crucial in getting my photojournalism career off the ground after college.

Life-changing opportunities are rare, but they cannot actually change your life if you don't have the wherewithal to take them. I'm not just talking about jobs or degrees. I'm talking about taking any ameliorating step in any better direction whatsoever, be it leaving a bad marriage, moving to a new city, or having the time and means to acquire new skills. Even Friedrich Engels, defender of the working class, was the son of a wealthy capitalist who funded his and Karl Marx's criticisms of the very capitalism that offered them the time and means to speak out against it.

So many of the people I know who've succeeded wildly, particularly in the arts or journalism, have done so because they had an economic cushion, whether from family money or a wealthy spouse. It's the dirty little secret to which few will admit, with rare exceptions. Novelist Ann Bauer, in an essay in *Salon* entitled "'Sponsored' by my husband: Why it's a problem that writers never talk about where their money comes from," described a reading at which an audience member asked a well-respected nonfiction writer how he'd been able to spend ten years writing a single book. His answer was hard work and magazine writing, which infuriated Bauer, because his answer left out an important fact: that he is the heir to not just millions but to more millions than his interlocutor could have ever imagined. Many of the young journalists in

New York right now, earning journalism's increasingly meager starting salaries, have their rents, mortgages, and cellphone bills paid in full by Mom and Dad. The book-publishing industry has long been a bastion of young, privileged, white Ivy League grads, whose parents subsidize their early years as they climb up the poorly paid rungs at the bottom of the ladder.

Sharky's *no* to my twelve-week leave of absence to work on the next season of *Younger* will also cost me more than $12,000 a year in health insurance premiums, as I'll now have to switch to the PR company's $1,000-a-month plan instead of paying $150 a quarter for my more comprehensive Writers Guild insurance. It also means a change of in-network doctors. And that I can no longer see my shrink without going bankrupt. Absurd, our healthcare system. Insane, choosing between mental health and food. And no, the irony is not lost on me that my job is to help pharmaceutical companies earn enough lobbying millions to keep this enraging status quo thus.

The morning I pack up and leave L.A., I head to the check-out desk at the Standard hotel, where I've been staying for two weeks, assuming my room has been prepaid by the *Younger* production company, as previously agreed. Instead, I'm handed a bill totaling more than $6,000 for my two-week stay, parking, and meals. "I thought this was supposed to be prepaid?" I say.

"Nope, sorry. Just put it on your credit card and work it out with your company later."

"I . . . don't have a credit card," I say.

"Seriously?" he says, a look of imperious horror on his face. "Well, we take debit cards, too."

"Yes, but I don't have an extra six thousand dollars in my account." I have, in fact, checking my balance online, less than $1,000. I received a nominal income for consulting on the show, plus my vacation pay from the PR firm, but I've had to eat out for every meal while I was here, pay for gas and my car rental—without a credit card, they make you pay it up front—and then every month there's that sinkhole of medical debt, my children's college housing, tuition, and living expenses, monthly payments to Freedom Debt Relief, etc. It's been years since I've had my head above water.

I feel once again like Cinderella at the stroke of midnight, only instead of leaving behind an uncomfortable glass slipper and a besotted prince, I'm leaving behind a new spring in my sneakered step and a job with which I've fallen in love. I can't reach anyone in the finance department at the production company, and I need to get to the airport immediately, so I call Jill, my film and TV agent, realizing I will now have to admit to her, too, that I'm an adult without a credit card. Jill graciously volunteers to pay the bill with her own American Express card and get reimbursed by the production company, but I can tell I've fallen several notches in her estimation: never a good thing, with an agent, in a profession where appearances are everything. Goodbye, smoke. Goodbye, mirrors. Goodbye, respect and potential. Goodbye, eventually, Jill. I feel not only half shod and in rags, I feel utterly exposed, naked.

ENFP

APRIL–NOVEMBER 2016

Stepping back into the pumpkin of my PR job after two weeks of working in the *Younger* writers' room feels like heading back into prison after a furlough in Tahiti. The work feels as important as making license plates, if not less so. Worse, our department's not meeting its budgetary goals, so there's a new sheriff in town, McKenna, a thirty-something upper management type who's worked in marketing and public relations since college, unlike us rabble-rousing journalists, and now sits next to Sharky cracking the whip and speaking in acronyms. "I'll be OOO on Tuesday, so if you could get those KPI numbers from the AE for that new B2C campaign to put in the RFP, then talk to the guys in UX, see what they're planning for the rollout. Talk to key stakeholders, decide on a CTA that's impactful, then run it by their head of comms and circle back when you're done . . ." (Obviously not a real quote, but close.) I make the stupid mistake of asking McKenna, in the small talk of our first meeting, whether she and her partner have children. "Oh god, no! Please," she says, rolling her eyes.

To say she's a micromanager would be like saying Jack the Ripper enjoyed a little light shredding. She rewrites my copy, makes it worse, then blames me when the client is unhappy. Her communication set point is somewhere between passive aggressive and Marquis de Sade. During a staff meeting, when it's my turn to report on the status of my various projects, and I announce I've just had a meeting with our company's CEO about doing more speechwriting and op-ed work, she says, "And your point is . . . ?" One day, when the public undermining starts to feel untenable, I pull her aside and say, "I want to figure out how we could work better together. Are there constructive criticisms you could offer that might help ease the course of our interactions?"

"We're just different, you and I," she says. "Have you ever taken a Myers–Briggs?"

When I tell her I have not, she plans a mandatory testing day for our entire team. She gets ISTJ—introvert, sensing, thinking, judging—which is the exact opposite of my results, ENFP—extrovert, intuitive, feeling, perceiving.

But this test is absurd, I think. It asks binary questions requiring binary answers, which I could have answered either way, depending upon mood and circumstance. No one is all extrovert or all introvert, but the test leaves no room for grays. You're either one or the other, black or white, and then you get sorted by the MBTI sorting hat into sixteen categories, based on your results. Our test coordinator actually had us stand in different corners of the room, depending on our labels, with the mushy loud extroverts at one end of the wall and the buttoned up quiet introverts at the other. At one point, I catch McKenna's eyes from across the hypotenuse. She half smiles and shrugs: an "I told you so" made visible.

Psychologist Robert Hogan, in his book *Personality and the Fate of Organizations*, calls Myers–Briggs nothing more than "an elaborate Chinese fortune cookie," which leaves academics, who actually study such things using the data analytical tools of science, "baffled and annoyed by [its] astonishing popularity." Annie Murphy Paul, in her book *The Cult of Personality Testing*, writes, "As many as three-quarters of test takers achieve a different personality type when tested again, and the sixteen distinctive types described by the Myers–Briggs have no scientific basis whatsoever."

"See?" McKenna says, after the test is over. "We're just different. No hard feelings."

One morning, I get a call from my son's principal, saying there's been an accident on the school playground. Two boys have pushed my nine-year-old's face into a metal pole, which has knocked out his adult front tooth, and he's now bleeding so profusely that the principal has decided to rush him in her arms to the emergency dentist in Inwood herself, is that okay? I tell her yes, yes, please, go! My office is an hour away. I'll get there as fast as I can. On my sprint out, I stop at McKenna's desk to say I'm so sorry, I know today is an important meeting with a client, but I have to run.

She says, "Do you have a sitter who can deal with that?"

I cock my head. Take a deep breath. I need time, I know, to formulate a non-emotional response instead of an angry one. "Um, no," I finally say. "I mean, I do have a sitter, but she doesn't show up until 3, when he gets out of school. And this is not something I would actually leave in the hands of a sitter anyway, even if she were available. Plus she's even farther downtown from my son than I am right now. I'm really sorry. I have to go."

McKenna bites her lips, as if literally keeping herself from saying something she'll regret, raises her eyebrows, and crosses her arms over her chest. "Of course. You do what's best for you."

What's best for *me*? It's all I can do not to scream, *Fuck you! My son is bleeding on the fucking playground! Minus his front tooth! This shouldn't even be a discussion!* Instead I say, "Thanks for understanding, McKenna. I really appreciate it," and run out the door.

What am I missing by leaving the office? A meeting both McKenna and Sharky will be attending anyway with a giant pharmaceutical company to discuss creating a glossy magazine for the launch of their new eye drops to combat dry eye disease. This is what printing presses now do to stay solvent since the collapse of the magazine industry: They work with deep-pocketed corporations to create what looks like high-art, oversized, *Interview*-style magazines but are instead guerilla marketing tools with prosaic photography and anodyne articles on company-sanctioned themes: Technology! Innovation! Creativity! Wellness! Or in this case, Visionaries! (Get it? Eye drops/vision?) These magazines are then handed out at conferences and placed in hotel lobbies where conferencegoers gather, in order to elevate the company above their competition and to make a statement about who they are: Look at us, aren't we cool?

For the record, I tried those dry eye disease drops, and they are excellent. I still use them.

Soon after my son's playground accident—which costs unreimbursed thousands in dental reconstruction and eventually thousands more, when it all has to get redone a second, third, and then *fourth* time—my colleagues and I are asked to complete our yearly 360 reviews: a multiday, time-consuming task in which we are asked to solicit and write reviews of those above, below, and on equal footing with us. The previous 360s had taken place after I'd been at the company for only a few weeks, so I wasn't obliged to complete one back then. Which means I have no idea, when writing this year's reviews, that these reviews determine how much of the 2016 bonus pie each of us gets. In other words, it's in my best interest to denigrate my co-workers for my own financial gain.

Instead, I write glowing reviews, even for McKenna, whom I praise for her drive, organizational skills, and dedication, because while I definitely have my personal issues with her, professionally these attributes are true, and I believe in noting the good in everyone, even those who might make our lives difficult. My friend Tad likes to joke that I'm the kind of person who says, "Ivan the Terrible? Not so terrible."

I blame my father. "If you don't have anything nice to say about someone, then don't say anything at all," Dad always said. Perhaps your parents did, too. It's taken me an entire lifetime to unlearn this rule, golden as it may be, or at least to take exception to it when the occasion calls for it. Like in a sanctioned corporate version of a teen slam book.

After the results of the 360 are tallied, Sharky pulls me aside to say he's read complaints about my dedication to the job. "From whom?" I say. (From McKenna, duh.)

That's ridiculous, I say. The op-eds I've been writing for our various foundation clients have garnered us money, gratitude, praise. The hourlong, TED talk–style PowerPoint presentation I just produced for the CEO of a pharmaceutical company had their head of communications asking me if I'd be willing to jump ship and come work for her instead. The yearly internal company magazine, highlighting the outstanding work of ten employees, has just published a long feature, with photos, on me and my work. In other words, in my first year on the job, in a company with seven thousand employees, I've been singled out as one of the ten to watch. Sure, I don't love my job, but I am grateful for it and have been nothing if not 100 percent dedicated to it and to the company, to the point of having turned down an opportunity to be a staff writer on a hit TV show to prove my commitment.

"This is not about who," says Sharky. "Or about your work. It's about fit. Are you a good fit for this place?"

"Not a good fit" is HR doublespeak that can spell doom for older workers. At fifty, that's me. I am both the oldest person on our team and exactly the age at which phrases like "good fit" get thrown around. A year from now, a fifty-two-year-old Facebook employee will sue Facebook for age discrimination after he, too, is told he's a "poor cultural fit." In his suit, he will mention a 2007 speech by Mark Zuckerberg, in which Zuckerberg said, "Young people are just smarter."

But this time, for this job, I was careful when signing my employment contract. HR had tried to get me to sign another at will contract, but I'd refused, so the company has to prove cause for my dismissal if they want to fire me.

Sharky's job, I can sense, is on the line, too. Everyone at the company knows our 2016 numbers are in the toilet. The CEO has told us in a company-wide meeting. It's been reported in the news, too: an embarrassing 0 percent growth heading into 2017, compared to a high of 11.4 percent as recently as 2013. Our own team, or so I've heard, is over one million dollars in the hole. Which explains why the money guy is literally always looking over our shoulders and yelling. Plus it's an election year. Hillary Clinton is winning in the polls, and no one in the pharmaceutical and healthcare industry is sure what this means for their bottom lines—will the U.S. finally institute single-payer healthcare?—so nearly every one of our clients has been either tightening their belts or halting their marketing budgets altogether until after the election. "This is about McKenna, isn't it?" I say.

"It's not just about McKenna," says Sharky. "Leslie also said she had to pick up your slack when you were off gallivanting in Hollywood."

"Off . . . *gallivanting*?" I am shocked by this statement. Leslie and I sit next to each other. We are both single mothers, and we've bonded over this fact and its difficulties daily. I've edited all of her work without complaint whenever she's asked me to do so, which is often, and I've picked up her slack countless times. I take a deep breath, the shock of this *Et tu, Brute* moment settling in. "I took vacation days to do that job on *Younger*," I say. "I wasn't 'off gallivanting.' I was working. On my own earned time. And even if I *was* off gallivanting, Leslie would have still had to pick up my slack anyway, just like I pick up hers whenever she's out of the office or on vacation." It takes everything I have to go against my own nature and break my dad's golden rule about not maligning others. *Lashon hara*, we Jews call it, this "evil tongue" talking behind someone's back, and it is considered worse than idolatry, infidelity, and murder *combined*. "Who do you think did all the heavy lifting on her security system campaign? I did. On my own time." Her writing on that campaign was so bland, I was worried it would cost us the client. (It did.) I spent hours late at night, off the clock, editing and rewriting what I could.

"Then why did you write such a glowing review of her work?"

Because who shits on their co-workers like that? I want to say. *What kind of monsters do we all have to become in order to earn a living?* I think back to my first day of work, Leslie's weak handshake. "Because," I say, "up until this moment right now, I thought she deserved it."

Earlier that year, *The New York Times* had published an op-ed entitled "360 Reviews Often Lead to Cruel, Not Constructive, Criticism," in which the author highlighted such comments as "stop using your looks and personality to get things done," "I never really liked you," and, my personal favorite, "You seem to be constantly traveling all over the world. Is that really necessary?" aimed at an employee whose job was in international relations. Years earlier, the *Harvard Business Review* published a scathing indictment of 360s, which they called "at best, a waste of everyone's time, and at worst actively damaging to both the individual and the organization." The data generated from these reviews is not only bad, the author wrote, "It's always bad. . . . Why? Because your rating reveals more about you than it does about me."

There's also the thorny issue of LIFO, which is a management-speak acronym for *last in, first out*. Which, in my department, is me. I ask Sharky to level with me. Is my job on the line? Should I be polishing my résumé? He can barely look me in the eye. "Yes," he says.

I have lunch with Aaron, the account executive with whom I've been doing all of my foundation work and with whom I get along well. "I need to tell you something," he says. He'd written a glowing 360 review of me, without any criticisms, but McKenna had kicked it back to him, telling him he had to write something negative, too. Not knowing what to say, he made something up. "I said something like, 'Sometimes she can get a little overenthusiastic because she's still new to the job and learning.'" But now that criticism, he's since learned, is being used against me. He feels awful.

So that's why Leslie probably wrote something negative as well, I think. To save her own skin. I get it. She's a single mother, too, and she knows things are bad, and one of us has to go. I ask Sharky to show me Leslie's three negative comments, each of which I quickly debunk with written proof.

Thus begins several months of trying to simultaneously prove my worth at work while secretly sneaking off for other job interviews. "Where are you off to for two hours this afternoon?" McKenna asks, when she sees it blocked off on my calendar.

"Doctor's appointment," I say. The real answer is *Buzzfeed*. For an informational interview with Ben Smith, to whom I've reached out, among fifty others, hoping to jump ship before I sink.

Little Buddha

NOVEMBER 2016–FEBRUARY 2017

On November 11, 2016—two days after Trump's election—an email appears in my inbox from Ken Kurson: a company-wide missive, sent to everyone working or freelancing for the *Observer*. "As you have probably heard or will shortly hear, the Observer has ended the print edition of the New York Observer," it begins, making no mention of the fact that our owner, Jared Kushner, is now the president-elect's son-in-law, or what this will mean either for us or for the paper. "A few columnists, who were edited by Lorraine,"—that would be me—"will be assigned to new editors," he writes, along with a long list of other housekeeping minutiae, such as the fact that pizza day will be moved to Monday instead of Tuesday. He ends with this kicker: "Our future is brighter than it's ever been. We are hiring journalists and investing in storytelling."

Really? I think. Hiring? Why not me? I had by then written eight columns for the *Observer*, all of which have done well or gone viral, but here I am, still relegated to freelancing. I quickly respond to Ken's email: "Pizza day? How had I never heard of pizza day? When does the pizza arrive? How would one find their way to said pie? All sounds good and normal to me. Onward!"

---------- Forwarded message ----------
From: **Ken Kurson** <kkurson@observer.com>
Date: Fri, Nov 11, 2016 at 3:45 PM
Subject: Re: Observer print edition
To: Deborah Copaken <███████████████>

1 pm.

How come you never asked me out?

OBSERVER
Ken Kurson, Editor in Chief
212 407 9356 | kkurson@observer.com
1 Whitehall Street, Floor 7, New York NY 10004
Observer reaches over 6M influencers every month.

> On Nov 11, 2016, at 2:17 PM, Deborah Copaken <███████████████> wrote:
>
> Pizza day? How had I never heard of pizza day? When does the pizza arrive? How would one find their way to said pie?
>
> All sounds good and normal to me. Onward!

Email received from Ken Kurson, 11/11/2016

An hour and a half later, his pithy response lands with a sick thud in my inbox: "1 pm. How come you never asked me out?"

I start to hyperventilate. I can't catch my breath. I'm clutching my chest. My PVCs are going into overdrive. I feel like I'm having a heart attack. Sharky, who sits behind me, takes notice. "What's going on?" he says.

I show him the email. "Holy fuck," he says. "That's totally not okay. Are you okay?"

"I can't . . . breathe," I barely eke out. So that's why Ken never officially hired me. That's why I ended up working here at the PR firm instead of there in the newsroom. He wanted to fuck me, not edit me, but he knew if he hired me and tried to fuck me, he'd be liable.

Oh my god. It's all so clear now. I'm such an idiot.

That lunch, way back when, when he offered me the $65,000 a year to jump ship and then mysteriously took the offer away: all a ploy to get in my pants. It had nothing to do with my writing, my skills, what I could offer to the paper. I'm just a body. A cock hole. An amalgam of ladyparts. All of the skin-crawlingly icky emails and comments come back to haunt me, obvious breadcrumbs: *In another life, I'd be Mr. Copaken; I love your sloppy seconds!; Are you proposing marriage to me?; What would be*

my chances on the open market of finding a soul mate?; Pussy chase; Wow,
it's so weird—here we are talking about your story about your breast can-
cer while I'm staring at your breasts.

We're still a year away from Harvey Weinstein and #MeToo. Still in
the era when speaking up about such things can get you blackballed.
Plus, as a freelancer, I don't have the rights of an employee, so I can't
even go to the *Observer*'s HR department to report this. If my editor Lorraine is gone—my only other contact at the paper—to whom would I
even report his email anyway? And let's not forget who Ken's best friends
are: Rudy Giuliani, Jared Kushner, and our new predator-elect.

I feel on the verge of throwing up. This is no longer icky boundary
crossing. It's sexual harassment, plain and simple. From his company
email address, no less. And this nine-word email, on top of Trump's
pussy-grabbing election, on top of fretting every day over losing my third
job in three years—first for spending too much time at Sloan Kettering,
then for not "dumbing it down and making it shorter," now for a $1.2 mil-
lion budget hole and a toxic co-worker and god knows what else—turns
out to be too much for my body. Eventually, after rereading the email a
dozen times, I slump over in my office chair and pass out.

The next thing I remember, I'm in the waiting room of an emergency room. No, no one in my office called an ambulance to get me
here. I wouldn't allow it, afraid as I was of any surprise bills during a
moment when I might soon be out of a job. Instead, after I fell out of my
chair, Erin, one of my co-workers, apparently ordered an Uber and
helped me into the back seat, telling the driver to get me to the nearest
hospital. I have no memory of this other than the feeling of being gently
maneuvered into the back of a car by kind, female hands. The waiting
room is crowded. Noisy. I feel boxed in, alone. Still struggling to breathe.
This is no place for a woman having a panic attack or whatever the hell
this is. I google the nearest doctor's office, a few blocks away, and show
up without an appointment. He's not in my plan. I leave. I call my cardiologist's office from the street. Tell the receptionist it's an emergency.
Come right now, she says. We'll squeeze you in.

Now I'm half clothed on an exam table, sticky electrodes glued to my
chest. "You need to rest," says the cardiologist, seeing a dangerous level
of PVCs, "until we get this under control." When she asks about my
various stressors, about what happened in the seconds leading up to my

blackout, I tell her about Ken's sexually harassing email, about an admitted rapist winning the presidency, about the constant threat of getting fired with two kids in college. She can't do anything about the first two, she says, but she can at least make sure I'm not heading into the lion's den of a job in crisis every day for a little while, as my heart heals. She hands me a prescription for various medications that will stop my heart from skipping so many extra beats plus a note to my employers stating that I am not to go to the office for now.

I still put in dozens of hours for a big—oh, the irony—heart valve client from my bed, but this enforced month of recovering at home, followed by weeks of steady recuperation back at work, during which I'll faint two more times, once hitting my head on McKenna's desk on the way down, will ironically save me from getting fired before the end of 2016. Employment judges do not look favorably upon employers who fire their workers while they're on disability and/or still passing out at work, and HR knows this.

When I'm finally off the beta-blockers, well-rested, back in good health, and moving forward with a half a dozen marketing assignments, Sharky stops by my desk to say, "We have to talk."

I see the real pain in his face and know it's over.

My official termination meeting takes place on February 17, 2017. The firing happens, of all places, in our newly built meditation room, which is the only private room not currently being occupied by our colleagues when Sharky stops by my desk to do the deed. The meditation room has a single cushion in it, for reclining during the meditative breaks no one ever has time to come in here and take, as well as a small stone Buddha and a few sad-looking chimes.

I stare at the Buddha, as we walk into the room, realizing he will now become one of the thousands of visual memory scraps I keep in my mental storage box, recorded during moments of violation, pain, sadness, or fear, each begging for release into the world, transformed. A slice of pizza, for example, is now forever paired with receiving that sexually harassing email from Kurson. Any gun, whether noticed on a cop's belt or a movie screen, conjures my muggings. Bananas trigger the day after my hysterectomy, when I left a trail of blood on the stairs in search of sustenance. And from this day forward, whenever I spot a small Buddha, I am immediately brought back to this sunlit room.

Because I've walked in first, in front of Sharky, I wonder whether I should take the one floor pillow or leave it for him. It's a small room. There's probably not even room for two chairs if we wanted them. "You take it," he says, reading my thoughts. "I have bad knees."

I sit cross-legged on the meditation cushion, pushing my skirt between my knees so as not to flash my boss, and I suddenly regret this positional choice because here we are: Sharky, all in black, his pro-basketball-player-sized frame towering over my tiny body; me, self-consciously hiding my underwear behind the fabric of my skirt like a nervous kindergartner during story time, sitting so low to the ground, I can barely make out Sharky's facial features from here. He looks like a movie screen projection of himself that I'm trying to view, in vain, from the first row. Moreover, the sun's so bright, my giant boss appears backlit, a hulking figure in dark shadow. Even if I'd remained standing, the physical power imbalance between us would have been comical, but this?

"I'm doing you a favor," he says at one point. "Believe me. You don't belong in here. You belong out there"—he points to the outside world—"making shit that matters. One day, you'll thank me for this."

"That's not your call to make," I say. "I need this job. My kids need me to have this job. What ever happened to 'You're indispensable to the team,' when I asked for a leave of absence to work on *Younger*? That was two months ago." The *Younger* writers' room ironically starts this week, but the job is now no longer mine to reclaim. "Is there any way at this point to save my job? A pay cut? Part-time?"

"No," he says. He's sorry. He's really sorry. (I'm crying now.) This is the worst part of his job. I'll land on my feet. He knows it. There's nothing he can do. "It's about fit. You're not a good fit," he repeats like a mantra whose meaninglessness is the point. Apt, since we're in the meditation room.

"Not a good fit!" Rafe, a senior creative executive, had said to me, unable to stop laughing, when he'd heard my job was on the chopping block a month earlier. The two of us had done a lot of brainstorming together and got along well. In fact, whenever he had a thorny problem he couldn't solve, he'd come over to my desk and ask me to sit with him, quietly, as we took turns free-associating. "That's ridiculous! They knew exactly who you were when you arrived here, and you have never once disappointed us. They hired you because you're you, not because they wanted you to fit your square peg into a round PR hole. This is bullshit."

"So, please. Help me save my job," I said to Rafe.

"I'll try," he said. "But ultimately it's Sharky's call to make. You're on his team. I can't step on his toes."

A week later, Rafe pulled me aside and said, "I want you to know that, no matter what happens, this is not about you. You've done nothing but good work here, and we all know it."

"So if you're a bestselling author, like, what are you doing working here?" McKenna once asked, and I made the mistake of answering honestly.

"Because I have to," I said. Isn't that why we're all here?

The first rule in marketing is "Know your audience." To whom are you speaking? Why are you speaking to them? What is it you're trying to say? What do they want to hear? How will you make them hear it? In fact, more than any other factor, my not understanding my audience probably lost me my job or at the very least pushed it over the edge. It didn't occur to me, when answering McKenna's question honestly, that those four little words—"Because I have to"—would stand as a rebuke to her entire life story and her sense of self-worth.

"What about severance?" I say to Sharky.

"No severance," he says. "We don't have the budget."

"Please," I say, snot running out of my nose. "I've been talking to a million people, but I haven't nailed down an actual job yet. I've been too busy trying to save my job here. I just need a couple of months to land on my feet."

"Sorry," he says. I lock eyes with the Buddha and remember his four noble truths: 1) Existence is suffering; 2) Suffering has a cause; 3) Suffering has an end; 4) A path exists that leads to the end of suffering.

My sole job now is to find that fucking path.

Bloody Mother's Day

MAY 2017

I am lying on an exam table in my doctor's office, naked from the waist down. "Okay, so, here's the problem," says the physician's assistant. "We don't even have a pull-down menu option for whatever this is."

It's the beginning of Mother's Day weekend, 2017. My legs are in stirrups, toes curled inward, and the speculum that has just been yanked out of me is now covered in blood. As are my underwear, my jeans, and increasingly part of the floor of my primary care physician's office, where I'm being seen by the PA because I showed up here, without an appointment, after waking up in a red puddle. I've also been bleeding quite copiously—Carrie-at-the-prom level, all over the sheets—and feeling intense pain during sex with a new partner, a fact I attributed to the freakish size of him until this morning's deluge, which was unprompted by anything but a good night's sleep, alone.

"What do you mean there's no pull-down menu option?"

The PA is squinting at the various insurance codes on her computer screen, now with a nurse looking over her shoulder, too, plus someone else who has been summoned into the room, all of whom are squinting and searching and pointing at the screen, whispering words I don't understand. "I mean," she finally turns to me and says, "I can choose abnormal *uterine* bleeding—you know, miscarriages, pregnancy spotting, postpartum bleeding, stuff like that—but there's no option for abnormal *nonuterine* bleeding." She looks over her shoulder, back at me: "When did you say your last menstrual cycle was?"

If I had a dime for every time a doctor or nurse, staring straight at the word hysterectomy on my chart, or having just heard me say outright, "I had a hysterectomy," has asked me when was the date of my last menstrual cycle, I'd have enough dimes to buy a jumbo-sized box of tampons. Maybe two. For someone else. With a uterus. "I didn't. I don't have a uterus."

"Oh, right. Duh. Sorry."

"So what should I do?" I say to no one, feeling vulnerable with my diagnostic code–less cavity exposed, as the three medical professionals in the room focus all of their attention on the thorny issue of how to define my vaginal Vesuvius for reimbursement. Meanwhile, the PA's attempt at a Pap smear has not only failed, it has further antagonized my already aggrieved cervix, meaning blood is now geysering out.

"What you should do," says the PA, snapping off her rubber gloves and looking concerned, "is to rush over to the hospital right now. I'll call ahead, so you don't have to wait in the emergency room. Go straight to gynecologic oncology." She hands me a clown-sized sanitary pad.

Go straight to gynecologic oncology? Not exactly the words I was hoping to hear after this fun-filled week, which included but was not limited to the following:

1. Applying for unemployment, as I've done every Sunday now for two months;
2. Liquidating my 401K to pay for a few months of extra COBRA coverage;
3. Preparing the paperwork to represent myself at a custody hearing in family court, now that my ex is back in New York;
4. Receiving the unfortunate news that, since my executive at NBC was either fired or resigned, the *Shutterbabe* pilot I co-wrote with Eddie will not be produced or shot.

"Do you ever wonder why so many bad things keep happening to you?" friends with household incomes twice the GDP of Tonga ask during this period. The subtext being: *What are you personally doing to cause this bad luck?* Everyone else—particularly those of my friends recently downsized from the publishing world, all of whom, back in the pre-digital '90s, had no reason not to assume that the lavish book parties and magazine budgets and publishing contracts wouldn't go on forever, if you were disciplined and shrewd and put in the sweat equity—keeps their mouths shut. They know, because they know, and because watching my one step forward/two steps back health and employment tango has reminded them: *There but for the grace of God go I.*

Let's do some on-the-dole math, circa 2017: If unemployment brings in $403 a week, but your rent has risen from $2,300 a month to $2,701 a month (the precise amount of money at which a landlord can flip a rent-stabilized apartment into market rate, so now the landlord is really doing nothing to maintain the apartment, as he wants to force you out); family COBRA is $2,314.20 a month; you just paid $12,000 to cover your ex's tax bill—money you were saving to pay a lawyer to divorce him; your daughter's college tuition and housing fees are due imminently; you have a $600-a-month repayment schedule to the debt relief scammers; and you also need food, a phone, electricity, etc.; how much money is left over after a $30 taxi fare to the hospital? Ding ding ding! You are correct: Less than zero. Hence the draining of your 401K, with all the financial penalties that this entails. What about the $2.75 subway fare, can you afford that? Depends if you can find a new permanent job in the next three months, instead of this patchwork of gigs, before your 401K dries up. Given that you're now bleeding, and that this blood might cloud future employment plans, we'll call that a tentative no.

But wait. There's still a doctor waiting for you in gynecologic oncology at Columbia/Presbyterian, eighty-three blocks north. Do you briefly contemplate walking? Yes. Because walking, as you've discovered, is not only an excellent antidote to the absurd cost of a modern-day gym membership—one gym quoted you $200 a month, and you literally lol'd—it's also a stopgap solution to the rising cost of public transportation, which recently jumped from $2.50 to $2.75 a ride. So now you're standing on the sidewalk on the corner of 85th and Madison, in front of a gleaming store selling designer yoga pants for $128 a pair, under an apartment listed at $28.5 million, crunching more numbers in your head. If twenty blocks equals one mile, and it takes you, on average, approximately fifteen minutes to walk each mile, how many minutes will it take you to walk to the hospital? The answer is a little over an hour, plus you'll have to walk several blocks west through Central Park as well, so add on approximately fifteen more minutes. Not so bad, an hour-and-fifteen-minute walk, under nonemergency circumstances, particularly if it involves a stroll through blooming trees on a spring day. But the clown pad between your legs is growing soggier, and the 86th Street crosstown bus has just appeared a block away, and the ladyparts oncologist is waiting, so do you walk to the hospital to save the $2.75 or run to catch the bus to the subway?

And the answer is . . . twelve: the number of seconds it takes you to sprint to the bus.

Once on the bus, that great American equalizer, I glance around at my fellow passengers and wonder what hidden blood they bleed. A body breaking down is normal. That's the fate to which all living creatures eventually succumb. But rushing to a hospital on a city bus, in the richest country on earth? No. Not normal. Or at least it shouldn't be.

Thankfully, I'm seen by the oncologist immediately. He takes one look through the speculum and orders an immediate cervical biopsy. "This will hurt," he says, and I am both grateful for his honesty and flattened by the pain: imagine a foot-long needle followed by a set of pliers up your vaginal canal, yanking off a bite-sized chunk. He then places a pasty substance up there to stop the bleeding until we figure out what's going on, which feels like a definite step in the right direction.

The eventual diagnosis? HPV 16 and 18 and precancer of the cervix. HPV 16 and 18 are what are known as the "bad" HPV, meaning they cause 80 percent of all cervical cancers and lesions. They are also the main reason Gardasil, the HPV vaccine I was helping to market at the PR firm, was developed: Alas, too late for me, but all three of my children have been vaccinated, so let's hear it for small mercies.

By the time I receive this diagnosis, a few days after the biopsy, the cervical putty has fallen out, and I'm waking up in puddles of blood again. I meet with Dr. June Hou, one of the two gynecologic oncology surgeons at Columbia/Presbyterian who's been trained in performing robotic trachelectomies (removal of the cervix). A date is set for an eight-hour surgery a week and a half later.

"Why, if I may ask, did you choose not to have the cervix removed when you got your hysterectomy five years ago?" says Dr. Hou. I'm now dressed, sitting across from her, a desk between us.

"I was told that it is believed to play a role in sexual pleasure," I say.

Dr. Hou, whose bedside manner has been as smooth as a glassy pond on a windless day, suddenly bristles, her mouth pinching into a line. "That's been debunked," she says.

"*What?!*" I sit with this information, shaking my head and blowing air out of deflating cheeks. "Of course it has," I finally say. "So now I have to undergo another eight-hour operation when I could have just had the whole thing yanked out five years ago and been done with it. All because my doctor gave me bad advice?"

"Don't blame your doctor," says Dr. Hou. "We've all been in the dark. *All* of us." Almost everything about women's health, she says, has been conjecture up until now, and we're only finally just scratching the surface of what's actually going on inside of us. It was only a year prior, after all, that a 3D model of the clitoris was finally produced. Modern science has been either neglecting the study of women's bodies or getting us wrong, over and over again, and every day, right here in her office, she sees the havoc wreaked by that ignorance.

Dr. Hou and I both sigh. And then break into the laughter of exhausted soldiers who've been sitting together in a lifelong trench. Wars don't have to be sparked by a gun-toting aggressor to be fatal, demoralizing, inhumane. Neglect and willful ignorance of the bodily mechanics of half of earth's population are equally destructive and deadly.

I fall a little bit in love with Dr. Hou at this point. She's young. Smart. Passionate. No nonsense. She doesn't wedge unnecessary words into the hard silences or rush me out of her office. She allows me to sit and take it all in before speaking. "I promise," she says, "you will feel the full range of sexual function after this surgery. In fact, sex might even be better, now that you're no longer bleeding and in pain. You'll have to wait the requisite twelve weeks post-op, of course."

"Of course."

"*Nothing* can go up there, understand? Not even your own finger. You'll also need a caretaker after surgery for about two weeks or so. Do you have someone in mind?"

Ah, yes. The dreaded emergency contact/caretaker issue when you are single. It rustles up that quinfecta of uncomfortable feelings: sadness, self-loathing, failure, abandonment, and fear. What kind of woman wakes up at fifty-one without an emergency contact? You do, you think. Take responsibility for the mess of your life, and figure this out.

I think back to the situation at home after my hysterectomy. The blood on the stairs, the hernia popped, the begging for food that never came, my son in the taxi after midnight, three flights down, waiting twenty minutes for help with the fare.

I cannot relive that experience, in any form.

"I'll figure it out," I say.

I run through the possibilities close to home. My older son is living abroad, teaching English in Thailand, so he's out. My daughter's away at college and about to head to Israel on an all-expenses-paid trip, and I will not deny her that experience. My little one, ten, is still too young to be a proper caregiver, plus he's leaving for summer camp anyway. My mother does not feel comfortable either in my neighborhood or in my home. If the elevator goes out while she's here—as it so often does—she won't be able to deal with the stairs, she tells me. As for my friends, they're all in the sandwich generation, dealing with ailing older parents and young kids while holding down full-time jobs.

Which leaves Eddie.

Hospitals Are Not My Thing

JANUARY 1, –JUNE 2017

Five months before my cervix blew a gasket, Eddie, my *Shutterbabe* screenwriting partner, called from L.A. on New Year's Day to tell me that he'd moved into one of his extra houses. He and his wife were getting separated, he said, and I was the second person he'd called. "Who was the first?" I said.

"My sister."

"Huh."

So my Spidey-Sense was right. He did have feelings for me that went beyond collegial. And I could tell by the pregnant pause in our conversation—highly unusual for our particular verbal gymnastics— that he was waiting for me to speak first.

I'd never thought of married Eddie that way, except to once wonder, when we were on one of our many walks, why I couldn't find someone in my age range with whom I could feel as simpatico as I so easily felt with him. He was not my usual physical type: over a foot and a half taller than me and ill-at-ease in his body. And yet we worked well together professionally. We were already good friends and had been for several years. And I was the second person to whom he'd reached out after calling his sister to say he was getting divorced. Could I make the mental paradigm shift, after nine years of platonic friendship and now a professional partnership, from colleague to romantic partner? I'd made a vow to myself to keep an open mind when it came to finding love. Kindness, empathy, and honesty were nonnegotiable. Everything else was window dressing.

Thus began a daily email, text, and telephone correspondence between us, during which feelings were admitted and dissected, all with a welcome lack of reserve and coyness born of an already well-constructed work dynamic and friendship. As with our screenwriting index cards, everything was immediately laid out on the kitchen table, to be sorted and arranged in whatever logical narrative arc we chose. Sometimes we'd speak several times in a single day, particularly on weekends, for hours at a time. It was decided that Eddie should come for the long President's Day weekend in February, when my son would be with his father. The idea was to see if the two of us were as compatible in a hotel room without a script as we were with one.

The answer was yes, with several caveats. First I had to tell him I just got fired in the meditation room, an hour before his plane landed: not the most auspicious start to our first romantic weekend. Then I had to leave to attend a memorial gathering for my friend and former neighbor Marco, who'd just died of lung cancer. His widow is one of my best friends, and their children, who are my children's age, had grown up as much in my home as in theirs.

Marco, who'd cooked some of the more memorable Sunday meals of my family's lives, was the Italian journalist who'd coaxed Nora into telling him all about her secret plans for *Julie and Julia* at one of my dinner parties. Much to Nora's delight, Marco had also quickly identified both the Ligurian town and the name of the cheese inside the focaccia she'd once eaten and loved but had never been able to locate again. Later, Marco would memorialize their exchange in Italian *Vanity Fair*, a few days after Nora's death:

> "That town is called Recco," I say. "Stracchino is the name of that cheese; it's better known as crescenza," and she smiles again. And I am happy, and so is everyone else at the table, because then we can talk all evening about cheeses from Vermont and cheeses from the Ligurian Apennine Mountains, and about the joy of discovering that you have things in common with one another, such as finding the

perfect dish in just the right restaurant, and about how some things cannot be separated from the place where they belong, because they'll lose their flavor. A bit like cheese focaccia eaten far from Recco. Or New York without Nora Ephron.

Now New York was suddenly without Marco, too. My grief over this was both brand-new and guilt-plagued: I'd been so busy trying to hold on to my job, I'd visited only once during his final days. He'd slept through the whole thing as his wife and I lay on their bed, holding hands and free-associating.

"I'm really sorry, but I have to go pay my last respects to a good friend," I say to Eddie, minutes after telling him I got fired. (*Boy*, I can imagine him thinking, *I did not sign up for* this.) "But you're more than welcome to come with me?" (*Please come with me*, I thought. *It would be so nice to have someone to lean on right now.*)

It didn't feel like any of his business, Eddie said, plus he was tired from the flight and needed a nap.

Fair enough. It would be slightly weird to have him tag along. Then again, I'd accompanied Gio, at his request, to a memorial gathering for one of his good friends I'd never met, and I'd found it both moving and inspiring. The point of remembering the dead is not just to pay tribute to the life lost but to lend succor to those shattered by the silence. My friend, Marco's widow, had practically begged me to bring Eddie along. "Kicking off your first romantic weekend with a new beau at Marco's memorial? Oh my god, Marco would have *loved* that. Please bring him. I insist!"

Eddie and I made a plan to meet up afterward.

Back at the hotel, utterly depleted by Marco's gathering and feeling more in need of a platonic hug than a first sexual encounter with an old friend, I then had to—caveat number three, and I know this sounds petty—overcome my revulsion to thick back hair. Caveat four was the structural delta between us: A man who shops only in big and tall stores versus a woman who often shops in the boys' department, size fourteen, turns out to be a complicated issue of mechanics. The third night of our inaugural long romantic weekend together was the first time my blood splattered all over the sheets. "Did I do that?" Eddie said, looking horrified.

"I dunno," I said, feeling all kinds of physical pain down there I'd never previously felt plus embarrassment over the blood bath. It wasn't like a menstrual blood accident from my pre-hysterectomy days. That I could handle: It goes with the territory of being born with a uterus. This was straight out of a horror film. The sheets were so soaked and splattered, I was worried the housekeepers would think we'd murdered someone. "That's never happened before."

Everything else about our rapidly budding romance, however, felt nourishing. We could talk for hours without getting bored. When we were apart, FaceTime stepped in to keep us connected. He loved to gallery-hop as much as I did, and visiting a camera store was at least as big a thrill for him as it was for me, if not more. Biking, my preferred mode of urban transport, was also his favorite way to explore the city. Because money was never an issue for him, thanks to a bottomless cup of TV residuals, his frequent cross-country visits and their associated costs—he liked having dinner out, staying in nice hotels, seeing Broadway shows—were neither a financial nor logistical burden. And it was relaxing for me to get a break from a life of constant impecunity.

It had never occurred to me that one could order both an appetizer and a main course plus a full bottle of wine followed by dessert and coffee without panicking over paying rent. In fact, eating out with friends had become so stressful of late—*If I order just the cheapest appetizer and nothing else, will they still make me split the bill evenly?*—I'd simply stopped accepting invitations that involved menus and credit cards.

So, yes. Of course. The thought did cross my mind, after Eddie and I had been dating for several months, and I still hadn't found a new job, that, should we work out as a couple, the financial anxiety keeping me up every night, leading to frequent suicidal ideation, would end. I could write novels again, all day, without worrying about selling them first. I could write magazine articles and scripts, essays and op-eds. I could have healthcare, go on a vacation now and then.

I should also add that I hated myself for thinking this way.

"Have you actually thought about how you would kill yourself?" my shrink had asked when I brought it up again, before I no longer had the proper health insurance to keep seeing him. My Writers Guild health insurance, unlike any other health insurance I'd ever had—all of which had limited the number of times you could visit a mental health professional to thirty sessions per year—paid for 85 percent of *unlimited* psy-chiatric treatment. A lifesaver while I had it. Literally.

"Yes," I said. "And it's always the same scenario. I throw myself out a window. And I can't get that image out of my head. It feels . . . constant."

"Is there anything that quiets it?"

"Yes. Getting out of bed and looking at my sleeping child."

"And when he's not home?"

"That's a problem."

The phrase "deaths of despair"—deaths related to alcohol, drugs, and suicide—had begun appearing in newspapers and magazines around this time, thanks to Princeton economists Anne Case and Angus Deaton's groundbreaking paper published in 2015, followed by another in 2017. The alarm bells were stark: The U.S. population had "a marked increase in the all-cause mortality of middle-aged white non-Hispanic men and women in the United States between 1999 and 2013." This sudden uptick in white people deaths, they wrote, "reversed decades of progress in mortality and was unique to the United States; no other rich country saw a similar turnaround."

And what age adult was primarily affected by these American deaths of despair? As of 2014—the precise year I was suddenly on my own and finding it impossible to keep my head above water—it was Gen Xers, like me, in the thick of midlife. Why? Exactly what you might think: income inequality, lack of living wage job opportunities, and the rising cost of housing and healthcare as either our wages grew stagnant, or we were downsized and/or suddenly facing age discrimination. We'd all played the game by the rules, throughout our adult lives, but you can't win a game rigged against you. The math doesn't work. The numbers don't crunch. They crush you.

So when Eddie called, wrote, and texted me every day from L.A. to say, "I love you," or when we were out riding bikes in New York, or when we were standing in front of art we both loved or having dinner with friends or walking hand in hand, and I was feeling more grounded and at peace than I had in years, I did slowly allow myself to imagine a future in which kindness prevailed, healthcare costs didn't make me sicker, and daily thoughts of suicide were muted. By the end of March, I'd in-troduced him to my kids. Yes, yes, the accepted rule of thumb is that you're supposed to wait at least six months to introduce your children to a new love interest, but since the younger two had already met him as my friend and then, more recently, as my collaborator, I figured this was different. I knew this man.

Or so I thought. Suffice it to say, there's a reason why marital vows include the phrase "in sickness and in health." It's easy to love a healthy partner. The real test is when someone you claim to love gets sick.

After leaving my meeting with Dr. Hou, nearly six months into my relationship with Eddie, I call him in L.A. to tell him about the decision to remove my bum cervix and to ask him, please, to be my postsurgical caretaker. "I realize it's a lot to ask," I say, but only because I'm still not used to asking for help. It's a tic, this throat-clearing preamble. I do realize it's a lot to ask. But I also know it shouldn't be.

"Sorry," he says. "Hospitals are not my thing." His mother died in a hospital when he was in college. It's too traumatic for him. "I'm not good at hospitals."

I am nonplussed by this response. "My dad died in a hospital," I say. "That's often what happens in hospitals. People die. And it's traumatic. How did you deal with the birth of your son?"

"That was really hard for me."

I picture his wife, having just finished the painful work of labor, having to comfort him instead of vice versa.

He asks for time to process. It's a lot to take in. Sure, I say, trying to show him the empathy I myself am asking for, by seeing my request from his point of view: the annoyance of having your first postmarital girlfriend get sick six months into a new relationship; a visceral fear of hospitals. I google "fear of hospitals." It has a name. Nosocomephobia. And it's not only apparently quite common, the internet is rife with advice on how to get over it.

The following night, he doubles down. "Look," he says. "I talked to my shrink, and he says I do not need to go."

"Your *shrink*?" It is our first major fight, over the phone, and it gets ugly.

Hospital trauma, Eddie says, is real. And I should respect that. My bum cervix is real, I say. And he should respect that. What does he think the rest of our lives are going to look like, now that we're in our fifties, rainbows and unicorns? I'm pretty sure that hospitals will play at least a recurring if not starring role. ("Enjoy this time of your life," Nora once told me, when I was complaining about the vapidity of a recent holiday party. "By the time you get to my age, your entire social life will revolve around hospital visits and shivas.")

"Let's talk tomorrow," I say. "When we're both less angry." I hang up the phone and cry myself to sleep. How can a man who tells me he loves me, several times a day, not be able to show it by showing up when I need him? Does every man lack empathy? My ex's Asperger's shrink had posited that all men fall somewhere on the autism spectrum. It was just a matter of where.

The next morning, I call my friend Tad to get his male perspective. Tad has met and liked Eddie. A lot. And he has known both me and my romantic history since college. He didn't trust Gio. Thought Durkheim and I were mismatched, energy-wise. Was wary of Santi's intentions: love or a green card? A writer of brilliant and often hilarious profiles for *The New Yorker*, each drilling down to the essence of his subjects by filtering out the noise and noting only the telling details, Tad has a preternatural ability to read humans. "Am I asking too much?" I say, starting to cry again.

"No," Tad says, "but give him time. He may come around."

I wish Eddie could understand my needs without my having to spell them out, beg for care, or shift my limited focus—during this particular moment of real fear—onto his irrational ones.

"I know," says Tad. "But for him those fears are not irrational. They are as real as yours. You either have to accept him for who he is, faults and all, or . . ."

"Or?"

"Or not."

That night, I write Eddie a long email, in which I say, as kindly but as bluntly as possible, that his not showing up at my bedside will be the end of us. In a sense, I'm almost glad we've had to face this challenge early on. Better now than several years from now, when I've moved out to L.A. or he's moved here to New York, or whatever it is we would have decided. "My needs, vis-à-vis a potential partner, are clear," I write. "Whomever I choose next as a life partner has to be able to show up, as best he can, even if his best is flawed."

Begrudgingly, after many more discussions with his shrink and me, he agrees to come. But not to the hospital itself. Only to my apartment after the surgery is over, and only for a couple of days. Following more tears, professions of love, and negotiations, he finally agrees to come to New York the day before my surgery to join my daughter and me at the hospital, but he will go only as far as the waiting room. When they call us into the pre-op room, with its curtained pens of humans awaiting excision, he has to leave, he says. He can't see me in a hospital gown. It will be too triggering.

My daughter's jaw drops to the floor as he waves goodbye and heads downtown to see the Rauschenberg exhibit at MoMA. "He's going to a *museum?* While you're getting *surgery?* Mom, seriously. Fuck this dude. You deserve better."

"I know," I say. Dating in middle age, I tell her vaguely, as we wait for the anesthesiologist to arrive, has been . . . challenging.

When I awake from having my cervix removed, my daughter is standing over me in the recovery room holding my hand: a nice change from my hysterectomy, when I awoke to the sounds of the nurses whispering, "Where's the husband? We can't find the husband."

"Where's Eddie?" I say.

"Being a tourist still, I guess?" says my daughter.

"I thought he'd somehow see the light and come around."

"Mom, seriously?" She rolls her eyes. "How are you feeling?"

"Like shit," I say. "Like I'm about to pass out from the pain. Thanks for being here."

"You're welcome," says my daughter. "You have a morphine button. Use it." She sleeps in the chair next to my hospital bed that night, both of us periodically awoken by loud beeps when the saline solution runs low. The next morning, she helps me dress, pushes me in a wheelchair, and helps me into a taxi.

When we arrive back in Inwood, Eddie helps me into bed. I can sense his discomfort in witnessing my pain, but still, he's here. That's something. And I'm grateful. I ask him to please pick up my pain meds at the drugstore. He seems relieved to be given an errand outside the apartment. "Sure!" he says. "Do you need anything else?"

I stare down at my torso, still pumped full of air from the surgery and crisscrossed with incisions where the robot arms had diced and dismantled my cervix before pulling it out through a port in my belly button, bit by bit. One of the incisions hurts far worse than the others.

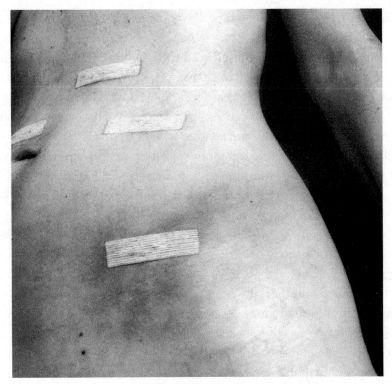

Infected incision, June 2017, © Deborah Copaken

In fact, it feels as if it's burning. "Does this look infected to you?" I say to Eddie, pointing to it. It's warm to the touch, tender and snot-colored.

"Yes," says Eddie, barely able to look at my ravaged body.

I tell him to wait on fetching the pain meds until I text the above photo of the incision to my surgeon, as I might need antibiotics now, too. This was the right call. My surgeon's office immediately phones in a second prescription to the drugstore as well.

My mother has sent a bunch of containers and bagels from Zabar's, the famous Upper West Side food mecca, just like back when my daughter was born and she drove up with my dad to help out with cooking, cleaning, and errands for the first week of the baby's life: a true gift, grandparents who show up like that and help out with the infants and fill the refrigerator with deli salads. But that was when I was married and living a middle-class life around the corner from stores like Zabar's and the Gap, instead of dollar stores and pawn shops, and not living hand-to-mouth on $403 a week in unemployment and the rapidly dwindling scraps of my 401K, most of which are going to pay the COBRA bill and a slumlord.

The contrast between these two me's, when the familiar containers of cream cheese and egg salad show up twenty years later, feels stark. Back then, in 1997, I had a brand-new baby, a working uterus, my parents' physical presence and care, a marriage, a half-decent if modest home, a job with benefits, and a father who loved to take my toddler out for bagels at Zabar's while my mom stayed home to keep me company as I nursed the infant. Now I have hospital-averse Eddie, who announces he's leaving in two days; five fresh holes in my torso; an infection; a new stack of bills I can't pay; a void where my reproductive organs once resided; a holy health hazard of a home; weeks of solo recovery stretching far ahead; and a custody hearing six days away, at which I'll be representing myself.

If I were my mother, it would make me sad to visit 2017 Deb, too. Which I think is the main reason she's not here but her food is, though I'd give anything for the obverse. The tearful fight we will have about this after Eddie and my daughter leave in two days—when I beg her to come up and help me out, but she says she can't—will be heartbreaking for both of us. Weeks will go by when we won't speak, then months.

"It's not written anywhere that you must have a relationship with your mother," my shrink will tell me, when I ask for an emergency session over FaceTime, "if it causes you more pain than good. Estrangement is an option." Normally Swiss neutral on every topic I broach, he'll seem visibly angry after I make my wishes to be cared for clear, and they go unheeded.

"But I love my mom," I'll say. I was done being angry. I have learned to accept her as she is, not as I want her to be or wished she would have been. Isn't that the whole point of therapy? To come to some sort of peace with the unmet needs and traumas of one's past in order to move beyond them?

My mother came of age, I remind my male shrink, in an era even more inhospitable to women than mine. She was told she couldn't go to medical school. Talking back could get her hit. She went straight from her father's home into her husband's, without any transitional moment to figure out who she was or what she might have achieved on her own. She got married at twenty, had me at twenty-three, my sister at twenty-five, my twin sisters at twenty-nine. That's four girls under the age of six before she turned thirty, during a period when women still didn't have a right to their own credit cards and wouldn't until she turned thirty-two. She had no help at home, a spouse who traveled four months out of every twelve, undiagnosed anxiety, depression, and most likely premenstrual dysphoric disorder, which wasn't even a clinical diagnosis until well after her reproductive years, plus she must have had some unresolved anger from her own childhood traumas.

Yes, I've often had to mother myself. But my mother gave me life; she sends Hanukkah and birthday presents every year; she loves my kids; she shows up at happy milestones (the grandkids' shows, graduations, bar mitzvahs, etc.); she giddily hosts my children and me every summer in Bethany Beach; and she loves me, I know, in her own way. The past is the past. And that past is both my millstone and my superpower: a black hole of sadness and a wellspring of resilience, forever intertwined. "The law of compensation," the teacher in Truffaut's *L'Argent de Poche* calls it. That film made me weep when I first saw it in high school French class, for reasons I was still too young to grasp.

"Then forget estrangement," my shrink will say. "But you *must* make sure not to fall prey to emotional neglect or abuse in future romantic relationships. Just because it feels familiar does not mean it's good for you. It's okay to ask for help. And it's normal to get it."

One morning, my friend Cindy shows up with a craniosacral therapist, who practices what I can only describe as restorative dark arts on my skull, and when the two of them leave I make a decision: I need an actual caretaker. Now. All of this trash-lifting and dish-washing and dog-walking and grocery-shopping and camp-packing for my son are taking their toll. My body *hurts*, and I'm not giving it the proper time and freedom from chores to heal.

I look into the cost of a home health aid, but it's prohibitive. I call Eddie and beg. What if I fly out to L.A. after my son leaves for camp, and you can help me recover during the four weeks he's gone? The cost of a flight is essentially the same as the cost of one day of a home health aid. "I can't do that right now," he says. It would be too awkward if I stayed at his house, which is next to his wife's, plus his son is out of school and about to head off to his first year of college.

Got it, I say. Totally understand. What if I come out for only a week or two then, and we can just hole up in a hotel in Ojai or something, chilling by the pool? I just need a chunk of time when I'm not doing chores. When someone else is scrubbing pots and taking out the trash.

"No," he says. It's not possible for him to be with me at this time, he's sorry.

What I don't yet understand is that there's another woman back in L.A. Eddie and this other woman have planned a romantic weekend getaway to . . . Ojai. I do not know this at this point in the narrative. I only know that on the morning he left New York, three days after my surgery, he placed my hand on his penis. This felt . . . shocking? Yes, shocking. In my post-op, Percocet haze, still wracked by pain, I thought about saying, "Postsurgical hand jobs are not my thing," but I didn't.

I'm embarrassed by this version of me. Ashamed to even describe her. She is fifty-one years old and still putting up with quid pro quo caretaking.

Finn, the young Texan who used to live in China, calls me from Guangzhou, where he's now based again, to see how I'm doing. I'm at a loss, I tell him. I can't seem to take care of myself and recover simultaneously.

"Can you get to Nepal?" he says, and I start to laugh. Hahahahahahaha! Very funny. No, no, he says, he's serious. If I can get to Kathmandu, he'll take time off from work to be my caretaker for two weeks. Nice hotels run around $20 – $30 a night. Nepalese food is healthy, delicious, and dirt cheap. The Nepalis themselves specialize in the healing arts: sound therapy, massage therapy, meditation, yoga, Reiki, hikes in the great outdoors. It's the perfect place for him to meet me and take care of me and for me to heal.

"You're serious?" I say.

"Would I joke about something like that?" he says.

No, I realize. He wouldn't.

I'll think about it, I say, and do the math: hiring a home health aide or even a housekeeper to help out with the chores will cost $200 a day minimum. I need to heal. The twenty-hour flight will be horrific in coach, but once I arrive, I can rest. Finn, I know, is a selfless caretaker. It's part of his DNA. When his brother arrived home from several tours of Iraq and Afghanistan a changed and troubled man, Finn flew home to rural Texas to take care of him and to argue tirelessly with the U.S.

government until they found him proper psychiatric treatment. When Finn's brother was later thrown into jail, on a minor misdemeanor sparked by PTSD-induced rage, Finn flew back to Texas to bail him out.

Over the next week, he'll send me eight gift packages, one by one, including a portable travel hammock and a slim book I loaned him, *How to Love*, by Buddhist Zen master Thich Nhat Hanh, which he has annotated with memories of our time together. Each gift arrives with its own note: "Deb, Nepal is an excellent place to recover from surgery, or so I hear . . ."; "Deb, Roses are red, Violets are blue, Nepali foothills are waiting on you . . ."; "Deb, I hear there are great deals on international flights right now"; etc., signed with private joke nicknames.

I check my airline points and realize I can get to Kathmandu for free with a small service charge. I put a pin in this thought until I get through my custody hearing, which takes place six days after I'm sprung from the hospital.

THIRTY-TWO

My Day in Court
(My Afternoon in Hospital)

JUNE 16, 2017

This is taking too long," says my still-not-yet-ex, in the waiting room of family court. We've been sitting in the middle of this fluorescent-lit holding pen for more than an hour, watching men and women who'd brought children into this world together acting worse than toddlers fighting over the one shovel in the sandbox. But I'd told him it could take all morning, and it's already taken us four years to get from waving goodbye in front of our house in Harlem to this inner sanctum of family court, plus he's not the one lying flat on a wooden bench to keep from passing out from pain.

"Excuse me, ma'am, get up! You can't lie down like that!" shouts one of the bailiffs. I pick up my shirt, and show her the still-fresh incisions, the infected one still oozing. "Oh my god, I'm so sorry. Sure sure, lie down, lie down. What is that, a hysterectomy?"

"Trachelectomy," I say, "but same neighborhood."

Today—on what would have been my parents' fifty-fourth wedding anniversary—we are here, without lawyers, dealing with issues of child custody only. Child support will be determined on a future date, with a separate judge; and then the divorce itself will take place in a completely different courtroom with a third judge. Again, all without lawyers. This is all on the advice of Antoinette, a charity divorce lawyer with the non-profit New York Legal Assistance Group. She's a friend of a friend who told me, at a recent Yom Kippur break fast, that a pro se divorce ("pro se," Latin for, "Fuck it, I'll do it myself") is not only possible, she has no idea why more people who are struggling financially but are capable of reading up on the law don't do it. Once custody has been agreed upon, she explained, then child support is decided via a strict formula, and the divorce itself is then usually a piece of cake, particularly in situations like ours where there are no assets to split. Antoinette is not my lawyer. I wish she were, but she can't be, because even though I'm currently unemployed and paying for rent, food, and health insurance out of my dwindling 401K, my 2016 taxes show too much income to be eligible for charity law services in 2017. Nevertheless, she is a font of good information and has been coaching me through the process via email. I've also been spending hours a day reading up on New York divorce law online and watching YouTube videos explaining the family court system.

I look around, wondering if anyone else is here on their own. But we seem to be the only divorcing couple in this hell pit of angry exes who are here by ourselves, without lawyers. Which means I have no intermediary as hand-holder, rule-enforcer, or buffer.

"I'm leaving," says my ex. "This is ridiculous. I have to get back to work." He's now working at another start-up that will collapse in a few months.

"You cannot leave," I shout-whisper, struggling to sit up. "Today is our court date. This is how family court works. We wait until we're called in front of the judge, who has us on his docket today. If you leave, we'll have to reschedule, and it could take another month or more. I told you we might be here all morning. Do you know what it took for me to get down here today?"

Several weeks earlier, in order to avoid paying child support, he'd made a fuss about wanting precise 50/50 custody, and now we're here to have the judge sign off on our original agreement. I'd begged him at that first hearing: Please! I have surgery coming up that same week! Had we just settled on the custody schedule we'd already successfully had in place for over a year, since his return to New York, I would not have had to come down to family court less than a week after having my cervix removed.

I have custody of our son Sunday night through Wednesday mornings, plus every afternoon after school; he has him Wednesday and Thursday nights, then we switch off every other weekend. Our son's bed sits in his father's living room, so he prefers to come back to my place after school, as I also have snacks for him and either myself or a sitter to keep him company until dinner. He's now eleven, so he does not technically need an adult to watch him after school, but study after study points to the adolescent's desire to have a "potted plant" parent around in the afternoons not as a babysitter, but as a benign presence in the home between the end of school and dinnertime. So when my ex, at the last hearing, had suddenly and surprisingly announced no, he did not agree with the schedule as is, he'd changed his mind and wanted precise 50/50 custody, the judge had ordered a three-week trial run of a new—and logistically untenable—schedule.

You're right, my ex had emailed me, one day after the new schedule was imposed. He couldn't actually accommodate 50/50 custody. It was impossible with his hours and housing situation. He wanted to go back to the way we had it. That was working well.

At stake is $608 a month in child support, which will be calculated by a new judge, in another couple of months, as a percentage of our joint income. Until now, I have not received child support, though we've been apart for four years. Instead, I've been shouldering the burden of our children's expenses: of having a large enough apartment for all three kids; of paying for camp and clothes and college and food and music lessons and shoes and health insurance and haircuts and uncovered medical bills and computers and MetroCards and all three of their cellphone bills, etc.

$608 a month, which in three months will be garnished from my ex's salary and placed on a debit card, to be used for our younger son's monthly expenses, will hardly make up for what I've already carried for the family and will continue to carry, but it's something: a symbolic gesture acknowledging his fiscal and legal responsibilities as a parent.

I am not asking for alimony, although I am technically and legally owed it. Yes, I've had to continually adjust my career to be the default then-solo parent, and he hasn't. Yes, this has hurt my bottom line, not his. And yes, women in America still earn 80.5 cents, in 2017, for every man's dollar. But I am not—at least I hope?—incapable of landing a new job after recovering from surgery. More critically, I cannot stomach the idea of my ex-husband paying for any part of my personal living expenses or even believing that he does. This feeling is neither logical nor fiscally sound. In fact, it's idiotic, as I could just use the extra money on the older kids, who have aged out of the child support formula, even though their college expenses (books, housing, clothing, food, tuition) are far greater than their little brother's. But I value my financial independence more than I value whatever drops of blood I might squeeze from a stone. $608 a month in child support for our little one is a sufficient acknowledgment of a burden I've been bearing alone. It's something. Replacing nothing. "Good," said Antoinette, when I told her this. Forgoing alimony will make the whole divorce process simpler if I'm doing it without a lawyer. It's one less battle to fight.

"Precisely," I said. The less fighting I have to do to complete this divorce, the better. I just want this whole thing to be over. To fast-forward to the part where we might even be friends again. (This happens. Like a Hanukkah miracle, it happens. Within three years, each of us will find storehouses of goodwill toward the other we can't, on this day, imagine we will ever be able to tap. I will even join him and our kids when he— having finally switched career gears, midlife, to computer coding, a job he loves—signs the lease on a two-bedroom apartment.)

My ex, tired of waiting, stands up and announces he's leaving. But just as I lose it and shout-whisper, "Are you fucking kidding me? Sit down!"—hardly the worst utterance we've heard in this waiting room today—the bailiff calls our names, and we are ushered into the courtroom. Or, rather, the bailiff calls the married name I no longer use but to which I must still officially answer, as my ex still hasn't notarized the paperwork granting me permission to change it back. The entire process in front of the judge takes less than ten minutes, after which my ex zooms out while I wait another hour for the final documents to be drawn up. By the time my no-longer name is called to retrieve them, my still-infected incision is now bleeding on top of oozing, and I'm feeling something else inside my vaginal canal: a painful tugging, if I had to describe it. The pain is so intense right now, in fact, I can barely stand up. "You don't look so good," the bailiff says, helping me stand. "Do you need help getting downstairs into a cab?"

I wish. Alas a cab home will set me back at least $40, if not more.

"Nah, I'm fine, thanks," I say, but when I exit the courthouse and start walking to the subway, I feel like I'm going to pass out. I hail a taxi and tell him to take me to the nearest emergency room, which is luckily only a $7.50 ride from family court and in the same hospital group as the one in which I had my operation.

Because I look basically fine on the outside—the curse of womanhood, with all of our ladyparts neatly tucked inside like Marie Kondo'd T-shirts in a drawer—I'm placed on a stretcher in the hallway of triage in my courtroom clothes and ignored for four hours.

"Hey, sweetie," I text my son, at the end of the first hour. "I might be late coming home today. Just fix yourself a snack, and I should be there by dinner, okay? Sorry."

I use these hours on the stretcher in the triage hallway not to sleep or rest, as I should, but to answer emails. There's no such thing as sick leave or disability when you're out of work. Since having been laid off from the marketing and PR firm, I've managed to cobble together a few gigs here and there, but nothing permanent. I've been emailing everyone I've ever known or met tangentially who might possibly have job leads, alerting them to the fact that I'm available to do any work at any time, no matter the scope.

One of the dozens of people I emailed that week before surgery was my sixth grade boyfriend, David. David is now a successful TV executive. When he comes into New York for work, we have dinner. "Do you have a script that needs to be written, polished, or given a new draft?" I wrote him. "Do you have a show that's staffing up? Do you have an idea for a show you'd like to see implemented in an outline or script? If so, I would really appreciate having the opportunity to do any of these tasks." If I can earn $38,302 in screenwriting income from a WGA signatory company this year, I can re-up my low-cost union insurance instead of paying $2,349 a month out of pocket for COBRA. "Not asking for a hand-out," I wrote. "Asking for honest wages for honest work."

Unfortunately, he wrote back, he knows of no job or script opportunities right now, although he'll keep his ears open. In the meantime, he said, he and his wife Andrea are sending me a check for $10,000 to cover my COBRA payments for four months. "Please accept; it's really my pleasure to give it."

Wait, what? *What?*

I bawled when I read this. He was a kind and mature sixth grade boyfriend, it must be said, putting to shame many if not most of those who followed. In fact, we never officially broke up. The school district lines sorted us into two separate junior high schools, and that was that. Our mothers remained friends, and his identical twin sisters kept passing their hand-me-downs to my identical twin sisters, but I would not actually see David again in person until I was living in Moscow with my soon-to-be-husband in the early '90s, and he was also passing through. Then he met and fell in love with Andrea, my close friend and former ABC News colleague, and finally I had the good fortune of having David back in my life.

David and Andrea's generous gift out of the blue will help me survive my recovery from surgery, until I land a new job with health benefits as head writer at the World Science Festival: one of the hundreds of jobs to which I will apply, both from this hospital gurney and afterward. "That's a . . . truly life-changing gift, David. Thank you," I'd said to him on the phone, immediately after receiving his email. Just imagine, I joked, if the U.S. government would step in when its citizens got sick, like they do in nearly every other first world country, so that friends and GoFundMes didn't have to.

"Yeah," he said, "that would be nice, but in the meantime please. Take care of yourself! Andrea and I are worried about you. We wanted to take at least one burden off of your plate."

Hopefully, I told him, I'll be in L.A. in a year or so to thank him in person, as I've been asked by Darren Star to help him flesh out a new show.

I spot a nurse rushing by. "Hey!" I shout. "Do you have any idea when I'll be seen? My son is at home by himself."

"We don't have a room for you yet, sweetie, so sorry," and she rushes off before I can ask a follow-up.

I dive back into my phone to apply for more jobs on the LinkedIn and Indeed job boards and to see if there's any news from Darren on the show. He'd invited me to see a production of Lucas Hnath's A Doll's House, Part 2 on Broadway two nights before my surgery, and it had rattled me. A follow-up to Ibsen's original, it takes place fifteen years after Nora slams the door on Torvald. In this version, she's back, a successful feminist novelist, but she needs Torvald to sign their divorce papers.

"What'd you think?" Darren asked afterward.

I shook my head and laughed. "I mean, I loved it," I said. "Obviously. But it also hit a tad too close to home."

Our plan is to start working on a pilot for the new show in earnest again after I recover.

He'd come to me with his proposal soon after I left the PR firm. He'd sold a concept for a show to Paramount about a young American woman who moves to Paris, but in the present day, he was quick to add. Not 1988, like *Shutterbabe*. And she'd have a normal nine-to-five job in marketing or something like that instead of being a war photographer. He asked for my help with the pilot—since I'd both lived in Paris in my twenties and worked in present-day marketing—in exchange for $5,000 out of his own pocket and a promise that, should the show get made, he would guarantee me a job in the writers' room and a script of my own. Both were critical, I knew, to landing another job in scripted TV, which is my goal.

In fact, writing for scripted TV had always been one of my dreams growing up, but when I spoke to other female friends who'd graduated from my college and tried to get work in that field back in the late '80s, when TV writers' rooms were predominantly filled with white, male writers from *The Harvard Lampoon*—the college humor magazine that had rejected me three times—it gave me pause.

I had written, directed, shot, and edited several short films for my college degree, but I figured I'd have a better shot as a woman of breaking into war photography when I graduated college in 1988 than of landing a job in scripted TV. Not that the statistics are much better three decades later, the year I'm lying on this gurney: According to a 2017 report, 80 percent of TV showrunners are male.

Was I concerned that working on a show about a young American ingenue who moves to Paris would kill any chance of *Shutterbabe* the TV series ever getting made? Of course. But Darren has clout in the TV world, I don't, and the promise of an actual paid job in a TV writers' room plus an actual script of my own—both of which would allow me to get back on my WGA health insurance for at least two years and give me an on-ramp into a new career—is too good to pass up.

At first we were calling it *The Paris Show*, before it had a name, then, for a while, *Ex Patty*, figuring we'd name the protagonist Patty or Patricia to fit the title. Soon Patty will become Emily. Gabriel, her downstairs French love interest, will grow out of Alex, an American friend of mine who worked as a chef at Taillevent when I lived in Paris and cooked dinner for a whole group of us expats every Sunday night. Emily will have worked in pharmaceutical marketing, just like I did, and her brand manifesto for Vaja-Jeune, a fictional French vaginal moisture ring, will be cut and pasted directly from the actual brand manifesto I wrote that first week in my PR job. Emily will rail against the idea of the French word for vagina—*le vagin*—being masculine, just as I had one of my characters do in *The Red Book* years earlier. This will give Emily her win at work and the pilot its ending when she tweets out, at my suggestion, "*Le vagin n'est pas masculine*" ("The vagina is not masculine"), and Brigitte Macron retweets it.

Darren will take a first pass at the script, folding in my dialogue, ideas, and character and plot suggestions, then we will pass the script back and forth several times, during which I'll add in the appropriate French turns of phrase and cultural idiosyncrasies I still know from my four years of living in Paris and my many trips back since for work or to stay with my friend, Marion, whom I will keep texting, calling, and emailing during the writing of the show to make sure our present-day Paris remains accurate.

Three years later, the show will air as *Emily in Paris*: the number one international hit series on Netflix the weekend it opens. A few months after that, it will get nominated, dubiously, for two Golden Globes.

I don't really understand why we can't just draw up a contract, I'd said to Darren, so my income could be official, since he's being paid to write the pilot by Paramount, a signatory company. Couldn't he just ask MTV studios to pay me, too? When I co-wrote *Shutterbabe* with Eddie, I was paid $80,000 by a signatory company (NBC/Universal): income that I then reported to the WGA, allowing me to pay dues on it, join the Writers Guild, and have affordable health insurance for two years. But Darren insists he has to pay me out of his own pocket for now, for reasons he doesn't elucidate, but he promises he will make sure I have both my own episode to write and a job on the show once the pilot is approved for production. He's a good enough friend that I trust he both knows what he's talking about and would never deliberately keep money out of my pocket or a credit off my résumé.

"I just want to write TV for a living instead of having to sell my soul to the pharmaceutical industry to feed my kids and cover their health insurance," I tell him. "So if working with you on this pilot can lead to that, I'm in."

"It will lead to that," he says. "I promise. If they like it, and it goes into production, this will become your new career."

Later that fall, during his kitchen renovation, he will also offer me the unused Wolf stove that came with his apartment when he bought it but doesn't match his interior designer's new color scheme. I really want and need that stove, since I cook all of my son's and my meals at home, and my 1950s-era clunker still leaks gas from its pilot light, which keeps extinguishing. But first I have to come up with $500 to pay the movers to remove it.

A year after it's installed, I will sell the stove on Craigslist for $2,500 when I move, which I will immediately hand over to my daughter's college bursar.

"Please!" I shout into the void. "Please, I'm in pain!"

My son texts me for the fifth time. "When are you coming home?" He's been home by himself for hours. I'd meant to stop by the grocery store on my way back from the custody hearing to pick up food for dinner.

I call him on the phone. "Whatever you do, when it gets dark, do not touch that kitchen light," I say. These days, to avoid being shocked, I turn it on only with a thick rubber oven mitt, but I don't trust him to do this alone. "I'll be home soon," I say. "Fix yourself a bowl of cereal before it gets too dark in the kitchen."

"There's no milk," he says.

I text my ex to see if he can feed our son tonight or just bring him some food, but he's out for dinner with friends. My daughter has left for Israel, so I can't ask her. My older son is in Thailand teaching English. I text a fellow mother who lives nearby, but this is her night to see patients. I order pad thai from my phone and call my son to tell him to press the left button on the buzzer to let in the delivery man when the food arrives. He's afraid of answering the buzzer with its still-broken intercom. What if it's another crazy person trying to set our building on fire? "You can do this," I say. "Just give the guy three dollars in quarters from the change bowl for a tip. That's twelve quarters."

"Okay," he says. His voice sounds scared and small.

"Hello!" I shout once more into the void. "I've been here for four hours! I've got a kid sitting alone at home!"

Nada.

By the time I'm finally seen in the hallway of triage, not in a room, I've had it. "On a scale of one to ten?" I'm asked by a harried physician. Always a trick question, when you're a woman. Whatever number you state, it won't be believed. You have to game it, like the stock market. I want to say ten, but the last time I said ten, a few minutes before collapsing on the floor of my former doctor's office in 2006, her male partner—whom I'd never met until that day—stood over me, arms crossed, eyes rolling, and said, "Come on. Get up. It's just gas! It can't be that bad," and sent me on my way. Three hours later, I was undergoing emergency surgery for a ruptured appendix.

Ten, I decide, is too risky. I'll short it. "Eight?" I say. Eight is a solid number, implying enough pain to be taken seriously but not enough to be called hysterical. Will it work?

The physician prescribes a new antibiotic for my still-infected wound.

"Don't you have a speculum to look inside me? That's where the real pain is," I tell him.

That would be a job for a gynecologist, he tells me. They don't have a gynecologist on call in the emergency room right now, but if I come back tomorrow—

"You . . . don't have a gynecologist. In a hospital. What if there were a gynecological emergency?"

He mumbles something about how women are better served seeing their own gynecologists in their offices during business hours and sends me home without looking inside me with a speculum. Had he done so, he might have noticed that the closure at the top of my vaginal canal, which is being held together by fraying stitches, has already started to split open.

I want to scream. Instead, I hop off the gurney, sign some papers that will result in a new medical bill, and make my way to the subway, bent over in pain. I ask a businessman who is sitting in one of the disabled seats on a standing-room only train to please trade with me. "Why?" he says, still sitting. Because I can't actually show him the fraying flesh at the top of my vaginal canal, or the blood suddenly pooling in my underwear, I lift up my shirt and show him my still-fresh scars. With an annoyed harumph, he gives up his seat.

In two weeks, on July 2, 2017—exactly four hours after my daughter arrives home from Israel, otherwise I would have been alone in my apartment and died from blood loss—the stitches at the top of my vaginal canal will come completely undone, and those eighteen large clots ("A *chai!*") that started this book will eventually shoot out of the cannon of my vaginal canal. After the first of the eighteen clots emerges, I will photograph it in the palm of my hand for scale, and I will call my surgeon's answering service three times over the course of one hour.

No one will return my call.

Why? In the chaos of the emergency, I won't find out. And I have neither the time, energy, nor inclination to push for an answer or to sue the hospital. But I suspect it's because the two robotics surgeons who perform scheduled trachelectomies and hysterectomies at the hospital— the only two surgeons who can actually save my life right now—are not usually summoned for post-op emergencies and vaginal cuff dehiscence tears. So no one is actually on call right now to look at the photo of the giant blood clot in my hand as three more shoot out, and I head to the kitchen in search of a glass Tupperware container to contain them.

Instead, my daughter is gently trying to convince me to just go to the hospital at 1:30 A.M., as I wander the apartment in an ashen daze, holding tight to my container of clots, which have grown progressively larger as the tear inside me widens, like a ghost cervix, to birth them. As I leak copious amounts of blood up and down the hallway, on my bed, on the kitchen floor and all over the bathroom tiles, I will actually yell at my poor daughter when she suggests calling 911, because an ambulance, right now, is "not a good fit" for my unemployed budget.

If I ever make it through this alive, I think, my soul hovering over my dying body as it's rushed into the operating theater to save it, *I'm flying this sack of cells to meet Finn in Nepal.*

PART VI

BRAIN

2017–2019

Empty Brain

JULY 2017

O utside the window, red-robed Tibetan monks are circumambulating the Boudha Stupa, spinning prayer wheels with outstretched hands. "*Om mani padme hum, om mani padme hum . . .*" they chant, over and over. Inside, I am lying on the ground of a tiny second-floor singing bowl shop in full view of Buddha's eyes, which are framed in the window, watching.

Floor-to-ceiling shelves groan with heavy copper bowls, several of which have been placed around my body for a session of sound healing therapy. Each bowl is a different size, for producing different vibrational tones. "Close eyes," says one of the two Nepali men about to perform the therapy. "Empty brain."

Empty brain? Hahahahaha. Yeah, right. But I'm willing to try anything at this point, in the name of healing. Or at least in the name of eliminating both the pelvic pain and the traumatic images of clots and chaos that keep intruding into my daily thoughts. My first few days in Nepal, after wheelchair airport transports on either end and a cramped nineteen-hour flight punctuated by a wheelchair-aided layover in Guangzhou, China, I could manage nothing more than to lie in the hammock Finn had set up on the balcony of our room at the Kathmandu Guest House, overlooking a courtyard garden below, the Hima-layas above. There I swayed, back and forth, back and forth, absorbing the sounds of birds in the morning, *bansuri* (a Nepali flute) at dusk, birds in the morning, *bansuri* at dusk. Several days passed thus, watching the clouds form and reform, the sun rise and set.

But now I'm ready to get intentional about my healing. To switch from being a passive patient to becoming an active participant in my own revival. To this end, I will have to drop my smug cynicism over step-ping outside the rigid confines of Western medicine, which has now failed me several times, and stay open. I have committed myself to seek-ing out and trying whatever ancient Eastern therapeutic modalities pre-sent themselves in this city, such as this tiny singing bowl shop we've stumbled upon by accident while searching for shade from the sun.

"You want?" the shop owner had said, pointing to the purple mat on the floor. "Twenty minutes."

Yes, and . . . I think, checking the rates of the various sessions, which are negligible. "How about thirty?" If nothing else, it'll be a nice midday nap. When he tries to put a bowl on my newly repaired pelvis, I wince, and he immediately takes it off. "Sorry," I say. "I just had surgery." I lift up the bottom of my shirt, show him my scars.

"Ah," says the man. "So sorry."

I wonder if the healing doesn't work without a bowl on the pelvis. Wait, what am I even saying? As if this would ever heal me. Stop, maybe it will. No, it won't. You don't know that. Stay *open*.

My brain is at war with itself, both apostate and believer.

Finn sits on a stool in the far corner of the room, which is near enough for me to still make out each whisker on his face. His hair and beard have grown to Jesus-length since last I saw him eight months ear-lier, when we ended things because he was moving back to China for work, and because we knew, eventually, we would have to anyway. He stands up and steals a few noisy shots with my SLR before the session begins.

An editor I know at O, *The Oprah Magazine* would not promise to cover my expenses for this trip—gone are the days when one could pitch and get fully funded for a foreign story, especially on such short notice— but she did offer to take a look at any images and words I might bring back. And Finn is eager to assist with making sure I have good photos not

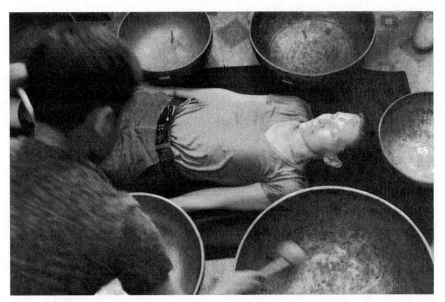

Singing bowl therapy, Kathmandu, Nepal, July 2017, © "Finn"

just of what I see but of what he sees: a woman seeking the terms of a ceasefire with her own body.

Would I rather simply live this experience instead of having to take notes in order to have my $29-a-night hotel room covered plus some cash in my pocket after I get back and write it? Yes. Absolutely. I'm exhausted. In pain. In no mood to focus on words or to lug around the heavy camera, though to be fair Finn won't let me lug anything. He carries all of our stuff, including water bottles and passports, in his backpack. Plus, according to the rules of my unemployment benefits, I can't actually take time off, even to heal after my second major surgery in three weeks. I have to be actively looking for work or doing freelance work every week in order to qualify.

In the freelance writer version of David Mamet's *Glengarry Glen Ross*, ABC—"Always be closing"—would be ABP: "Always be pitching." I'd emailed several magazine editors from my hospital bed on the third morning after the emergency surgery, when I made the final decision to come here. Writing about and shooting photos of my search for healing seems like a logical solution to the conundrum of working while recovering, since writer and photographer are the two professions I always jot down on my tax forms.

Nevertheless, I will end up having to represent myself in unemployment court a few months later to prove this, after I make my weekly online application for benefits from my hotel room in Kathmandu, which triggers an IP address tripwire and puts me in a catch-22 welfare purgatory. Any travel outside the U.S. is read by the NY Department of Labor algorithm as non-work-seeking vacation, so my benefits are immediately cut off.

The website suggests hiring a lawyer to represent my case at the hearing, and when I read this I'll laugh. A lawyer? To recoup $403 a week? Hahahahaha! No, thank you, dol.ny.gov. If I can figure out custody, child support, and divorce by myself, how hard can it be to explain to a judge I'm not a welfare cheat?

Kind of hard, as it turns out.

"No," I'll tell the judge, "I was not on vacation." I'll show her photocopies of the emails with several editors, written from my hospital bed; plus paperwork from the hospital; plus more emails and résumés sent from Nepal, looking for work; plus scans of the resulting stories in both Oprah.com and *Business Insider*; plus my six books; plus copies of the many previous stories I've written and shot abroad to prove my bonafides as a writer and shooter of international stories. "I was taking notes and shooting photos in a foreign city in the hopes of turning the story of my healing into a remunerative asset. As I've done many times. I am a writer and photographer. That's how I earn my living."

"So you were working. And someone was paying you in Nepal. Which means you are not entitled to U.S. benefits for those weeks."

"No," I'll explain again, as patiently and calmly as possible. "No one was paying me. I did it on spec." Repeating the story out loud, it will, admittedly, sound sketchy and nuts—going to Nepal to heal, because it would have been too expensive in the U.S.; turning that experience into a search for work, so as not to lose unemployment benefits—but everything about the U.S. health and labor situation is sketchy and nuts, which is not my fault except insofar as I blame myself for not using my outdoor voice over the years to scream loud enough. "Think of it as a job interview in another city," I'll say. "You get on a plane and travel to that interview in Cincinnati because you hope to one day get that job, not because you're sure you will. You take a leap. Pray to land. That's what freelancing is."

The lawyer representing the New York State Department of Labor will come up to me in the elevator afterward and say, "Well, *that* was a waste of everyone's time and energy today. I'm so sorry we put you through this. But I look forward to reading whatever you write about it." Then he'll wink. And walk away.

Challenge accepted, government lawyer dude.

In the end, I will have presented the judge with enough hard evidence of the trip's intent as a generator of income to provide reasonable doubt over the government's charge of "willful misrepresentation" that she will reinstate my benefits from the day I arrive home from Nepal until the day, a few weeks later, when those benefits will run out anyway. But I will still get docked $806 in unemployment benefits for being away "on vacation" during those two weeks in Nepal when I should have been searching for paid work, despite *two* published articles proving otherwise. The fact that I'd nearly died the week prior and needed time to recover from surgery, the fact that I'd had my cervix removed three weeks before that will be immaterial. Both the algorithms and humans in charge of calculating unemployment benefits in the U.S. make no accommodations for illness, near-mortal or otherwise, nor for attempting to find work, as required by unemployment law, by doing that which you have always done since college to earn money as a freelancer: to seek out and report some story out there in the world, on a wing and a prayer, in the vague hope that someone somewhere will want to publish it. Which is just so American it will make me laugh until I cry.

"You ready?" says Finn, snapping one last photo of me lying between the bowls.

"As I'll ever be."

"Just breathe," he says and winks. Our own private mantra, born of a Pearl Jam song we played once and then every day thereafter when we were together, sometimes several times in a single hour. During the song, I was not allowed to fret over money, kids, or work. Or to get up to do chores or to respond to electronic beeps and buzzes. It was an enforced three minutes and thirty-five seconds of quiet breathing, often in his arms.

Finn, born into the kind of rural American poverty that produces childhood memories of the tap of rain on tin roofs and the thwack of men slamming doors, sees it as his god-given duty to connect with and lessen the burdens of others. From the evening we met in front of that bar on Bleecker Street, and I spotted him crossing Cornelia as if in slow motion and thought, "Who is the lucky woman who gets to hang out with *that* man tonight?"—before suddenly realizing, staring down at his photo on Tinder, that that person was me—I've felt as if I'd dreamed Finn into being.

"The bar's way too noisy to talk," I'd said. "Wanna go to John's Pizza instead?" The restaurant, one of the few untouched and still-reasonable gems of old New York, stood across the street.

"Twist my arm," he'd said, all Southern drawl, which was another ironic Finnism. You never had to twist his arm to do anything. Earlier that day in Kathmandu, he'd found us a houseful of blind masseuses. "They see with their hands!" he said. "How cool is that? It *has* to feel good." Of course, he was right.

A line from the Pearl Jam song hits me, as the bowls start vibrating. *Yeah, I don't wanna hurt, there's so much in this world to make me bleed . . .*

Earlier that morning, a Hindu priest guarding the dead at Pashupatinath Temple had walked up to me, without asking, and smeared a red *tika*, made from dried turmeric, onto my forehead. "Protection," he'd said. *Not from you*, I thought, as he held out his hand for rupees. Nor from the sadness of seeing a boy weeping over his mother's corpse on the banks of the Bagmati just prior to her body being set aflame. How had she died? I asked. One of the boy's relatives mimed illness in the area of her reproductive organs, and I had to hold in my tears. I pictured my own young son, safely ensconced in his miniature bunk bed at camp. A counselor walking in, had his older sister not been home that bloody night, to tell him . . . what? How had this sobbing boy learned the news of his mother's death? Was he there when it happened? Or did a grown-up have to tell him? Her feet, I note, are unusually small, dainty, like a child's.

The *tika* on my forehead was placed, like all *tikas*, between my eyebrows on the *ajna*, the sixth chakra and "third eye," the so-called seat of concealed wisdom. The *ajna*, according to Hindu tradition, marks the point at which creation begins, which makes sense with its proximity to the brain. Its role is intuition, intellect, and imagination: picturing that which you cannot see with your own eyes, so you must "see" it with your

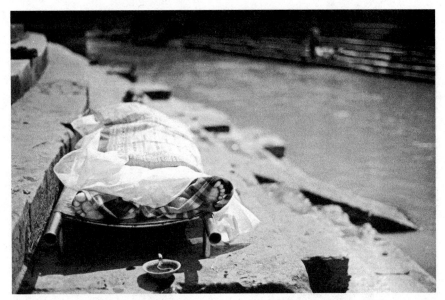

Woman's corpse, Pashupatinath Temple, Kathmandu, Nepal,
July 2017, © Deborah Copaken

third eye. Such as a book, as yet unwritten; my father's face, now that
he's gone; a boy at the moment he is informed of his mother's last breath.

Forgetting the red mark had been placed on my *ajna*, I wipe the
sweat from my brow, and now my Jewish forehead is smeared in Hindu
turmeric as my Christian caretaker and I wait for the Buddhist ceremony
to begin.

I'm an equal opportunity mender.

As is Nepal, with its long history of religious tolerance. Hindu remains the primary religion, but signs and acceptance of other beliefs
flutter in the wind everywhere. Earlier that morning, Finn had stood in
a shaft of light, dressed in his tai chi clothes, arms outstretched to the
sun, with striped shadows of Tibetan prayer flags fluttering behind him.
He looked so much like the embodiment of Nepali tolerance—Taoist
Jesus in Buddhist Hinduland—I yelled out, "Don't move!" and snapped
a photo.

The only major world religion missing from this particular moment
in the bowl shop, I realize, is Islam. But back when I was covering the
war in Afghanistan, the mujahideen had taught me to recite the opening
lines of the Koran (*Bismillah ir-Rahman ir-Rahim, la ilaha illallah mu-*

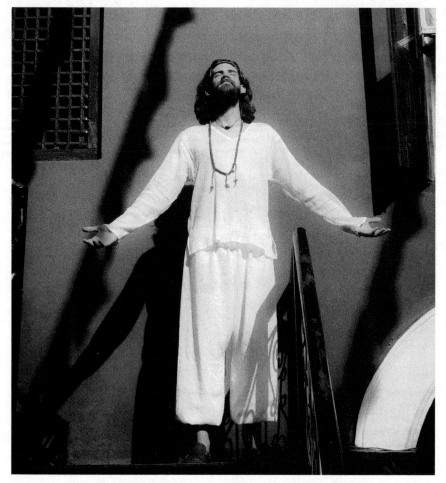

"Finn" in Kathmandu, Nepal, July 2017, © Deborah Copaken

hammadur rasulullah . . .) while we shivered in our mountain cave, hiding from Soviet bombs, and this ability to speak the *kalima* out loud apparently automatically makes me a Muslim. It also makes me popular with Muslim cab drivers.

Wait! I think. That cave. That freezing, foodless, fetid cave, with the frozen drip castle of shit out front, and the photos of the Ayatollah Khomeini and Kalashnikov lining the walls inside, in which I slept and starved and hid during those first few months of 1989. That cave was also in the Himalayas, a thousand miles northwest of here.

Duh. Of course.

The previous morning, Finn and I had wandered into a used bookstore in Thamel and found a dog-eared, annotated copy of *Shutterbabe* facing out, exactly at my eye level, part message in a bottle from my former self, part rebuke. And though Finn had insisted on shooting a souvenir photo of this odd little moment, my brain *still* hadn't made the connection until just now.

Pain, I guess, will do that. It scrambles everything in there except the hurt.

As the singing bowls start to vibrate all around me—what an odd and lulling sound, I can actually feel the vibrations entering my body, as if I've suddenly atomized into mist in a belfry—it finally dawns on me that I've returned to the same stretch of tectonic plate subduction in which Act I of my adult life began: at war; in the snow; my twenty-two-year-old brain filled with Hollywood fantasies of how the story of my life might unfold, none of which came true. I did not remain in the field of war photography: Words became too urgent, my need for roots too strong. I did not marry the young man I met in Jamaica and would later visit in

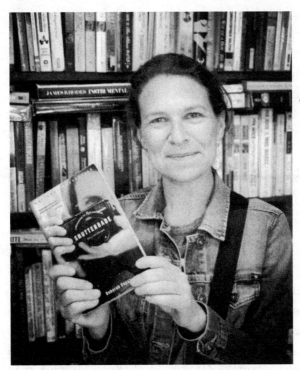

Used bookstore, Thamel, Kathmandu, Nepal,
July 2017, © "Finn"

London; fate intervened to make him lose that scrap of paper with my phone number on it when he came to visit me in Paris. I did not live happily ever after but rather as we all do: in fits and starts of joy and sorrow.

My body, back then, had not yet produced three humans or been carved up by the vicissitudes of womanhood. Now, three decades later in these Himalayan foothills, it is summer, not winter. Peaceful, not war-torn. Technicolor, not the blacks and whites of night and ice. The vibrations entering my chest originate from bowls not bombs. I'm no longer eager and unlined and throwing myself at danger, but rather circumspect, cautious, corrugated, crisscrossed.

How ironic, I think, that covering actual wars produced only one tiny wound in the webbing of my right hand while existing in the form of a woman's body has produced an entire constellation of scars. "There's a war going on, and I'm bleeding." That was the first line of that first book, about my years covering those wars, but only a few readers noted the subtext, and none — not even I — could have predicted its foreshadowing.

Yes, back in Afghanistan I got my period in a minefield, and one of the mujahideen sat on my backpack, crushing a bottle of rubbing alcohol all over my one box of tampons, and that was less than ideal, hygiene-wise, but the larger point I was trying to make was not about actual menstrual blood in an actual war but about how living in a woman's body, too, can feel like war. But now, deep in middle age, my body bears so many actual scars from what I once wrote off as metaphor, I've lost count.

Linguistic clues teach us that, for early humans, any number beyond two was known as *many*. Three, as a concept, was the same as four, five, six, or a thousand. So counting went something like this: "One, two, many." I stopped counting my scars after three as well, except when I'm forced to reckon with their existence while filling out medical paperwork before a doctor's visit. I've actually had to jot down all of my surgeries in alphabetical order in the notes section of my iPhone, otherwise I can never remember them all: adenoidectomy (1972), appendectomy (2006), D&C #1 (1983), D&C #2 (2000), frenectomy (1988), hysterectomy (2012), inguinal hernia repair (1997), meniscectomy (2018), Morton's neuroma repair #1 (1995), Morton's neuroma repair #2 (2020), trachelectomy (2017), vaginal cuff dehiscence repair (2017).

It's telling, I think, that my iPhone doesn't even recognize the word *trachelectomy*, the only surgery on my list with a red dotted line under it, as if challenging me to prove such a common ladyparts excision actually exists because, yes, even spell-check is sexist.

One day, just out of curiosity, I typed in *prostatectomy*: prostate removal. Yup. My iPhone knew that one. Then I tried some of the rarer male reproductive surgeries and ailments, such as *seminal vesiculitis*, *preputial diverticulectomy*, *penile hematoma*, *inguinal herniorrhaphy*, and *phallorrhaphy*.

My iPhone knew those words, too.

My surgery list also does not take into account the many biopsy scars (five in 2013; one in 2015; another in 2017); or my three episiotomies from giving birth (1995, 1997, 2006); or the stab wound on my right forearm (1989) when I caught those drug dealers in Zürich ransacking my hotel room.

Nor does it take into account all of those moments that became "indelible in the hippocampus," as Christine Blasey Ford will later call her assault by Brett Kavanaugh, from the multiple assaults I've also endured: the policeman in Mexico who grabbed my prepubescent breast while I was asking him for directions (1979); the older teenage boy who placed my young hand down his pants (1980); the large stranger who broke into my college dorm while I was in it typing a paper and threatened to rape me (1985); the combat boot kicked into the left side of my skull from an unseen assailant on my way home from the library (1986); the two classmates in my documentary film class who mistook my enthusiasm for our film for consent to have both of their hands under my clothing (1986); the first thief who robbed me at gunpoint (1987, probably crack-related); the second thief who robbed me at gunpoint (also 1987, also probably crack-related); the group of drunk college boys who collectively assaulted my body outside the video store near my dorm before I beat one with the hard plastic shell of *A Clockwork Orange*—homework for a seminar on men and violence—and escaped (*also* 1987, when I was twenty-one, a bad year to be in my body); the fellow student who raped me on the night before our college graduation (1988); the white-bearded rabbi in Israel who stuck his tongue down my throat and placed his hands on my breasts when I was interviewing him (1988); the Frenchman who took advantage of a Métro strike in Paris to fondle my ass

(1988); the businessman, in an angry rush, who pushed me down the subway stairs when I was seven months pregnant (1997); the countless frotteurs I've had the not-so-unique displeasure of witnessing (1985–present day); and the creepy older dude from Tinder who followed me home on the subway and felt it was his tongue's right to enter my mouth without asking (2015).

Women, maybe you know what I'm talking about when I lay it all out like that. Maybe you, too, have your own laundry list you pull out now and then to gape in horror before re-interring it under memories of birthday parties and beach walks. Men, if you don't know what I'm talking about, talk to the women in your midst: your mothers, sisters, daughters, wives, and friends. Ask them for their lists. Theirs might not be as long—being five foot two perhaps makes me an easier target?—but be ready to be appalled by their answers.

This was the original idea behind #MeToo, which was coined back in 2006 by Tarana Burke, a sexual harassment survivor and activist who believed that breaking the silence would elicit change. The movement will go viral soon after my return from Nepal, when two *New York Times* journalists, Jodi Kantor and Megan Twohey, break the story of Harvey Weinstein's multiple assaults on the women in his orbit. Like so many other women, I will use the #MeToo moment as my own hour of reckoning with the collective burden of having bodies that make us targets for sexual abuse and harassment.

In May of 2017, I'd sent Ken Kurson's "How come you never asked me out?" email to the only other contact I had at the *Observer*, my newly assigned editor, Sarah. "I felt it was my duty to send this to someone," I wrote, "just so the *Observer* understands what happened to one of its columnists."

My new editor's response? "I am baffled by the pizza emails and not quite sure what I am looking at but it doesn't feel like any of my business."

The "pizza emails"? Minimizing takes all forms. Yes, even by women. No, sometimes, unfortunately, *especially* by women. Patriarchy does not discriminate against whom it infects. Male, female, trans, nonbinary: We are all the unwitting hosts of its systemic toxins.

I shot back: "I'm not sure why that's baffling. Even reading it now feels icky." I took a screenshot of his email and pasted it into the body of mine, just to remind her what it might feel like to be the recipient of the words "How come you never asked me out?" from your boss.

She never responded.

A few days later, I entered the cervical mystery tour, and those emails submerged under a torrent of blood.

Bong! Bong! Bong! The vibrations from the bowls grow stronger. I sneak a peek at how they're produced: a man on each side of my body, in perpetual movement. Each has two felt-covered gong mallets. They place one mallet in the center of the bowl to steady it while striking the outside of it with the other, bowl by bowl, until all the bowls are vibrating at once.

I am now just bowls, brain, and body, the latter of which is slowly letting go. But not so the brain. The brain is still gripping tight to its swirl, either trying to think its way out of what's happening or willfully holding on to the sight of blood, the smell of bleach, the sound of that anesthesiologist counting backward from ten. *Go away, brain!* I think, then my brain immediately starts thinking about what it means to think about wanting my brain to go away but not being able to stop it from doing so.

It's been a week and a half since the life-saving surgery that has repaired and hopefully permanently reconnected the frayed tissue at the top of my vaginal canal. "Good thing your daughter was home," every doctor and nurse in the hospital kept saying, shaking their heads as they checked my vitals. My *vitals*: a word whose meaning I'd never really noted until its definition nearly no longer applied. Latin root: *vita*. Life. Did I understand how rare it is to hemorrhage like that after cervix removal?

"No. How rare?" I kept asking.

"*Very* rare," I was told vaguely.

But "very rare" for others means nothing when it happens to you. Winning the lottery is also "very rare," but if you win, you're no longer focusing on how often it doesn't happen, you're just trying to get your relatives to stop asking for money. The parallel with vaginal cuff dehiscence is that you're just trying to wrap your brain around what just happened, since you've never heard of this malady before, while simultaneously managing the PTSD of bloody gore and near death. Meaning, each time your daughter stepped out to go to the bathroom or to get food, you googled the thing to death.

Vaginal cuff dehiscence: I had to ask the medical staff to repeat this combination of three words several times before it sank in and became a permanent groove in my cortex. *Vaginal*: Okay, that one was easy enough to remember. *Cuff*: That's the incision that was supposed to be sutured closed but came undone. *Dehiscence*: A surgical complication in which the edges of a wound no longer meet or tear apart. Here's what else Google explained to me: "Vaginal cuff dehiscence after hysterectomy is a rare, but potentially devastating complication. If it is not corrected in a rapid fashion, there is significant potential for morbidity and mortality."

Yes, but *how rarely* does it happen? And how significant is the potential for disease and death? And how many hours after it ruptures do you have, more or less, before you die? And why had no one warned me of the risks of this particular bloodbath either before or after my trachelectomy or before or after my hysterectomy five years ago? Is there a greater chance of vaginal cuff dehiscence if they have to go in there multiple times, as they did with me? And what are the chances of all of this happening again one day?

Surely someone out there has studied the mortality rates of this thing and knows the answers. But every article I read had a different answer with a similar caveat explaining that we don't really know how often it happens, because it doesn't always get reported. Sometimes women just bleed out too quickly and die. Or their bowels and/or intestines protrude through their vaginas and they die. Or their viscera fall out, and then they die instead of being rushed to the hospital for an emergency surgery that can be counted as part of the data set and recorded.

One study I read said, "Despite being rare, VCDE"—the acronym for vaginal cuff dehiscence and evisceration, meaning the cuff comes undone and viscera falls out—"can carry a lot of morbimortality if not treated on time." A lot of death? Cool. Define a lot. Another study went so far as to say, "The incidence of this condition is not clear, ranging in the literature between 0% and 7.5%." Wait, what? Zero percent to 7.5 percent? That's a huge statistical range for the risk of massive, deadly hemorrhaging following the second most common procedure (the first is cesarean) that women of reproductive age undergo. In the U.S. alone, an estimated 600,000 hysterectomies are performed every year. And 7.5 percent of 600,000 women a year is—I open my calculator app—45,000 women.

45,000 women? How could the statistical chance of a complication that could potentially affect 45,000 American women a year not be clear and, more important, why are we not told to look out for it when we leave the hospital? Men are told that the incidence of erectile dysfunction after prostate surgery is 60 percent, and that's not even death. And yet those studies get funded. Men are *informed* of the risk before they go under the knife. I know the risks of erectile dysfunction after prostate surgery, and I don't even own a penis.

Then I read this phrase, so common in women's health: "missing data." Ugh! Missing data! Again! To really study the percentage of women who nearly die after hysterectomies and trachelectomies from VCD would require a deliberate gathering of data. Which would mean collecting that data from multiple hospitals. Which would mean investing money and time in the answer. Which would mean actually caring about the answer. Which would mean making sure that at least half of those holding the science purse strings in one hand are not holding their cocks in the other.

No one is funding these studies. Even though the *American Journal of Obstetrics & Gynecology* wrote, way back in 2012, the year I had my hysterectomy, that more research into these dangerous outcomes is both needed and necessary if we are to prevent them from happening in the future. In fact, they called for the development of a national reporting system or registries for vaginal cuff dehiscence, while also noting that such a system and study "would be quite costly and time-consuming."

Several hours after her partner finished sewing me up, my original surgeon, Dr. Hou, paid a visit to my hospital room with her young daughter. It was July 3, 2017. A Monday during the Fourth of July weekend. Clearly she was not planning on being in the hospital that day, and her daughter looked none too pleased to be dragged along. "I'm so sorry," she said, on the verge of tears. "How are you feeling?"

A bright future, this woman has, I thought. Her empathy runs deep. And she showed up with her kid on her day off. So unusual for a surgeon, in my now extensive experience. "I'm fine," I said. "And please don't blame yourself. You told me to get a caretaker. But mine flaked."

"Your boyfriend, right? Eddie?" I was shocked she'd remembered his name. It's rare for a medical professional not only to listen to their patients' stories of illness and woe but to retain the seemingly (but not) superfluous information such as a partner's name.

"Narrative medicine": it's the new battle cry on the front lines of healthcare. Every illness, like every novel, tells a unique story with its own plot, characters, conflicts, and metaphors. These days, it's no longer enough to ask, "Where does it hurt?" A good doctor, like Dr. Hou, will conduct both a close reading and a deconstruction of the entire narrative arc of her patients' lives, including the telling silences between utterances. Why? Because we are not just our illnesses. We are every plot twist leading up to them, whether chosen or imposed.

"Ex-boyfriend," I said, after a long pause, telling her how Eddie had left me to fend for myself, three days after surgery. About how in my daughter's panic the night prior, when I was out cold, she'd group texted him along with a bunch of others she found in my phone—basically the last ten people I'd texted. His first response, when he called me that morning to see how I was doing, was to fret over how my emergency had affected his evening. It had ruined his experience of seeing his friend's play in Portland, he said. It was quite upsetting.

"I'm sure it was," I'd said, and hung up the phone.

My daughter pushed off the start date of her summer internship with a brain surgeon to take care of me during the first week after the VCD. Dr. Hou gave me her tentative blessing to fly to Nepal where Finn awaited starting the second week, provided I remained in the hospital for the next two days to be monitored and that I returned for a check-up in one week, the day before my flight. It would be good to get out of the four walls of my bedroom, she said. A change of perspective is always useful, a caretaker even more so. "But no sex!" she reminded me. "Until at least the beginning of October, when I'll check the cuff again." As if I needed reminding. I couldn't imagine, in that moment, having sex ever again.

"Go ahead," I tell the men in the bowl shop, miming putting the missing bowl back on my stomach, between ribs and scars. "It might not hurt here?" I'm right. A smaller bowl on the part of my torso without the incisions feels fine and also closes the loop so that every surface of my body is now pulsing with vibrations and sound.

Bong! Bong! Bong! Bong! At some point, I can feel my whole body giving in to vibrations, and then my brain, too, finally shuts down. No more thoughts of blood. No more memories of the smell of bleach. Now I'm only sound. Now I'm only vibration. It's not that I've run out of thoughts to think, it's that through some alchemy between cacophony, tone, and sound oscillation, my brain has grown quiet. It's still there in my skull, ready to spring into action, but it feels as if it has been placed, like a laptop, in sleep mode. Without actually being asleep. I'm both aware and not aware. Awoke but not awake. Corporeally on earth and also just a collection of atoms.

The last conscious thought I have between chimes, before my mind shuts down completely, is simply *Here I am*. Which are the same words Abraham spoke to God—הנני (*hineni*)—when he was called upon to prove his surrender to an almighty being. In Judaism, it is an expression of total submission to faith, as God asks Abraham to bind and slay his firstborn. I would never slay my child for anyone, let alone some wrathful godperson I don't believe in, but somehow—the brain is so weird—that lesson from Hebrew school stuck and popped up at the moment of my own surrender: *Hineni. Here I am.* A surrender not to an almighty being but to just . . . being. To breathing. To life. *L'chaim.*

When the final chimes finish vibrating, I open my eyes and stand up. Without any help. And with vastly reduced pain in my pelvic area, which, I know, seems crazy, but apparently it's not. A year earlier, researchers at the University of California San Diego had conducted a study into the effects of Tibetan singing bowl vibrations on anxiety reduction. On a hunch, they also asked participants who were currently feeling pain to rate their pain on a scale of 1 to 5 both before and after sound bowl therapy. To the researchers' surprise, they discovered that those suffering from pain found a statistically significant relief of that pain after the sounds and their vibrations ceased.

Ted Kaptchuk, a Harvard Medical School professor who studies the effects of placebos on physical health and well-being, compared conventional Western medicine, acupuncture, and Navajo chantway rituals, the latter of which involves tribe healers leading storytelling ceremonies for the sick. Each modality, he realized, had its own set of rules and rituals, and it was, he posited, perhaps *the ritual itself* (going to the doctor, getting the needles, telling the stories) that was healing, curative. "Rituals trigger specific neurobiological pathways that specifically modulate bodily sensations, symptoms and emotions," he wrote. "It seems that if the mind can be persuaded, the body can sometimes act accordingly."

In a nutshell, what Kaptchuk discovered, in his many studies using both fMRI brain scans and other surveillance techniques, is that our bodies have a biological response, on a molecular level, to a ritual act of care. Many cancer treatment centers these days, in fact, now provide mindfulness therapies derived from Eastern practices such Reiki, a Japanese form of healing touch; Buddhist meditation; Tibetan singing bowls; and Navajo-style storytelling—the root of today's narrative medicine and long considered, in nearly every society, as an important path to physical and mental healing.

"Hey, do you wanna go on a hike tomorrow?" I say to Finn as we walk out of the bowl shop. I haven't felt this calm, energetic, or pain free in weeks.

"Do *you*?" he says, looking baffled.

I stare up into the giant Buddha's eyes, squinting at the glint of sun on its gold-flecked face. I get it. Just let go. Be. That's the path out of suffering: a radical acceptance of it. The body is mortal, a simple container for the soul/essence/whatever you choose to call the nameless *I* of you. The body will keep getting sick. It will keep breaking down. It will die. The point is to brush it off, after each new knockout, and keep going.

In other words, the Nora Ephron School of Life.

I smile. She would find it amusing, my equating her with Buddha. Preposterous that I had to fly halfway around the world for the epiphany. And yet it's so clear to me now. All those lunches. All those times she allowed me to—no, *urged* me to—laugh at life's pain. All of her exhortations to just yank out the damned uterus already and keep living. What was the point of holding on to something painful when you didn't have to? Cut it out! Chop chop. *How's the chicken salad today, good? Great. We'll take two.*

I take Finn's hand. "Yeah, I do. I really do want to go on a hike tomorrow. I mean we can try? And if I get too tired, we'll stop." Every morning in the Kathmandu Guest House, a large and ever-changing group of climbers gathers in the lobby with their waterproof duffels on their way to hike the Himalayas. I obviously can't scale a large mountain in my condition, but I've read that some of the nearby foothills are worth a gentle day's hike.

"Twist my arm," says Finn with a wink and a smile, and the next morning, after breakfast, we head out in search of ascension. Though I have not been able to walk more than a few blocks on flat ground without pain since the day they yanked out my cervix, today I put one foot in front of the other at the bottom of the hill, and we start to climb.

Along the winding path skyward, we find a woman with a cow, a

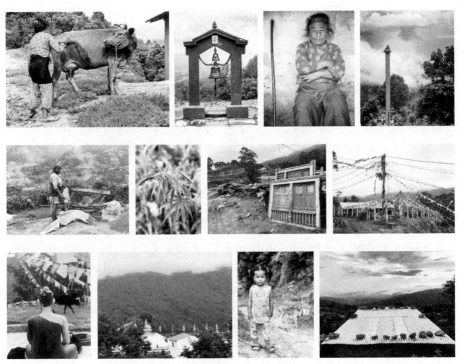

All images of the climb up the Himalayan foothills outside Kathmandu,
© Deborah Copaken

Hindu *ghanta* bell, a lady with a stick, an arrow pointing up; a woman bagging ash, a field of cannabis, a blue discarded door, a string of faded flags; a Buddha with big ears, another on a roof, a little girl with a goat, a tin roof held with rocks.

This! I remember this. This finding. This seeking. This looking. This seeing. This turning a blind corner and not knowing what you'll find. This stopping and noticing. This pausing and saying, "Hey! Hello! Yes, you over there. Please tell me: How do you see the world?" This listening to the answers. Actually listening, not just nodding. This connection of eyes. This melding of minds. This collecting of these small scraps of humanity and chaos and finding a thread onto which to string them so that maybe—just maybe—an organizing pattern will emerge.

This. This is who I am.

Hineni.

This is what I've been missing as each organ was removed, as my marriage crumbled, as I struggled to earn a living, as the medical bills piled up, as my will to climb broke.

At the top of the foothill, which feels more like a small mountain than I would have presumed, I check the altitude on my phone: 6,301 feet. I google the altitude of Kathmandu: 4,593 feet. So we climbed 1,708 feet. Not bad. A good start, 1,708 postsurgical feet into the sky. I check in with my body: It's winded and tired, but fine. "You doing okay?" says Finn, and I nod. He wants to shoot a photo of me at the top of the hill to mark the end of one climb and the beginning—I'm sure—of many others.

"Wait," he says, plucking a pink flower and placing it in my hair, "you need this."

And though it seems comical to pose for a tourist photo at the top of a hike with the flower of youth in my middle-aged hair, I give myself over to Finn's gauzy lens vision. In my mind, I'll always be that twenty-two-year-old setting out in the world, ready to climb it. It's only my body that keeps doing what all bodies eventually do—getting sick, breaking down—until it eventually returns to the soil from which it sprang.

"Come on, smile!" he says, snapping off a couple of shots, being his goofy, game self. I break into a genuine smile.

"Okay okay!" I say.

"Will you even remember me, if I'm not in the shot?" He knows how much I hate selfies. How every time I see a couple shooting one I can't help but offer to take it for them.

"I'm looking at you," I say. "How could I forget?"

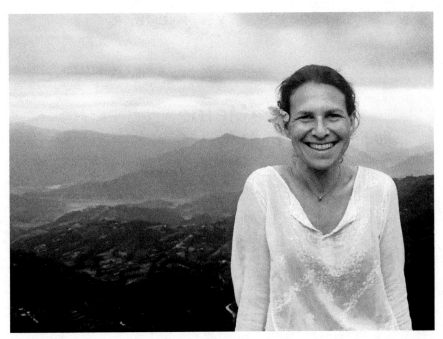

Himalayas, Nepal, July 2017, © "Finn"

THIRTY-FOUR

#MeToo

SEPTEMBER 2017–JULY 2018

U pon my return from Nepal, feeling emboldened by reading about the women speaking out publicly against Harvey Weinstein, I email Sarah, my new *Observer* editor, once again and ask her to please send me the name, phone number, and email address of a contact at Human Resources, so I can report Ken Kurson's sexual harassment. She never responds. I forward the "How come you never asked me out?" email to her again with this note: "Resending this in case it got lost in the shuffle. I need this information, please. I'd like to make a formal report. And with both Ken and Lorraine gone, you are my only contact at the paper. I can of course call the operator and try to figure it out from there, but I would hope you could help me with this. Thanks."

Again, no response, though I'm able to see, via HubSpot, an extension my son put on my computer, that the emails have been opened by someone dozens of times. Sometimes several times within a single hour.

I call the *Observer* switchboard. Ask to speak to Human Resources. I leave multiple messages.

Again, no response.

With no other recourse, I do what I've always done when faced with solutionless problems: I write it down. But how? An essay in the form of an ironic listicle seems like the right approach, so I do that. Afterward, I send my listicle out to the editors of those magazines and newspapers for which I still have contacts. *The New York Times* op-ed editor turns it down. A male editor at *The New Yorker* writes: "First of all, and above all, I am sorry you had to suffer this. No one should, and, maybe, after this moment, fewer will. I dearly hope so. But I am going to pass on this one, Deb; we have a lot of material on this in and coming in from staffers. I am sure you will find a place for it, though, and I hope you do." A deluge of similar rejection emails follows, from *New York* magazine, *The Washington Post*, and others, many of whom will cite the legal ramifications of going public with the story: They don't have the resources, should they get sued, even though in my original essay, I do not name Kurson. I just call him the "Big Important Male Editor."

Before throwing in the towel, I email the essay to Caitlin Flanagan, an *Atlantic* columnist whom I've never met but whose work I admire, and I beg her for a contact. What happens next—thank you, Caitlin—is a lesson in the power of sisterhood. Of women working together with common purpose rather than tearing one another down. This stranger writes back to me, "What a devastating piece. I'm so very sorry you had to endure that. What a loss . . . I am going to send this to Adrienne La-France, who is my *Atlantic* web editor. I am pretty sure that if they want to publish it—which I really think they should—they would want it to go up very soon."

"Very soon" turns into three months of careful vetting by lawyers and editors, who insist I publicly name my perpetrator, though I fight against this. It's not just about this one male boss, I argue. He's a stand-in for every male boss who abuses his position of power.

"You should name him," says Will. Will spent three decades as a magazine editor, the last ten as the boss. Bosses, he says, need to be held accountable.

Several weeks after returning from Nepal, I happened upon a photo of Will laughing in a sunny kitchen on my phone and swiped right. This was on Bumble, the dating app that requires the woman to make the opening salvo within twenty-four hours, or you lose the match. In the career section of his profile, Will had indicated that he worked in magazine publishing, so I texted, "Magazine publishing, huh? How's that going for you?": a quick inside joke to let him know I was both in on it and in the same sinking boat.

"About as well as can be expected," he wrote back, and we began chatting amiably. His wit was sharp, his mind agile: a file cabinet, I would later learn, overflowing with primary sources, doorstop books, and yellowed newspaper clippings, all as easily retrievable to him as mine are buried under dust and trauma. He was a few years out of his two-decade marriage, separated but not yet divorced. Same, I wrote back. He reminded me that we'd met once before, back in 2001, at a mutual friend's birthday party for one of their kids.

Wait, what? From my own brain's file cabinet, way in the back in a hard-to-reach drawer, I plucked a vague memory of looking up at a tall man with an angular, welcoming face and having a fifteen-minute discussion about . . . something. Right. Of course. *That* Will. Got it. Once I'd merged the photo of salt-and-pepper-haired Will in the palm of my hand with the auburn-haired version in my mind, the memory expanded. I could picture us laughing, standing next to a dining room table stacked full with my friend E.B.'s always delectable offerings. *Shutterbabe* had just been published that week, Will reminded me, on the day we'd met. Remember? He'd been trying to ask me a bunch of questions about my years covering wars, but we kept getting interrupted by screaming toddlers.

Yes. Yes! I remembered. Not the specifics of our small talk, exactly, but rather my thought bubbles as he spoke: What a kind man behind that boyish smile. His friends must feel lucky.

Will texted again the next morning while I was at the end of a bike ride with my friend Rebecca. "I'm not sure if this is the right way to do this," he wrote, having never been on an app date before, "but would you like to meet for coffee . . . now?"

Rebecca and I had just stopped in Harlem to buy sandwiches at Fairway, a grocery store off the Hudson River bike path, after pedaling for several miles. The courtyard of The High Line Hotel, where Will wanted to meet for coffee, was six miles south and (I checked Google Maps) a thirty-one-minute bike ride. "Should I go?" I said to Rebecca. "I mean, look at me." I was wearing my bottom-of-the-pile, frayed white T-shirt with the outline of a black tree I'd bought at one of those outdoor Christmas craft stalls in Union Square. I thought it would look good under a leather jacket, but I was wrong.

Rebecca laughed. She'd just finished many years of training to be a therapist. She'd also borne close witness to the pain in my marriage. She was the one, in fact, who was there the night my ex had stood up from the dinner table, right after the four of us had sat down to eat, and announced he was going to the gym. "I mean, it'll be a pretty good test of who he is if he takes off points for the way you're dressed to go on a Sunday-morning bike ride, right?"

I warned Will, via text, that I was unshowered, wearing the ugliest T-shirt I owned, and that I'd be drenched in sweat from biking, but if he was fine with that, so was I.

A year later, despite the ugly tree tee, we will set down roots together and split the cost of a mold-and-cockroach-free apartment *with a dishwasher* we'll find a block and a half from the East River in Williamsburg, Brooklyn, with a view of the old Domino Sugar factory out the back window—where Kara Walker once placed her giant ten-foot vagina— and the Empire State Building out front. Before moving in together, not wanting the bad juju of my wedding ring hanging over our bed, I'll use an X-Acto knife to chip away at the superglue holding it in place in the center of the lotus flower painting I made with it, in the wake of my separation, before taking a solo walk to the top of Inwood Hill forest, where I will toss the ring, unceremoniously, into the woods and say goodbye both to it and to my beloved canopy of leaves.

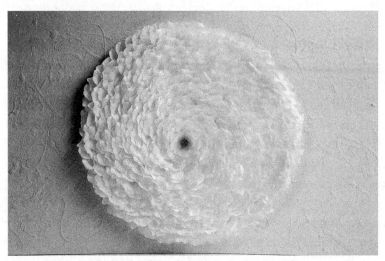

Circle #1, 2014 (house paint on wood, acrylic petals, glue, nails, wedding ring), © Deborah Copaken

Will will accompany me through two new surgeries (knee, 2018; foot, 2020) with a steady hand and outstretched arm. Hospitals, it turns out, are not only his thing, he'll admonish me for constantly thanking him for his help and apologizing for asking for it. "Stop saying sorry. That's what people do for one another," he'll say, bringing me a pillow to elevate my foot or some water to take my pain meds, utterly baffled that this has not been my experience in love thus far.

"But how can I name him in a public essay in *The Atlantic*," I say to Will—it's now early January, 2018—"after he wrote that email saying he comes 'from a grudge-holding desert people'? His best friends are Jared Kushner and Rudy Giuliani! He calls them by their first names. You don't want to fuck with those people."

"Because you have to," says Will. Will, like Nora, is frustratingly right, most of the time. "Sorry. If you're going to go public with your story, you have to have the courage to name names."

"Okay, okay," I say. I email Adrienne and tell her I'm willing to name my harasser.

The Kurson edit drags on and gets meticulously fact-checked. The fact-checkers even call Melissa, my friend and colleague from *Cafe*, to find out what frame of mind I was in when I came back to the office after my first lunch with him and whether I happened to mention the weird breast commentary to her (I had). Meanwhile, I double down on my search for a new salaried job to stop hemorrhaging four-figure monthly COBRA fees. After sending out over a hundred more letters and résumés, I land a decently paid, relatively fun six-month gig as a senior writer/producer at the World Science Festival that comes with health insurance, and I breathe a sigh of relief.

On March 9, 2018, while I'm sitting in my World Science Festival office in New York, researching the link between the microbiome and the brain, my editor Adrienne hits the publish button from her office in D.C. on my first story in *The Atlantic*—"How to Lose Your Job From Sexual Harassment in 33 Easy Steps," which immediately goes viral.

Within days, dozens of readers—men and women both, but mostly women—contact me with their own tales of woe not just at the hands of men but *specifically at the hands of Ken Kurson*. In fact, two days after its publication, Will drives my sons and me upstate for a hike in the woods for my fifty-second birthday, and all I'll remember about what should have been a peaceful walk through snow-covered trees will be the hundreds of notifications—mostly from strangers, but also from colleagues and friends alike—blowing up in my pocket every second: So many, in fact, that I turn off the phone and create a spreadsheet when I get home that night, to separate out the more troubling first-person accusations from the random missives of solidarity, rage, and "I saw Ken Kurson be a dick to so-and-so, too"s.

"The Others," I name the Google doc, in honor of the TV show *Lost*. It has twelve people on it, carefully organized by name, email, phone number, accusation, and source of the incoming message.

Here are a few excerpts from some of those messages, which arrived via the usual channels: Facebook, Twitter, my website, email, text, etc. I think it's important to note that this is the first and only time a personal story I've written has elicited such a flood of private missives from strangers wanting to share not only their "eerily similar experience"—this happens often enough, particularly when you write about the fruits of sexism—but their eerily similar experience *featuring the same person*:

> "I had an eerily similar experience with KK. Not that I was sexually harassed, but he put me in a position that left me unemployed with three kids."

> "Ken Kurson invited me to a professional lunch in 1999 and sent me an email about my breasts later. I was just starting out as a writer, in my 20s."

> "Did you know you're not the only one he offered a job to, then revoked the offer and acted like the person who'd just quit their job was the one in the wrong?"

> "Ken told [redacted], 'Why are you here? A woman like you doesn't need to work' and said she should just marry some rich guy who'd pay her bills."

> "I also have a creepy Ken Kurson story that can be summed up as: 'I may have told your colleague I wanted to interview your boss/feature

you/your organization in profile but I really just wanted a date and that's why I set up the meeting.'"

"Ken was a creep to me, condescending as well . . . I got paid more for being receptive to him. He doubled my pay for taking the flirt."

"He was a creepy guy who would send inappropriate messages from his Observer work email address."

"I had a similar experience w Ken Kurson . . . Ken very specifically targeted me."

"Your frightening experience with him gave me flashbacks . . . The way he spoke to me haunts me to this day . . . Drag the ogre into the daylight."

"His only job was to get Trump elected. Once he'd done that, and his 'best friend' Jared wasn't working with him anymore, it was no fun."

"In addition to Ken's $325K salary, he was compensated by being allowed to invest relatively small sums in Kushner real estate deals."

Those real estate deals—which, if my source is correct, have made Kurson a wealthy man—were made possible via Cadre, a New York–based real estate company founded by Mr. Kushner and his brother, Joshua. Cadre was funded in part by Yuri Milner—a Russian oligarch who himself is funded by the Kremlin—and others who to this day funnel money through the Cayman Islands, which was technically legal but not, for Kushner, necessarily ethical, due to both perceived and real impropriety of foreign influence over our government.

All of this troubling information about Cadre, Kushner, Trump, and Russian oligarchs pours into my inbox in the middle of the Mueller investigation, and I grow downright paranoid. Is my phone tapped? Is anyone reading my emails? Can they hack into my Google Docs? Who are "they" anyway? The U.S. government? The Kremlin? Trump's lackeys? My friend Virginia Heffernan, who writes about technology and politics and personally knows one of the victims Kurson targeted, calls me on my phone early one morning, out of the blue, while I'm toweling off from my shower. "Download Signal right now," she says, "and never speak to anyone about any of this ever again over normal channels. Do you understand? You are not safe. Call me back on Signal when you can."

Meanwhile, three days after my story is published, the *New York Post* runs a headline under Keith Kelly's byline that reads, "Ex-Observer editor joked about my breasts: writer," followed the next day, March 13, 2018, by, "Observer fashion editor denies knowing about freelancer's sex harassment claims" over a risible stock photo, more amateur porn screenshot than workplace harassment illustration, of a disembodied woman fending off staged advances from a disembodied man.

"Oh, for god's sake, look at this!" I yell half at my screen, half at my co-worker Nils, after digesting both stories. Nils, like me, was fired from *Health Today*, and I helped him land this position as my officemate because he's always been incredibly good at his job, kind, and ethical. "Sarah"—the aforenamed fashion editor of the *Observer*—"responded to my emails with, 'It doesn't feel like any of my business.' How can she claim she never knew about the harassment? And I fucking *sent* those emails between Sarah and me to Keith Kelly, when he called me for a rebuttal. You were here. You heard me!"

"I did, indeed," Nils says.

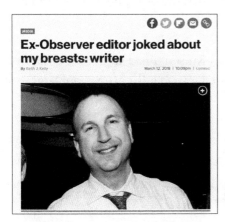

New York Post, March 12, 2018

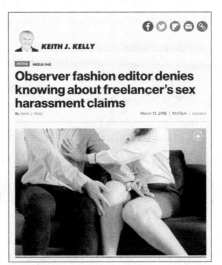

New York Post, March 13, 2018

But now I'm on a holy tear. Can't stop. I feel like I've been harassed all over again. "I debunked Kelly's story with proof before he even wrote it, and he ran with it anyway, under a staged photo of sexual assault and a headline calling me a liar? Fuck him. Shame on Sarah. Shame on all of us. This is not about my boobs! It's about a multi-step, manipulative, and calculated campaign of sexual and professional harassment—not 'sex harassment,' what the fuck is *that*?—during which the boob comment barely registered as anything but yucky awkwardness before I even understood what was happening. Sexual harassment is not about tits and ass! It's about power! This man dangled a salary and a full-time job in front of my face then yanked both away like a dime-store sadist when I showed no interest in fucking him. *That's* the real crime of sexual harassment. Stealing a woman's financial future and hijacking her power!"

But headlines about boobs and photos of women's disembodied bare legs garner pageviews that sell ads. A woman's body will always be viewed as a commodity, even in the very reporting of its illegal commodification. Lost wages, lost potential, stolen power? Who'd want to click on those?

"I don't envy women," Nils says to me.

The next afternoon during my lunch hour, determined to get to the bottom of the various Ken Kurson stories that continue to arrive in my inbox, while also keeping up with my full-time job, I download Signal and speak on the phone to a woman—we'll call her Pam—who wrote the most troubling message of all, as well as the only one that mentioned the word *criminal*.

> "I woke up to your article about Ken Kurson. I had an insane, if not criminal, experience with him that I'd love to talk to you about—off the record at first."

I quickly realize I am in over my head.

"What was *that*?" says Nils, when he hears my end of the conversation. "That sounded bonkers."

"You don't even want to know," I say.

"Do you have security?"

"No."

"Seems like you might need some."

Pam's story goes something like this: One day, Ken's wife, Becky—

yes, the same Becky to whom Ken allegedly showed my photo of Durkheim in Inwood forest wearing the *Observer* T-shirt; the same Becky
about whom I received multiple emails from Ken, saying she was going
to leave him if he didn't change his ways—spoke to her friend Jane, a
doctor at Mount Sinai hospital. Jane was a mutual friend of both Becky
and Ken's as well as, supposedly, Ivanka Trump's.

Jane, based on the information Becky told her, apparently urged
Becky to leave Ken. This was around the same time Ken was emailing
me, both about coming to work for him and about his wife wanting to
leave him.

Ken, per Pam, blamed Jane for breaking up his marriage, so to take
revenge—"I come from a grudge-holding desert people," indeed—he
concocted two pseudonyms, "Eddie Train" and "Jayden Wagner," to
email Pam, a media company employee who was married to Jonathan,
Jane's colleague and boss at Mount Sinai. In his first email to Pam,
"Eddie Train" claimed he had direct knowledge that her husband and
Jane were having an affair, and he threatened to reveal it publicly.

Stick with me here, I know it's complicated and sounds nuts, but
Pam's story will not only turn out to be completely consistent with criminal charges that will be brought against Kurson in a 2020 federal cyberstalking complaint, the whole thing will prove to be even creepier, more
calculating, and deliberately fear-inflicting than she'd had time to re-
count over the phone. Here are the characters again, just to keep them
all straight: **Pam,** the stranger who emailed me and was married to **Jonathan,** a Mount Sinai doctor; **Jane,** also a doctor working with Jonathan
at Mount Sinai; **Becky,** Jane's friend and Kurson's wife, who will eventually divorce him; **Eddie Train** and **Jayden Wagner,** Kurson's nom de
plumes in his emails to Pam; and **Ivanka Trump** and **Jared Kushner,**
the president's daughter and senior advisor respectively, who are also old
friends of Becky's, Kurson's, and Jane's.

When Pam went to find the threatening Eddie Train email again to
show her husband, it had, she says, mysteriously disappeared from her
inbox. (A few years later, *The Intercept* will publish a story about government surveillance and apps that provide disappearing message features,
but back then she didn't understand how this could happen. How could
a threatening email replete with a claim of her husband's infidelity
just . . . disappear?)

Meanwhile, Pam continues, Ken began to stalk Jane throughout the hallways of Mount Sinai, not realizing that his stalking was being recorded by CCTV cameras. He also, under his pseudonyms, started posting dozens of negative reviews of Jane on websites such as Yelp and RateMDs.com. All of these shenanigans made it up the chain of command at Mount Sinai, until the powers-that-be realized they had a PR and security nightmare on their hands. They hired K2 Intelligence, a private security firm that employs ex-CIA and ex-Mossad agents, to protect Jane, and the situation magically disappeared.

For Pam, however, the situation had not disappeared. In fact, the fear, harassment, and massive life upheaval she'd experienced at Kurson's hand, in an effort to denigrate the reputations of her husband and his colleague, was, she was sure, a federal crime. And no one was looking into it.

"Jesse, I need help," I say to my acquaintance, Jesse Drucker, an investigative journalist at *The New York Times* who covers this kind of stuff. "I want to help this woman, but I feel like I'm out of my league." I forward him my Google doc, "The Others"—redacted to remove the name and story of one particular source, who was scared for her life—with the obvious caveat that it was highly confidential and he should not share it further. As Jesse starts looking into each allegation that has come in over my transom, President Trump suddenly nominates Ken Kurson to a post in the White House.

Because of course this happens.

"Oh, for fuck's sake!" I say. "The White House?"*

---

* Kurson, at this point, will be working at the consulting firm Teneo, which is run by Declan Kelly, whom I'd met years earlier, when he called my phone out of the blue to say that I was single-handedly responsible for his happiness. I'm putting this here in a footnote because, though it's not relevant to the story of Kurson as predator, it is nevertheless such a weird coincidence. Declan's wife, Julia—the source of his happiness—was seventeen years old and known as Yulia when she tutored me in Russian in 1991. This was during the months leading up to the Soviet coup, after I'd relocated to Moscow to start shooting for *Newsweek* and others, and realized I could not do my job without at least some basic proficiency in Russian. That spring of 1991, Julia was admitted to the University of Pennsylvania, and we celebrated her monumental achievement. But then she was told by the Soviet government that she could not leave the country, because her refusenik Jewish parents had once applied for and been denied asylum. As a corrective, I offered to accompany her to the American Embassy in Moscow to sponsor both her and her parents myself, which meant I would be financially and materially responsible for the whole family, which was crazy, since I was only twenty-five at the time and dirt

Jesse's story, "The Trump Administration Considers an Old Friend: Ken Kurson," appears in *The New York Times* the following day, and it mentions my story of harassment in *The Atlantic* as well as Kurson's denial of wrongdoing: "Concerning Ms. Copaken's account, Mr. Kurson said, 'I categorically deny any claim of inappropriate behavior.'"

In response to his categoric denial of impropriety, I write a Twitter thread presenting all of the written evidence of it, email by icky email.

At the end of the thread, I write the following tweet, never expecting the FBI to actually contact me. I don't even @ them. I'm just in such a

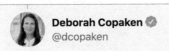

Deborah Copaken ✔
@dcopaken

Replying to @dcopaken

It always amazes me when someone categorically denies something for which documentary evidence exists. I've only ever posted the "How come you never asked me out?" email, but in light of Kurson's denial of inappropriate behavior, here we go.

12:13 PM · May 12, 2018 · Twitter for iPhone

---

poor, but I did it anyway because you would have, too. Julia's parents were doctors. They'd find their way, I was sure. Declan found me just prior to Julia's fortieth birthday to say he wanted to reunite the two of us as her birthday present. Up until then, I'd had no idea what had become of Julia, and I hadn't seen her at all since she left Moscow for the U.S. when she was seventeen. We had a wonderful fortieth birthday celebration at my house in Harlem, and then Declan offered to help me find work at Teneo when I lost my job at the PR and marketing company, but ultimately neither of us could figure out a place for me there. When I heard through my friend Eric Alterman, a professor and journalist, that Kurson A) was still was going around town, saying he wanted to get in my pants; and B) had landed a job at Teneo, I called a friend of mine who also coincidentally works for Declan, to warn her about Ken's behavior, as I feared he might target her next: We are around the same age, both Jewish, we look enough alike that we could be sisters, and she was in the middle of her own marital free fall. But I did not call Declan because I did not yet have a multipage Google doc of other accusations against his newest employee, and this was pre #MeToo, when we women worried more about reprisals for speaking up. I regret that decision. I should have formally called Declan, too, not just my college friend as a part of the women's whisper network. This, to me, is the most useful part of the #MeToo movement: allowing us to name and call out sexism in the workplace out loud. The next step should be its criminalization. A stolen career, income, and future should be punished at least as harshly as a stolen flat-screen TV.

blind rage at having been called a liar by Kurson in the paper of record, I want to set the record straight:

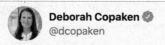

Deborah Copaken ✓
@dcopaken

Replying to @dcopaken

Also? Many more women and two men have contacted me about similar fuckery. So FBI, if you're vetting, call me. I know things.

12:15 PM · May 12, 2018 · Twitter for iPhone

Soon thereafter, Mateo Gomez, who says he is an FBI agent conducting a background check on Kurson, contacts me via cellphone to ask if he might come to my apartment in Inwood. Frightened that I'm being set up by either Kurson or someone else in the Trump world—*How did he get my cellphone number? Can the FBI just . . . do that?*—I call my friend and neighbor MaryBeth Williams, a journalist for *Salon*, to ask her to please be my "plus one" for my alleged FBI investigation. *What if he's not who he says he is?* we wonder. *How do you actually know the FBI is the FBI when they show up at your door?*

On Monday, June 4, 2018, Agent Gomez arrives at my apartment with his partner, Special Agent Emily Eckstut, who's young and kind-faced and wearing sensible flats. Somehow, it's her shoes that immediately win me over, make me feel at ease, but not before I make both agents show me their badges at the door. Not that I would necessarily know what a fake FBI badge looks like anyway, but it feels like the prudent thing to do. "I figured I'd bring a woman along, since I know this stuff is hard to talk about with men," Gomez says, and I think, good on you, FBI! That is correct. I definitely do feel better with a female special agent present, thank you. Although I'd feel much better if you hadn't had to come at all.

After going over every major and minor thread of my own story itself plus each similar allegation reported to me from "The Others" in the wake of its publication in *The Atlantic*, the FBI agents head back to their desks with my Google doc and start hunting down each lead.

Jesse Drucker, along with his colleagues Emily Steel and Danny Hakim, continue to do the same from their desks at *The New York Times*.

Two months later, Jesse's second story appears: "A Kushner Ally Was Up for a Federal Post. Then the F.B.I. Began Digging":

"In November 2015, Mount Sinai began an investigation into allegations of harassment made by two of our doctors against Ken Kurson," the hospital said in a statement. "We also took measures to protect our staff and the alleged harassment ceased shortly thereafter. We are cooperating with the F.B.I. on their current background check of Mr. Kurson."

Mr. Kurson said in an interview last week that he withdrew from consideration for the government post around early June, citing the amount of paperwork involved in the vetting process.

"The amount of paperwork!" Will laughs, reading it out loud.

"I know," I say. "It's all so crazy."

In his story, Jesse identifies me as "a journalist who accused [Kurson] of commenting on her breasts as she sought a job at The Observer," which, though I admire Jesse's work, I find frustrating once again. The breast comment was but one tiny aspect of a much larger gender-based violation. My accusation was not about his boobs comment alone but about a step-by-step chain of grooming, manipulation, and harassment that denied me both income and dignity. And which, granted, is hard to express in an identifying clause, which is yet another scourge of sexual harassment in the workplace: how difficult it is to describe succinctly. But how about just "a freelance journalist for the *Observer* who accused Kurson, her boss, of sexual harassment"?

Once again, to set the record straight, I add to the Twitter thread on this topic I'd already started. "It wasn't the breast comment that rankled," I wrote. "The reason I wrote my story in the *Atlantic* is because I LOST MY COLUMN after not capitulating to this email." I attach a screenshot of the "How come you never asked me out?" email. "More saliently," I continue, "the doctor in question here had HER career threatened, via the online Yelp reviews. What this shows me is that #MeToo is often just the tip of a very ugly iceberg. And that those who engage in sexual harassment are often harassers in other ways, too.

What's at stake is not only bodily autonomy and freedom from sexual harassment. What's also at stake for women—what's always been at stake for women—is financial autonomy & financial control. Or rather the freedom from having our careers threatened by controlling men."

In the midst of all of this, just as my World Science Festival gig is winding down, and I'm once again starting to worry how I'll pay my rent and have health insurance when the festival is over, I receive an email from Elli Kaplan, the CEO of a Silicon Valley–based tech company aimed at the prevention of Alzheimer's, which to me is one of the scariest illnesses out there. Who are we without our brains?

"I'm reaching out," Elli writes, "because at the risk of sounding a bit stalkerish, I read everything you write and am always blown away by the beauty of your voice and the importance of your work." Now you've got my attention. Have there ever been sweeter, more alluring words to a writer than these? No. There have not. We are as shallow about compliments to our brains as social media influencers are about likes on their butts.

After describing what her product does—using eye-tracking software to assess individual risk for Alzheimer's, then putting those at risk for the disease on a six-pronged program to improve cognition (diet, exercise, sleep, social engagement, intellectual engagement, and stress management)—Elli asks if I might consider coming to work for her. "Let me know if you would be open to a conversation. Look forward to hearing from you."

When the student is ready, the teacher will appear, indeed. I've been noticing my own brain going on the fritz of late: words forgotten, appointments missed, names of friends—good friends!—unretrievable. Why? I pick up the phone. And dial Elli's number.

Cognitive Health

MAY 2018–JUNE 2019

O kay, so cognitive health," I say to Elli. "Tell me about your company." Earbuds in, I'm rushing from the World Science Festival offices to the 116th Street subway station on Broadway, an hour later than usual. The festival is in three weeks. Work is heating up. It's raining, windy. My five dollar umbrella has just concaved into a tulip with an errant gust. My son needs empty soda cans for a science project, he texts. And black sweatpants for the performance tomorrow. (*What performance tomorrow?*) Also, we've run out of snacks. When am I coming home? I make a mental scan of what's left in the fridge to cook for dinner. Nothing. So now I'm crossing 116th Street to pace in front of Morton Williams, a small grocery store near the subway, engaging in just one of a million private conversations that take place on the public streets of New York City at any given minute between sirens and blares. *He hit her? Oh, no, it's cancer? How can you say you love me if you're fucking her, too?* "Sidewalk snippets," my kids and I call them: prompts for short stories whose endings we'll never learn. "*Two* of your grandparents died of Alzheimer's?" I say, adding to the cacophony of snippets. "That's awful. I'm so sorry."

Elli started her company, she tells me, after these two grandparents, one on either side, succumbed to the memory holes and devastations of Alzheimer's. In other words, this is more than just a business for her. She's trying to save both her own brain as well as millions of others' before they go dark. Stress, for example. Did I know that stress is considered one of the leading causes of cognitive decline?

I laugh. "No," I say, "but I'm pretty sure I'm living proof of it." I'm now standing under a scaffolding to avoid getting drenched, my brain churning with pressing tasks. "So wait, just out of curiosity, how did you happen upon my writing? Why me of all people?"

"I read one of your novels," says Elli, "the one about the mother who kills herself and her children? I loved it."

"*Suicide Wood.*"

"No, that wasn't what it was called. What was it?"

"Oh, right, duh," I say. "Sorry. I meant *Between Here and April.*"

"Yes! That one."

"The publisher changed the title at the last minute, and I can literally never remember it. Unfortunately, neither can anyone else."

We both laugh. Elli's laugh is warm, generous. "Well, we're all about saving memory!" she says. She mentions two friends of hers, Joanna and Sharon, who are also friends of mine.

"I love Joanna and Sharon!" I say. A good sign: If she likes them, according to the transitive property, I will like her.

The two of us agree to meet in person when I fly out to California for my sister Jen's surprise fiftieth birthday the following week.

I hang up the phone, oddly excited by this unexpected plot twist. *Shutterbabe* brought Nora Ephron into my life. Now a novel based on the murder of my friend Connie by a mother who gave up was about to give my children and me a new reason to live.

I picture little Connie Hummel, on our first day of first grade — September 5, 1972 — two months before her mother killed her. She was standing by our shared cubby and putting on a pair of red gym shorts under her dress: a moment that has not only stayed with me, it was the memory prompt for the entire novel. "What are you doing?" I'd asked, visibly alarmed. I was a rule abider. A goody two-shoes. Shorts under a dress? *Who does that?*

"I like going on the monkey bars," said Connie, with a shrug.

"That's allowed?" All of our mothers made us wear dresses and Mary

Janes on the first day of school. I had not yet learned that a girl could say no to the strictures placed on her.

"Who cares if it's allowed?"

Before that exchange, it had never occurred to me that you could jerry-rig your girl fate with boy shorts. How many other tricks to surviving femalehood without flashing your underpants to get from one side of the monkey bars to the other could Connie have taught me, had she not been murdered by her mother?

Elli and I meet in her sunny, ground-floor office in Redwood City, California, the day after I watched my sister Jen walk into a restaurant in Carmel as fifty of us screamed, "Surprise!": a moment of shock and disorientation dissolving quickly into tears, love, and gratitude that never fails to choke me up whenever I see it in the wild. Her husband, Todd, beamed with delight, having pulled off the impossible: keeping a giant secret from my sister. He sprang for our hotel rooms as well. A godsend. I would have never been able to afford this trip otherwise. I brought Will as my date and introduced him to the whole family for the first time, as well as to Jen's college roommates, all of whom I've known for thirty-two years.

But when I tried to make the introductions to the roommates, my brain faltered. "This is Karen, Alison, and . . ." I was looking straight at Marcy, drawing a total blank.

"Marcy," she said.

"I'm so sorry," I said, feeling terrible.

But Marcy, who was in the middle of a divorce herself, laughed it off. "Please! No need to apologize," she said. She gets it.

Maybe a job delving into memory and cognitive science is just what my scattered, stressed, middle-aged, still-divorcing brain needs right now. I did my homework before this meeting. Neuroscience has reached a new threshold. Or at least a new understanding of the many outside factors affecting memory retrieval. Ever since the FINGER study in Finland was able to show significant improvement in the cognitive functioning of at-risk seniors through a program of sleep, exercise, diet, stress reduction, social engagement, and mental engagement—you need all six, you can't just have one without the others—it has now become plausible to attach the word *prevention* to the word *Alzheimer's* by focusing less on the brain and more on its scaffolding, the body.

Elli and I agree that I'll start working as a consultant at first, to see if I like the work and if she likes me. My title will be Head Writer. Over the course of that summer, I'll help rewrite all of the lessons in the cognitive health program as well as doing research on the brain, creating a company blog, ghostwriting Elli's op-eds, and generally being available to write any materials the company needs: our website language, marketing materials, Facebook and Twitter posts, public announcements of new funding, etc. I will enjoy this work, for the most part. The inner workings of the human brain are interesting, and I'll be able to do all of the writing on my own time, on my own schedule, at home. By mid-August, Elli will ask me to come on full-time, with benefits and a salary that will allow me to pay off the rest of my daughter's college tuition, some of my medical bills, and to be relatively stress free month to month for the first time in, well, ever. It'll mean flying out to Redwood City once every month or so, to meet up with the rest of my team, but otherwise I can keep working from my apartment in Brooklyn.

"Sure!" I say. "I'm in." This will give me more time to see my sister Jen and her family in Los Gatos, why not? And win-win for the company, since this will save them my hotel costs when I travel. I agree to her proposal and mention three caveats: 1) I want to be able to keep writing my *Atlantic* columns, whenever possible; 2) If *Emily in Paris* goes into production, which it's looking more and more likely it will, I'll need to be able to take a short leave of absence to work on that, but I will definitely find an interim replacement while I'm gone; and 3) I've been trying to sell a new book—this book—which I plan to write between 5 A.M. and noon, when the California workday begins.

"Of course!" says Elli. "I would be upset if you stopped doing your other writing. Welcome to the team!"

During the two weeks I still have my World Science Festival health insurance, I push off the start date for my new job so I can get a knee operation I've been needing for years, to repair a torn meniscus that had collapsed under the weight of my uterus when I was pregnant with my youngest. My knee, after twelve years of injury, is nonfunctional. "No more cortisone shots," Struan—my freshman year college boyfriend, now orthopedic surgeon—tells me. "It's time to fix this thing." I also need time during business hours, when courts are open, to tie up the last strings on my DIY divorce.

Divorcing without a lawyer has required much more legwork and confusing paperwork than I'd ever imagined possible. One hot summer morning, a week after knee surgery, I end up hobbling up the staircase of the Supreme Court building on crutches to file yet another stack of papers in yet another well-hidden office. Halfway up the wide stone stairs, I pause to rest. I remove the heavy grocery bag of documents from my shoulder and place it down on the step but accidentally drop one of the crutches. It slips with a clang down several steps, and I stumble trying to retrieve it. This all feels too symbolically on point, this slapstick climb toward the halls of justice. Too on the nose with the crutches and the bum knee, the pratfalls and Sisyphean ascent.

I should just come back when my knee feels better, I think. But I've made it this far, and my new Silicon Valley tech job starts in a week, so I have to get this done today. I keep climbing, one step at a time: First the bag of documents, then me. Bag of documents, then me. Now, finally three steps shy of the grand colonnade, my bandaged knee throbbing, I spot—at the top of the stairs, not the bottom—a sign for the disabled entrance around the corner.

"Oh, for fuck's sake!" I say. Then I burst out laughing.

"What's so funny?" says the policeman guarding the door.

I'm laughing so hard at this point I can barely speak. I point to the sign with my right crutch. Try to form words, but the laughter is winning. "Life," I finally manage, before heading inside.

Altogether, my pro se divorce will take four years: two and a half of them in a holding pattern of paralysis for lack of money and options; another year and a half of acting as my own lawyer and representing myself. It will cost $626.50.* Which is 99 percent less than the $60,000 I was quoted to do it with lawyers, so I guess all that climbing on crutches was worth it.

Or was it? Maybe we should do away with all those painful, conflict-laden steps that feed only the divorce industrial complex, not those getting divorced, and even the playing field in terms of cost, as they do

---

* I paid $210 for an index number. The final filing of the papers cost an extra $125, plus $57 to have the papers served, then another $57 to have another set of papers served. If you want to change your name, as I did, a new driver's license costs $12.50, and a new passport costs $145. Retrieving the final judgment costs $20 for three copies. When all was said and done, the grand total was $626.50.

nearly everywhere else in the world except the U.S. In China, it costs $1.30 to get divorced and it takes around a half an hour. In Denmark, you don't even have to go in front of a judge. You can pay $77 and do the whole thing online. In Sweden, it's $151 out of respect to those who might not be able to afford the expense of divorce otherwise.

When the official postcard arrives confirming my divorce has been filed and is complete, I feel not only elated and relieved, but an entire chunk of my brain feels finally freed up for more fruitful pursuits.

A few days later, hoping to start a *Medium* channel for Elli with interesting stories about the brain and Alzheimer's research, I interview Dr. Lisa Mosconi, a neuroscientist at Weill Cornell who studies the link between estrogen depletion and Alzheimer's in women. Why, she wondered, early in her career, do twice as many women fall prey to Alzheimer's as men? Her grandmother and two great aunts had all died of the disease, while her great uncle was spared. Longevity alone cannot account for this. Alzheimer's plaques and tangles can start building up decades before symptoms arise.

The key, Mosconi became convinced, is the loss of estrogen associated with menopause. But no one was really looking at the difference between men and women when it came to brains.

During our interview, I happen to mention offhandedly that: A) I don't have a uterus; and B) I've been having word recall issues: names of friends; an artichoke held in my hand as my brain draws a blank; a windshield, which I described as "that piece of glass between me and the world;" even just the word *wind* itself, gone with it. The thing that blows?

"We have known for a good ten years," says Dr. Mosconi, "that taking out the ovaries or the uterus increases the risk of dementia in women."

At this point I turn off my tape recorder. "Are you fucking kidding me?" I ask for a moment to catch my thing that lungs do.

"It's true," she says. "There's a strong association between induced menopause and a higher risk of Alzheimer's in women. And some studies indicate that oophorectomy before menopause, which is the surgical removal of the ovaries, may increase the risk up to seventy percent relative to not having your ovaries removed."

"Seventy percent????!!!!!" Why the hell didn't I know this? *Why don't any of us know this?*

Later, I type up our interview and publish it on *Medium* not just for

Elli, but as a public service announcement to the millions of women like me—600,000 of us in the U.S. every year—who were told nothing about the risks of cognitive impairment before having their ladyparts removed, even though that information has apparently been available to scientists for more than a decade.

That interview, published in the spring of 2019 with no paid promotion, goes viral, well over a half a million views as of this writing and counting. And at least once a week from henceforth, an apologetic stranger will reach out to me over Twitter or Facebook to ask if I could help her join Dr. Mosconi's study, which I also eventually join as a subject, because while I'd like to say I'm surprised we've been ignoring half our society when it comes to the study of the human body, decades of experience and multiple excisions have taught me otherwise. If I can be one tiny ladyspeck on a data graph, I tell the doc, count me in. Even if it means spending two days every year or so for the next decade, or however long I have left in this corporeal form, being poked and prodded, questioned and challenged, filled with radioactive isotopes and shoved in PET scans and MRI tubes. "Any metal in the body?" the MRI attendant asks.

"Yes," I say. "A couple of breast clips in my right breast and a tiny shard of shrapnel in my right hand."

"So two wars?" the attendant jokes, and I want to hug her.

"Yes." I laugh. "The others didn't leave any metal." What they did leave were neurological scars in the folds of my hippocampus, which I've been painstakingly wresting onto the page ever since. This is how my brain has always extracted and processed life's buckshot: shard by shard.

"Today was a good day because I got you," I wrote on March 11, 1972, the day I turned six and was given my first diary. This was followed seven months later by "Connie is dead and her mommy killed her." Adolescence produced "God, girls can be so, so, so MEAN!" and "Everyone already has boobs and their periods except for me," and "I wish I could ask David to go sledding with me, but apparently that's not allowed, because for some reason boys have to ask the girls, and that's just stupid." Yes, sixth grade boyfriend David who would decades later offer to cover four months of my health insurance while I recovered from vaginal cuff dehiscence. I eventually did ask him out to the movies, and he said yes, and the world did not end.

After my brain scans with Dr. Mosconi, Maria Shriver, founder of the Women's Alzheimer's Movement, who read my *Medium* post, interviews me for the *Today* show. "Have you looked at your brain scan?" she asks. "Are you scared?"

"Yes and no," I say. "Yes, because one is always scared—I don't want to find something in there—but no because I'm going to get this information, and it's going to give me more knowledge about how to treat my body, how to treat my brain."

Information. Knowledge. Data. Studies. Yes, please. When, please? *Now*, please. Use us. Probe us. Study us. Know us. Let's figure this shit out, once and for all, Dear Science, because we've had it up to here—up to our brains, yes, but deep into our vaginas as well—with being ignored. Knowledge is power, or so we've heard, and we want both so we can make measured decisions about what goes into our bodies and what comes out of them without turning our brains into . . . what's that word? Mush.

To wit: Did you know that if you're a middle-aged woman, you have only a small window of opportunity between the beginning of perimenopause and the start of menopause to start estrogen replacement therapy to protect not only your brain but also your bones and cardiovascular system? I did not, until I dug into the science, because as a woman who was diagnosed with a stage 0 breast lump, I was scared off like so many of us from the results of the Women's Health Initiative, which got blasted out all over the news and initially showed a link between estrogen replacement therapy and breast cancer, but guess what? That study had so many flaws, its findings are little more than useless and possibly harmful. Worse, women like me without uteri show a *decrease* in breast cancer with estrogen replacement therapy. But this information never made it either into the headlines or into our gynecologists' offices. I had to find it in scientific publications such as *The Lancet* online.

In fact, get this: Our medical system barely trains gynecologists in menopausal medicine. A recent study found that only 20 percent of obgyn residency programs in the U.S. provide *any* menopause training. Yes, any. Which means that 80 percent of all gynecological residents in school today are getting *no training whatsoever* in post-reproductive women's health. These are people whose job it is to know everything going on in our ladyparts, but they have not been taught the basic tenets of how to care for either us or our plumbing after we stop menstruating. And by "us" I mean 30 percent of all women alive on earth at any given moment.

Half of my middle-aged female friends deal with chronic urinary tract infections. Oh, well, we think, throwing up our hands in defeat and consuming far too many antibiotics than are rational or safe or even good for the future safety of humanity. It took Dr. Rachel Rubin, a urologist in Washington, D.C., reaching out to me over Twitter to explain that UTIs in menopausal women do not have to be recurrent. They can be mitigated with, yes, vaginal estrogen. Not once was I ever told this by my own doctors. Not because they're not good doctors or they don't care, but because no one ever bothered to do the studies or to teach this to *them*.

Fuck Your Dumb Fire

JULY 2018–OCTOBER 2019

One year to the day after my return from Nepal—July 24, 2018—I get an email with a subject header that reads, "exciting news for you." I almost delete it. Exciting news in my headers these days means my old friend Old Navy is trying to get me to buy pants, or a PR rep is urging me to write a story about a new brand of personal lube so natural, you can spread it on toast. Then I note that the email is from Dan Jones, the editor of Modern Love. Amazon, he writes, has decided to make a TV series out of the column. "They love 'When Cupid Is a Prying Journalist,'" he writes, "and intend to make it the opening episode of the series."

I gasp. My blood vessels immediately fill with the kind of warm ecstasy that normally leads to rehab, but this high doesn't come with rotted teeth or a hangover. It's real. It feels miraculous, except it isn't. It came about because one morning three years earlier, on a packed subway to work, I opened up my computer and entrusted my brain with the task of counteracting the shame of using my words to help opioid addicts poop by jotting down a few truths I've learned about love—a natural opioid derived from endorphins, which doesn't cause constipation—instead.

"Shooting will begin in NYC in late September," Dan writes, "so we are on the fast track; they are casting it now. Maybe this fall we can visit the set together and you can see yourself being performed!" Later that summer, I'll learn Catherine Keener, the actress I would have chosen to play me in my fantasy version of who-would-you-want-to-play-you, will actually play me.

I want to scream this exciting news from the rooftops, but I'm allowed to tell no one. I'm not even allowed to tell Will yet, but come on. I tell him.

Will I get rich over this adaptation of my essay? Hell no. I'll earn $4,990.47, minus my agent's commission, on top of the $250 I was paid for the original essay back in 2015. But validation-wise, the enrichment feels boundless. John Carney, the writer and director of both the show and my episode, is the writer and director of what is arguably one of my favorite films, *Once*, a love story about a love that is never allowed expression, except through the heartrending music it spawns. The film was subsequently turned into a Broadway musical, which—get this—I happened to catch with the long-lost lover I described in the essay, the one who lost the piece of paper with my address and phone number on it and wound up sleeping in a youth hostel and wandering the streets of Paris all weekend by himself, making me believe I'd been stood up. For twenty-one years. He'd traveled to New York the year of the Broadway premiere of *Once*, which he had to see for his work.

The missed connection and loss of this man—with whom I watched that show two decades later, while crying in sad recognition over its unlived love—sparked not only my Modern Love essay itself but also the wedding of my essay's main characters: Justin, the dating app CEO, to his own long-lost love, Kate, at which I was the sole witness after they decided to call off their big wedding and elope.

In fact, let's dive a league deeper: The theme of my essay was that when it comes to affairs of the heart, a love that cannot last in the traditional sense because of circumstance, nevertheless can live on in the brain as a memory whose generative powers are infinite. "Because real love, once blossomed," I wrote, "never disappears. It may get lost with a piece of paper, or transform into art, books, or children, or trigger another couple's union while failing to cement your own. But it's always there, lying in wait for a ray of sun, pushing through thawing soil, insisting upon its rightful existence in our hearts and on earth."

And now here was that same love once again, spawning an episode on Amazon Prime.

Later that fall, five years after leaning my head out the window of my Harlem writing studio, wanting to end it all because I could no longer write books, my agent sells the proposal for this book to Random House, where I began my writing career, on the same day another email lands in my inbox. This one's from Catherine Keener, who's about to play a slightly altered version of me named Julie, so Amazon can avoid paying my life rights. Which is apparently why no one wants Catherine and me to meet in person, even though we've both expressed interest in so doing: Meeting would imply that she is, in fact, playing me. Which she technically isn't. But really she is. And just because everyone else has bought into the delusion that she isn't, so that all of the Modern Love essayists can be denied payment for our life rights, doesn't mean Catherine and I have to. "I know, it's so dumb," she writes, of whoever's edict it is to keep us apart. "I just laughed cause I was going to find you anyway."

I love her already. So often those of us with ladyparts are told to follow the rules and stay in our lanes, to play the part society dictates instead of being our genuine selves. Or we're fed corporate pablum telling us to stand tall and lean in. But you don't get to become Catherine Keener by simply tilting your body toward the burning wreckage. You say fuck your dumb fire and use the shoulder to drive around it.

In *The Ladies' Book of Etiquette, and Manual of Politeness*, published in Boston in 1860, Chapter XVI, "Polite Deportment, and Good Habits," reads thus:

> Many ladies, moving, too, in good society, will affect a forward, bold manner, very disagreeable to persons of sense. They will tell of their wondrous feats, when engaged in pursuits only suited for men; they will converse in a loud, boisterous tone; laugh loudly; sing comic songs, or dashing bravuras in a style only fit for the stage or a gentleman's after-dinner party; they will lay wagers, give broad hints and then brag of their success in forcing invitations or presents; interlard their conversation with slang words or phrases suited only to the stable or bar-room, and this they think is a dashing, fascinating manner. It may be encouraged, admired, in their presence, by gentlemen, and imitated by younger ladies, but, be sure, it is looked upon with

contempt, and disapproval by every one of good sense, and that to persons of real refinement it is absolutely disgusting.

Yes, it was considered "absolutely disgusting" for a woman to be bold, tell stories, pursue traditionally male activities, speak loudly, sing funny songs, be funny in general, laugh loudly, gamble, brag, use slang, and curse. I wish I could say we've had progress since 1860, but really? I have scrapbooks full of anti-woman tear sheet vitriol levied against me proving otherwise.

Catherine and I meet for lunch downtown at the Odeon, where we split a giant chocolate sundae for dessert and proceed to engage in every single one of the "disgusting" activities listed in the ladies etiquette book except gambling and singing. I'm no gambler, but had there been a karaoke machine nearby, I can guarantee we would have belted one out without shame or compunction. My daughter and her son, it turns out, are a year apart at the same college. Her laughter is unapologetic and contagious. She curses freely and with great gusto. Shots of tequila are downed, stories of surviving single motherhood and a career in the arts exchanged. No, I explain, I do not—*cannot*—live solely off the fruits of my personal writing: I have a corporate day job writing for a Silicon Valley tech company to make ends meet and procure health insurance. She tells me about the ways in which Hollywood treats women of a certain age, just when you're at the peak of your acting powers. We shake our heads and roll our eyes at the absurdity of it all.

By the end of that three-hour meal, she already has my mannerisms down pat: The way I gesture wildly when I get excited; my nasal, unbeautiful voice; the line of my lips when I'm trying not to smile or show emotion, which only highlights the unhidden emotion even more; the precise angle at which I extend my torso when I want to make a point. It feels like looking into a mirror, watching her transformation. Her hands are big, beautiful, like a man's. I can't stop looking at them. Admiring them. Afterward, we'll walk up to Washington Square Park, where in a couple of days she will speak words I wrote in a last-ditch effort to be heard.

I tell her about two days prior, when I'd written more words seeking an audience, only this time it was an audience of one: a letter written to the fellow student who raped me on the eve of my graduation from college, sparked by going hoarse from screaming at the TV during the Kavanaugh hearings. It begins thus:

September 18, 2018

Dear [redacted],

You may not remember me from college. We didn't even meet until the night before graduation. But I have never been able to forget that night or you. The memory, over these past 30 years, comes and goes, but it always pays a visit whenever I hear or read stories of sexual assault between acquaintances. As you can imagine, that's pretty much all the time these days, and this latest Kavanaugh hearing is no exception. In fact, it's been the straw that finally broke this aging camel's back. I realized I could not go on with my life until I finally wrote this letter. I'm shaking, even as I type it. . . .

I read the letter in its entirety to Catherine, after she asks to hear it, off the screen of my phone as we walk: "Let me state it as simply as possible, for clarity's sake," I read. "You forced yourself on me and pushed yourself into me as I kept saying no."

"Whoa," she says, when I finish reading. "That's intense. Did he write back?"

"Better," I say. Within half an hour of my sending him the email, he picked up the phone and called to apologize. We spoke for a long time, maybe twenty minutes. He had no recollection of raping me, just of the party where we'd met. He'd blacked out that night from excessive drinking and soon thereafter entered Alcoholics Anonymous. But that, he said, was no excuse. The fact that he'd done this to me and that I'd been living with the resulting trauma for thirty years was horrifying to him. He was so sorry, he said. He just kept repeating those words, "I'm so sorry," over and over. Then he promised to pay it forward in some way, this horrible thing he'd just learned about himself for which he was never punished.

Suddenly, I tell Catherine, thirty years of pain and grief fell out of me. I cried. And I cried. And I kept crying for the next several hours, as I prepared for Yom Kippur, the Jewish holiday of forgiveness. And then, after all those tears, I was cleansed. Reborn. The trauma was gone. All because of a belated apology.

"Wow," says Catherine. "You should write about that."

"Can't," I say. "I'm too busy right now with my day job."

The next morning, I wake up and read Trump's tweet, which begins thus: "I have no doubt that, if the attack on Dr. Ford was as bad as she says, charges would have been immediately filed with local Law Enforcement Authorities by either her or her loving parents."

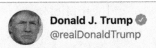

Donald J. Trump ✓
@realDonaldTrump
ooo

I have no doubt that, if the attack on Dr. Ford was as bad as she says, charges would have been immediately filed with local Law Enforcement Authorities by either her or her loving parents. I ask that she bring those filings forward so that we can learn date, time, and place!

9:14 AM · Sep 21, 2018 · Twitter for iPhone

21.1K Retweets   **21.8K** Quote Tweets   **94.1K** Likes

Fuck that guy, I think. And fuck staying quiet. Staying quiet has gotten us nowhere. Worse, it's made men doubt the veracity of our stories.

Driven by rage, I pound out the story of my rapist's apology in the hours between Trump's tweet at 9:14 A.M. and noon, when my day job in California officially begins. I write about the fallacy of our president's logic; about Kavanaugh, who is my age and grew up in my hometown, albeit on the wealthier side of it; about how hearing a real and heartfelt apology can literally change the way the brain processes trauma. I send it off to Adrienne, my *Atlantic* editor, with a closer that will echo into the future in ways I cannot yet fathom: "The life of my daughter is at stake. Her bodily autonomy is at stake. As a mother who grew up being groped at house parties in the '80s, I want to make sure that whoever is passing judgment on the next generation has, at the very least, judgment to pass."

Adrienne wants to publish my story the next day, after it gets vetted and copyedited. I'm not allowed to tell her that I'll be on set of my Modern Love episode that day, unreachable and often unable to talk, because I'm still not allowed to tell anyone about the show. So I just say, "Great," and pray I can use my cellphone as a hotspot to finish the edit.

Which is how I find myself, the next morning, sitting on a bench in Washington Square Park in front of Dev Patel, who's playing Justin, and Catherine Keener, who's playing me, as I furiously edit the new essay about my rapist's apology while hearing the words from my old essay coming out of Keener's mouth: "He was a senior in college, studying Shakespeare abroad, and I was a twenty-two-year-old war photographer living in Paris. . . ."

Words. Words are the one constant in my life and the only way my brain has found to make sense of it. No, they have not made me rich. But they have enriched me and, based on the evidence in my inbox, others. They've given me purpose; saved me multiple times from throwing in life's towel; sparked countless heartfelt letters from strangers; and allowed me to speak loudly, publicly, and decidedly unladylikely about topics that, for too long and to women's detriment, have remained private, particularly with regards to the female body: its health, its pleasures, its objectification, its violations, its blood, its clinical neglect, its autonomy.

After the rapist apology story is published in *The Atlantic*, thousands of women—and men!—write to tell me that they, too, have reached out

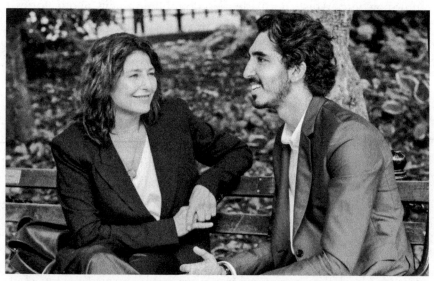

Catherine Keener and Dev Patel in "When Cupid Is a Prying Journalist,"
Modern Love, Season 1, © Giovanni Rufino/Amazon Studios

to their rapists and victims respectively for a necessary reckoning with the harm they've either experienced or perpetrated. Some of the women are disappointed and angry by either the lack of remorse or by the silence they receive from their perpetrators. Others are floored by the sudden healing of a true apology. Some men want to know if their past actions would be considered rape or simply dumb teenage fumbling. Others have suddenly realized what they did was wrong and want to figure out the proper way to make amends. All of them ask to read the letter I wrote, so I publish it on my otherwise mostly empty blog on my website with redactions for the sake of anonymity. This is not about calling out my rapist specifically or maligning his name thirty years after the fact for a crime he had no idea he'd committed. It's about calling out all men to hold themselves accountable for their actions.

Within hours of the story's publication, I am hounded by TV producers to come on their shows and continue the conversation my words have sparked. I speak live with CNN International; do a taped segment with Juju Chang on *Nightline*; reject an invitation to go on Fox News. "Call me when you stop lying and being the mouthpiece of the Trump administration, and then I might consider it," I say. I sit in either radio booths or my own living room, talking to disembodied reporters from all over the world, day, night, and sometimes in the wee hours of the morning, depending on the time zone of the live morning radio hour.

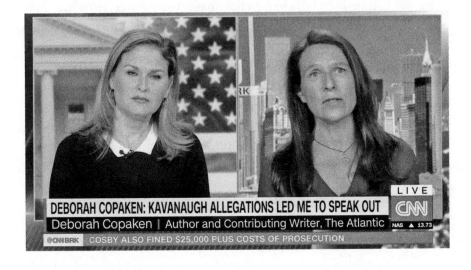

LIVE

DEBORAH COPAKEN: KAVANAUGH ALLEGATIONS LED ME TO SPEAK OUT CNN

Deborah Copaken | Author and Contributing Writer, The Atlantic | NAS ▲ 13.73

@CNNBRK COSBY ALSO FINED $25,000 PLUS COSTS OF PROSECUTION

Woman says she forgave her rapist after Kavanaugh allegations inspired her to reach out to him

"I have absolutely forgiven him. And it's the most beautiful thing..."

By **Claire Pedersen**, **Katie Muldowney**, and **Alexa Valiente**
September 27, 2018, 6:32 PM • 9 min read

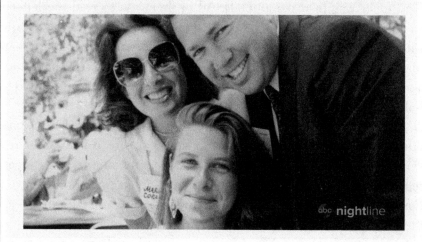

abc **nightline**

The ripples from this story will continue flowing outward. One of my sisters calls to tell me about the rabbi she runs into, whose husband teaches a philosophy course at UCSF about forgiving the unforgivable. For a week, this rabbi tells her, her husband used my essay to lead one of his discussions. Another sister tells me about the rapist who, as an adult newly confronted with his past violations as a teenager, has donated a large sum of money to fund research for the cancer that killed our father. Katherine Schwarzenegger reaches out to ask if she can turn my story into a chapter in her book on forgiveness. My own rapist will reach out, months later, to express gratitude over the way our private moment of healing sparked a growing number of others: "I wish you well in every respect . . . and I'm glad our interaction is creating good things."

Imagine how different college life would be, I think, for both women and men, if restorative justice were the norm in cases of campus rape, rather than these ridiculous Title IX kangaroo courts, in which no one's rights or mental health are well-served, neither the victims' nor their perpetrators'.

Catherine Keener will reach out to me again after a young woman she loves is later raped. She wants to know how best to talk to her. Just listen, I say, and let her speak. Don't offer palliatives or advice. She needs to work through the trauma herself, word by word. Your job is simply to absorb them.

On October 10, 2019—a year to the day after my divorce was finalized—I attend the premiere of the Modern Love TV series at the Museum of Love in SoHo, constructed specifically for the show, in which each of the nine episodes has been turned into an interactive experience for visitors. For my episode, you get to retreat into a confession booth and type your private secrets onto a public screen. Which is pretty much as on-brand for me as you can get. Will snaps a photo of me standing in front of it.

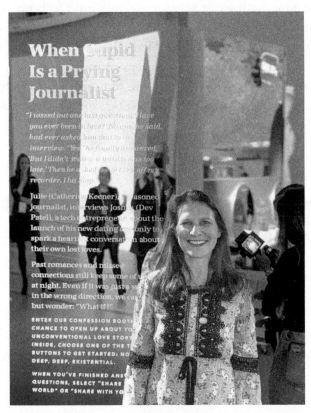

Premiere of *Modern Love*, © Will Dana

Justin and Kate are there as well, their brand-new baby strapped to Kate's chest in a red velvet baby carrier, which catches the eye of a hugely pregnant Anne Hathaway, who asks where she bought it. "I mean . . ." Kate says, shaking her head and hugging me. Justin tears up again, just as he did when he first told me about Kate, fearing he'd lost her forever. He opens his mouth to speak, but nothing comes out. This man is the normally extroverted CEO of a popular dating app. He's never, in the four years I've now called him my friend, been rendered speechless.

"I know," I say, feeling every word he's not saying. Dev Patel is standing behind us. Andrew Scott, the hot priest from *Fleabag*, and Andy Garcia, who played my long-lost lover, are both in my sightline. Ann Leary, an old friend, is standing with us as well, having had her own love story of playing tennis with her husband Dennis adapted by Tina Fey and John Slattery. "It's *crazy*."

And for a moment—just a moment—my world feels not only in balance but breathtaking.

Of course, balance never lasts. That's the recurring motif in each of our lives. Just as you have all three legs of your stool finally standing solid—work, love, health—one or more of them start to wobble. Or at least two of mine will, after the word *breathtaking* takes on a whole new meaning.

PART VII

LUNGS

2020–2021

Make a Wish

MARCH 11–MAY 6, 2020

"Stay in Cameroon!" I tell my daughter, who has now graduated college and is serving in the Peace Corps. "You'll be safer there." The coronavirus has swept through China. Italy is on lockdown, its hospitals overburdened to the point of breaking. We're next, that's clear to everyone except the U.S. government. My daughter lives in Kamba, a small jungle village of a thousand without running water or electricity, which means she's miles from the nearest big hospital but also from the nearest town and other humans who might infect her. My older son has been volunteering in Samos, Greece, doing laundry, cleaning dishes, and teaching war-traumatized refugees from Syria and elsewhere how to play guitar and record their own songs. His plan is to produce an album of these songs and pump the proceeds back into the organization after a quick jaunt through New Zealand to visit friends on his way back to the States. I urge him, too, to stay put in New Zealand, if he can afford to. "New Zealand has a female prime minister," I say. He'll be safe there. His job as the manager of a radio station near our home in Williamsburg won't be here when he gets home anyway. He should maybe even look for woofing (working on an organic farm) opportunities, if possible.

Official edicts for social distancing in the United States are still days away, and those that do come down from mayors and governors will be haphazard at best. Tonight, on March 11, my fifty-fourth birthday, New York City's bars are packed. My son's public middle school is still open. Everyone's still traveling back and forth to work on crowded subways, trains, and planes.

This morning, Will emailed our dinner guests and gave them an out if they felt uncomfortable showing up: "We've put Purell in the lasagna and Deb's wearing an outfit made of Clorox wipes. But if you don't want to risk it, we understand and won't be offended." Ten friends show up anyway to what we are all jokingly—but also presciently—calling the last supper.

"We're going to look back on this night," says my friend Al, "as the moment it all changed." She is right. "Cancel everything!" the head-lines will suddenly scream, as journalists fill in the leadership void. Can you believe Harvey Weinstein got sentenced to twenty-three years today, too? What a day. What a dizzying, crazy day.

It has become impossible to keep up with the news. One of my din-ner guests, Amanda Brainerd, served on the Weinstein jury. "What???!!!!" Every mouth at the table is agape. What a crazy secret to have kept for two months. "How was it?"

"Traumatizing," she says and leaves it at that. She is not allowed to say more.

While Will lights the candles on my cake, our phones start to buzz with notifications from various news organizations. Trump is apparently addressing the nation right now, calling Covid-19 a "foreign virus"; the NBA is canceling its season; the World Health Organization has de-clared Covid-19 a global pandemic; Tom Hanks and Rita Wilson have the virus.

"Make a wish!" everyone says. I ponder: What do I want? Last week, if you'd asked me what I really wanted, I would have said simply, "A string of normal days." Without qualification. Just a string of normal days. For *me*.

This week? Tonight? I look around at this circle of friends; at Will, holding the glowing cake; at my youngest, now thirteen, the last child still at home, gamely showing up to a tableful of grown-ups when all he wants to do is FaceTime with his friends. I think about my daughter tucked away under her mosquito netting in the jungle; about my older son, waking up on the other side of the earth. They are children of the world, my kids. I'm proud of them. None of them will ever be able to afford to take care of me in my dotage, but that's okay. Let them spend their limited time caring for others, if that's what drives them. When I'm old—if I'm lucky enough to grow old—I'll have somehow made it to being old, and that will have been enough. My candles will one day burn out like everyone's.

I close my eyes. Squeeze tight. Today's wish cannot just be about me.

I've already been all-but quarantined this past month, having undergone foot surgery to remove a Morton's neuroma from my right foot. Morton's neuromas are a thickening of the tissue around one of the nerves leading to the toes, which causes a shocking, searing pain in the ball of the foot every time you step on it. One of the major risk factors for sprouting a Morton's neuroma between your third and fourth toes, where mine is located, is walking in stiletto heels. I haven't worn stilettos since college, plus the occasional wedding in my twenties and thirties, but the damage from that small window of adhering to female beauty standards had already become permanent. I could no longer walk without feeling like I was stepping on a pebble with every step.

Morton's neuroma surgery is not nearly as bad as getting your lady-parts cut out. It was quick: in and out of the Hospital for Special Surgery in three hours. And it was paid, minus $800 in co-pays, by the affordable health insurance coverage now provided to me by my union, the Writers Guild of America. I qualified for WGA insurance this year by virtue of having been a staff writer on *Emily in Paris*, but my right to that insurance runs out after one year, not two, as I'd expected, and now I'm once again fucked.

I do not like this game of Frogger. I've been playing it for three decades, and yet somehow I still always end up missing the log by a fraction of an inch and plopping right back into the water. Then again, the game is rigged. That's the whole point.

As of 2020, the WGA requires nearly $40,000 in yearly screenwriting income, which can get carried over from year to year, to qualify for union health insurance. If I'd earned $80,000 from working on *Emily in Paris*—which I should have—I'd be okay. But I didn't. I fell $14,000 short of this number. Why? Because I did not insist on a written contract to help write the pilot in exchange for a job on the show and a script of my own. No, let's take that one step further. I should have never agreed to give away my intellectual property for the chance of a middle-aged lady on-ramp.

In other words? At least half of this is my fault for being shortsighted, naïve, and a patsy. Darren knew both my ladyparts and ladypurse struggles intimately. We were constant companions and confidantes during each of them. In fact, the two of us were having lunch one day during one of our *Emily in Paris* brainstorming sessions in New York when I received yet another difficult call from a doctor two months after my bleed-out—a bright spot on my rib on a PET scan, which showed the "uptake" of a tumor,[*] meaning the area on my rib that hurt was "hot" with cell division—and I broke down in tears in front of him. "It's too much," I'd said. "I can't catch a break."

Darren knew I wanted to transition into full-time TV writing, both to fulfill a lifelong dream and to never have to think about paying outrageous COBRA fees ever again. More saliently, he knew I'd do anything for him, just as I'd always assumed he'd do anything for me. We'd been close friends since our big fat gay honeymoon to Paris in 2002, on our *Shutterbabe* research trip. When my dad died, he sent food. When he was thinking of having a baby, I offered my ovum. When my marriage broke up, he was there. When each of his two serious relationships broke up, I was there. We texted each other on Rosh Hashanah, the Jewish new year, no matter where we were in the world, which is more a thing that Jewish family members do for one another: "*Chag sameach!*" I'd write—*happy holidays* in Hebrew. "I love you." I showed up at his ex-boyfriend's son's birthday, the one he helps raise. He showed up at my son's bar mitzvah. We'd taken hours-long walks on beaches, through the streets of New York City, all over Paris. When he moved to New York from L.A. in the fall of 2014, I'd thrown him that twenty-person welcome party to which I'd first invited Gio. It had taken me weeks to plan,

---

[*] Two weeks later, this alleged tumor was deemed to be my broken rib healing itself from the fall at the hospital during my bleed-out. I had no idea I'd broken a rib during that fall, as I was not conscious for its violence, so when I was asked if I'd broken a rib, I said no. The only thing I remembered from that night was the darkness that descended just prior to my fall, with a pastiche of broken shard memories after, and all I knew was that my rib had been hurting every time I took a breath since the surgery. Had I allowed my daughter to call an ambulance that night, instead of taking UberPool to the emergency room, my rib would not have been broken, as I would have been wheeled in on a gurney instead of walking from the car while leaning on her shoulder.

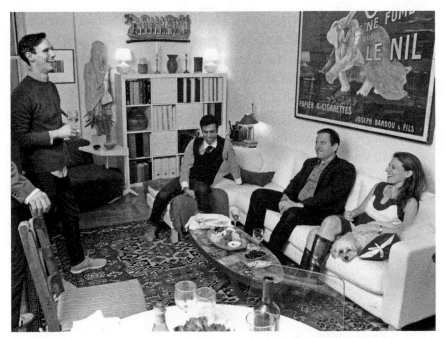

October 2014, welcome dinner for Darren Star, Deborah Copaken, © Cristobal Vivar

days to cook, right as I was starting my full-time job at *Cafe*, but I loved every second because I loved him.

Darren was, in essence, the brother I never had. The fact that we'd both grown up in the same hometown and had gone to the same high school; the fact that his little brother was once best friends with my little cousin, and therefore my aunt and his mother were friends: all just icing, when we discovered this, on our multilayered friendship cake.

He is conspicuously absent tonight as I stare at the flickering candles on my actual cake.

"Great news on *Emily in Paris*!" a TV executive friend will say to me, after the show once again hits the top five on Netflix. "Congratulations!" Not wanting to poison the well, I'll say a quick thank-you and try to change the subject, but my face will betray me.

In exchange for the nominal $5,000 I was paid to work on the pilot for *Emily in Paris* with Darren—instead of the $80,000 I was paid by a signatory company on *Shutterbabe*—I'd been promised two things: 1) a paid job in the writers' room; and 2) my own episode to write: Again, a bargain I'd stupidly agreed to, trusting those promises would be kept.

Darren had followed through on the first promise, but only after serious nudging from my agent and at the lowest and least well-paid rung on the TV writing ladder: staff writer. He did not follow through on the latter. I kept asking which episode I'd be writing. He kept telling me to be patient. Months passed. I remained both patient and scriptless. Later, when seven of the scripts came in needing extensive polishing and Darren panicked, he asked me to punch up all of them. I switched out wooden lines such as:

> EMILY
> I don't want half of you. I need all of you.

And turned them into . . .

> EMILY
> I'm not somebody who can share a crepe. I need the whole crepe.

. . . but without any "written by" credit on any of the scripts.

Two weeks before the show's premiere as the number one streamed show on Netflix, my best friend from Paris, Marion—the editor at *Paris Match* with whom I was constantly consulting while working on both the pilot and the show; the woman to whom I'd introduced Darren during our 2002 research trip as the best friend described in *Shutterbabe*—will send me the Netflix publicity materials in an email, with my name omitted from the credits. "WTF?" she'll write.

That same day, I'll receive an email from the WGA, reminding me that my health insurance premiums are about to go up from $150 a quarter to $2,398.39 every month—that's $28,776 a year—on October 1, 2020: exactly one day before the *Emily in Paris* premiere.

That night, I will sit down and write Darren a long email with the header "Some thoughts I needed to air." "Dear Darren," I'll begin. "I have been avoiding writing this letter for over a year, but I realized that our friendship is too important not to say hard things when they must be said. In fact, not saying these things has already hurt our relationship, at least privately, on my side of it, and for the two of us to share an honest friendship, hard truths must be aired and told." Over the course of the next several paragraphs, I will remind him of all of the work I did on the pilot that was supposed to have been exchanged for a "written by" credit on my own script: the key, for me, for procuring more work in TV. I will then ask for credit where credit is due.

A pilot has three different credits: "created by," "written by," and "story by," in descending order of importance. I will ask him for the latter, "story by," to at least acknowledge the story's origin in both *Shutterbabe* and in my own twentysomething expat life in Paris; in my subsequent position as an executive in pharmaceutical marketing at the PR firm; and for my dozens of all but unpaid hours of hard work in fleshing out Emily's world. "I'm not even asking for writing credit on the pilot," I'll write, "or for money. I just want an adequate acknowledgment, through a proper shared 'story by' credit, that I put my barely remunerated sweat equity into that pilot."

He'll apologize, kindly, for not keeping his end of the bargain. He'll tell the production company to fix their mistake and add my name as "staff writer" to the listing on IMDb. But he will also claim he cannot give me "story by" credit on the pilot. That's not how things work, he'll tell me over the phone. He will offer me a script for season two but not a job in the room, which not only makes little sense, it contradicts the terms of our oral arrangement: a guaranteed job on the show and a script, in each season, for my uncredited help with the pilot. "Will you put that promise in writing?" I'll ask of the season two script.

"No," he'll say.

Colleagues who worked with me on the show will urge me to take action. "Of course you should have story credit on that pilot!" one of them will yell at me. Several of them will urge me to contact the WGA: That's what you pay your dues for, they'll tell me. For situations just like this.

Distraught, I'll email the WGA and ask for help resolving this amicably. The next day, Darren will block me on Instagram.

"Don't take it personally," the TV executive will say to me.

"But I do," I'll say, holding back tears. "I'm actually more upset about the loss of the friendship than I am about the loss of credit."

The week before the show airs, when Darren and I should be high-fiving each other and sending congratulatory texts, an icy silence will descend. I'll read all of his interviews, in which Darren will say his backpacking trip through Europe as a nineteen-year-old was the origin story of the show. "Star studied French through college and used to imagine living in Paris," Alexis Soloski will write in *The New York Times*. "So it didn't take much effort to put himself in Emily's shoes, no matter how high heeled."

Darren Star is worth a purported $120 million. I'm still living paycheck to paycheck and paying $2,398 every month in COBRA fees.

Suffice it to say, the health insurance part of this is utter insanity, all of us having to figure out coverage through our jobs, which for many of us are constantly changing. Or in my case, sometimes you have no health insurance or obscenely expensive COBRA, because you're sick or recovering from surgery or you've been fired or sexually harassed; or sometimes you have four jobs all at once because feast or famine. During one twelve-week period at the beginning of 2019 my schedule looked like this:

4:00 A.M.—9:30 A.M.: Write this book
9:30 A.M.—10:00 A.M.: Walk to work
10:00 A.M.—4:30 P.M.: Work in the *Emily in Paris* writers' room[*]
4:30 P.M.—5:00 P.M.: Walk home from work
5:00 P.M.—11:00 P.M.: Alzheimer's and cognitive science writing
11:00 P.M.—4:00 A.M.: Sleep
Weekends: Catch up on all of the above plus *Atlantic* writing

Meanwhile, Harvey Weinstein's sentencing today felt less like a birthday present and more like a sad reckoning long past due. I do not celebrate his incarceration over the next twenty-three years, but I am glad for it. The next man in power who tries to use that power to steal a woman's dignity or paycheck or reputation for the sake of his own sexual gratification will have to think twice before dangling work he never plans to provide and promises he never plans to keep, should the target of his manipulation not submit to her own violation or mortification.

Actress Mira Sorvino, whom Weinstein blackballed to every director

[*] I was able to relocate to L.A. for those twelve weeks thanks to childcare provided back in New York by Will, my new partner, and by my son's father. The two shared custody while I was away. I think it's important to mention this here, that I was finally able to take a leap thanks to two men caring for my one child.

in Hollywood as being difficult after she refused his advances, performed in a lip-sync, rock opera version of *Wuthering Heights* with me back when we were both undergraduates. Mira landed a bit part in the chorus, as the wind on the moors. I danced around her half naked as Isabella. Despite having one of the smallest parts on that stage, Mira was hardworking, humble, kind, and collaborative: a team player through and through. Weinstein deliberately ruined this talented, dedicated, and brilliant woman's reputation. He went out of his way to destroy her career. She'll never get those years back. It pains me to think about Mira's loss of potential after her Oscar win. What other Oscar-worthy performances did we miss out on because she said no to this monster? How many future dollars did he steal from her children's mouths? And she's just one actress of many.

My friend Al is sitting across from me, next to Will, aglow with candles. A talented writer with a big heart and nimble brain, she started out as an actress, but found the casting couch intolerable. What performances did we miss out on from Al because men kept asking her to use her body as a conduit to success, and she said no? "Quick! Blow out the candles!" she says. They're dripping all over the cake.

"Sorry," I say. "I'm still thinking about my wish. Um . . . uh . . ." *A world in which #MeToo is no longer necessary? A string of normal days for all women?* I open my eyes. "Okay. I have my wish." *A string of normal days for all of us,* I think, looking out at my friends. Imagining all the other vulnerable bodies out there. Then I repeat it in my head a second time, in case the wish fairies require dedication: *A string of normal days for all of us.* I don't believe in wishes coming true, but hey, why not? It can't hurt at the beginning of a pandemic. To wish for my fellow humans not only to live but to live decent lives, free from unnecessary suffering, with their minimum basic needs met. That's all I really want.

The last supper, indeed. Tom Hanks has it! That's it. No one's safe.

But of course safety is an illusion during the best of times. My daughter just spent three terrifying hours, between midnight and 3 A.M., hiding from a home intruder. She barely escaped her tiny village on the back of a motorcycle, clutching her kitten. Suzi and Franklin, sitting to my left, just lost their twenty-three-year-old daughter, Maddy, to an icy road and an oncoming truck. One week to the day following their daughter's death, Franklin insisted on celebrating Suzi's birthday, because what else are you going to do? The wax is melting. It's the ritual itself that's soothing, curative. A reminder that life goes on until it doesn't. So you blow out the candles. Poof.

A week after blowing out my candles, I hand in this book to my editor. Or rather, I hand in the happy-ending version of this book I'd signed a contract to write a year earlier, which ended with Part VI, "Brain." To celebrate finishing, I go out for a bike ride with Will. The air is finally warm enough. My right foot finally feels strong enough, one month after surgery, to press down on a bike pedal without too much pain, as long as I favor the left foot. Lockdown in New York has just begun, but we are being urged to step outside every day for a little exercise if we can.

Usually, my elation over finishing the first draft of a book produces a kind of euphoria that lasts for days, but this ride lasts all of ten minutes before I feel a wave of fever and exhaustion and have to turn around.

I chalk it up to my latest UTI, which has been raging for more than a week: the last UTI I will ever have before going on estrogen replacement therapy,[*] which has, I'm happy to report, completely solved the problem of recurring UTIs while also—added bonus—lifting the brain fog of menopause, alleviating the severity of my migraines, and making me feel like myself again. But this last UTI is a doozy, and it is not going away without a fight.

I'd told the young, male doctor at the nearby urgent care that Keflex, the antibiotic he prescribed for it, wouldn't work. I even told him which one would work—Cipro—but he wouldn't listen. He knew what he was doing, he said. I'm sure he did, I said, and I understand why Cipro has to be the antibiotic of last resort. I even worked on a seminar about antimicrobial resistance for the World Science Festival, so I get it. But I also know my body and how it reacts to various medications, and after dozens upon dozens of UTIs, my urinary tract has become resistant to every antibiotic except Cipro. But the young doctor would not be swayed, no matter how vehemently I argued. "That can't be true," he said.

---

[*] I use Divigel, a gel you apply once a day to the inside of the thigh, switching thighs each day. If you're reading this, and you're perimenopausal and curious, I urge you to contact a gynecologist who specializes in treating women who are either in or heading toward menopause to discuss your options before you're on the other side of it. Your brain has only a small window of opportunity to benefit from estrogen replacement therapy. After menopause, it's too late.

"But it is true," I said.

Dear Medical Schools: Please teach your male doctors to listen to their female patients. We know a thing or two about what goes on inside us, even if we may not know why, how, or what to call it. We also definitely know which medications have worked and not worked on our bodies in the past, so please treat that information as valuable.

I took the antibiotic the doctor prescribed. It didn't work.[*] The infection worsened.

I call the urgent care on March 18, after my aborted bike ride, to get a new prescription. But their office, which does not yet have the means to test for Covid-19, has become so overrun with a surge of patients showing up with hacking coughs, they've stopped answering their phones. I can't visit my regular primary care physician, because that would mean taking the subway to see him, plus he's been stricken by Covid-19 and isn't seeing patients anyway.

Epidemiologists now believe that by March 1, 2020, roughly 10,000 coronavirus infections had already spread through New York City alone, undetected. My first visit to the urgent care, to be given what I knew was a useless antibiotic for my UTI, was on March 9.

On March 19, with a raging fever, I hobble over to the urgent care on my cane—yes, I'm still using a cane to walk for more than a block at this point, post foot-surgery—and open the door. "Hi," I say, peeking my head in, but standing firmly with my body outside on the sidewalk. There are several patients coughing violently into the reception area and struggling to breathe. No one is wearing a mask. "I came in here for a UTI a week ago, but the antibiotic the doctor prescribed didn't work. And now I have a fever. And you guys aren't answering your phones. Can you please tell the doctor I saw to send in a prescription for Cipro to the same Duane Reade as before? I'd rather not come in, for obvious reasons."

"You have to come in," says the harried receptionist. "We can't give you a prescription without a positive urinalysis."

"But you have my pee from last week!" I say, panicking. "Use that pee! Nothing's changed. It's just gotten worse."

---

[*] A year later, on February 24, 2021, *The Society for Healthcare Epidemiology of America* will publish a damning report showing that in the 670,000 health claims filed for uncomplicated UTIs between 2011 and 2015, nearly *half* of the women were prescribed the wrong antibiotic.

"Sorry," she says. Those are the rules.

At this point, I have two choices, both zonks. Behind door number one, go home and wait for a kidney infection to settle in, which will mean having to enter a coronavirus-inundated hospital later on. Behind door number two, risk contracting Covid-19 today by walking through this urgent care door right now and peeing into another cup.

Untreated UTIs are not only painful, they can kill. I choose door number two and spend forty minutes marinating maskless in Covid-infused air, hearing other patients in severe distress in various exam rooms. Meanwhile, patients continue to arrive, gasping and unabated. When the receptionist asks them what's wrong, they say, "I can't breathe," between labored breaths and hacking coughs. Many beg to be tested for Covid-19, but tests are still weeks away from becoming available to anyone who hasn't visited China.

In other first world countries (*are we even first world anymore?*), it takes four to six hours.

The immediate results of my UTI test are clear: It's still bad and getting worse. It feels like fire when I pee and smells like burning tire; there's blood in my urine; the compulsion to pee now comes every minute or so while producing only a pathetic stream with each visit to the bathroom; I have a fever.

I pick up my prescription for Cipro by standing in line with several unmasked pharmacy patrons who look at me as if I'm crazy for wearing the mask I nabbed at the urgent care.

Back at home, I wipe down my cane and face mask with bleach, strip off my clothes, and toss them immediately into a scorching hot wash. Later that day, Will comes down with a fever, as does my younger son. Then Will becomes violently ill with gastrointestinal distress, which at the time is not yet being reported as Covid-19-related. A few days after that, on March 23, while organizing my spices into new containers, I notice I can't smell them. I lose my sense of taste the same day and become too nauseated to eat. The next day, I have a raging sore throat. A day after that, wracked with body aches, I find I'm unable to breathe. I feel like a fish flopping on shore, gasping for each breath.

My hunch is that my two visits to the urgent care are to blame. And yes, it is not lost on me that had I known—or had any of my many doctors told me, as I entered perimenopause—that topical estrogen works well to combat UTIs, I would not have had to make that first visit to the urgent care, at the beginning of a pandemic. And had the urgent care doctor trusted my knowledge of my own body's reaction to various antibiotics, I would not have had to make the second visit to seek out a prescription for the antibiotic I told him to give me in the first place.

Sexism in medicine nearly killed me once, when a lack of understanding of the shape and mechanics of the clitoris and its gift, the orgasm, resulted in my being advised to keep my cervix during my first hysterectomy, which then led to the second major surgery to remove the cervix five years later. Which, in turn, led to my bleed-out. Now ignorance of estrogen's curative role in managing recurring middle-aged female UTIs, along with the medical establishment's abysmal track record on proper UTI prescriptions for women and lack of trust in my own understanding of my body, its ailments, and its drug resistances, has put my life at risk for the second time in three years.

I wonder if I were a man saying, "Keflex won't work," to the urgent care doctor, would he have listened? And why did it take a female urologist *reaching out over Twitter*, after reading my story in *The Atlantic* about the link between estrogen loss and Alzheimer's, to tell me what should be common knowledge among menopausal women with recurring UTIs? Or at the very least one of the recommended courses of action by our doctors.

Even migraines, the prevalence of which researchers have found can often intensify in women entering perimenopause, are still today being treated as unsolvable clinical mysteries at our neurologists' offices instead of as a possible side effect of hormonal fluctuations. I was "healthcare gaslit," in fact, by two neurologists, who told me hormones had nothing to do with my migraines, before finding a third who would both listen to my theory and believe me when I said I'd had intense migraines as a young child, prior to puberty, but then they went away completely until perimenopause.

Even so, it took a conversation at a wedding reception with a stranger to inform me that the migraines from which I'd been suffering sometimes daily could be eliminated—completely!—by a new drug she was taking called Aimovig, a monthly self-injection that contains a monoclonal antibody called erenumab, made from immune cells. This monoclonal antibody blocks the activity of calcitonin gene-related peptide

(CGRP), a protein that causes the inflammation and vasodilation in my brain that leads to severe migraines. She was living proof, she said, that it worked, and she was right. Since starting the drug in 2019, I had three migraines—instead of an average of fifteen a month post-hysterectomy—during the first month and zero every month thereafter.

My neurologist still had to argue with my insurance company to have this miracle cure covered, by proving that the three other medications we'd tried had all failed, two of which produced such intense brain fog, I could barely work. And yes, men have to fight just as hard as women to have the $603.18 monthly cost of Aimovig covered by insurance, minus their co-pays, but migraines are also three times more prevalent in women as they are in men. Why? Recent research suggests a drop in estrogen is believed to play a significant role.

We women also visit our doctors more often than men—33 percent more often, by some estimates, and that's excluding visits for pregnancy and childbirth—for yearly Pap smears and annual physicals, which are two separate visits (why?), as well as to have our prescriptions filled for medications that are either necessary for our survival or keep us from getting pregnant. Never mind that 76 percent of all doctors believe that oral contraceptives should be available over the counter, without having to first visit a doctor for a prescription, and that more than 100 countries worldwide already provide this benefit to their female citizens. We are also fourteen times more likely to get a UTI than men. And every time we get a UTI, instead of calling up our doctors and saying, "Got another one, can you please call in a prescription?" we have to pay an in-person visit and pee in a cup just to prove what our bodies already know. And when we pay in-person visits to our doctors, urgent cares, or hospitals for easily treatable UTIs, we are that much more likely to catch whatever bugs are floating around that day.

In the end, it doesn't really matter how I caught the coronavirus. Because now all three of us in my household have it, and we must self-isolate, my doctor tells us, to keep from getting one another sicker from viral load. My son's fever is mild. He feels better after a few days. Will's case is worse. He spends the next several months battling periods of intense fatigue. Me? I can't breathe. As in I literally cannot get enough oxygen into my lungs, just at the moment when New York City's hospitals have reached capacity. For three nights, my oxygen saturation dips below 90. This leads to hypoxemia, in the short term; in the long term, permanent lung damage. It also results in months of intense brain fog, fatigue, and POTS: postural orthostatic tachycardia syndrome, which manifests as a heart rate that suddenly spikes from resting to marathon level from the simple act of climbing a staircase, walking up a small hill, or even sitting up in bed. My fainting spells, in other words, have now increased from once every few months to several times a day.

The Zoom funerals, too, come fast and furious. Within one week, I lose an old friend, and three of my friends lose parents. But this plague is also as personal as it is ubiquitous, leaving scars on both of my lungs and on every family in the country. With zero national leadership and pitiful national stimulus—the governments of our wealthy allies pay their citizens a basic monthly income to stay home—American workers who are still lucky enough to have a job often face a choice between sickness or starvation.

Enraged and still febrile, I decide to reckon with this sudden calamity on the page, in *The Atlantic*.

I open my computer, where I have several stories open at once. First I finish the story about coming down with the virus. Then I hand in the one about the challenges of shared custody under quarantine. Then I write about the sadness of having to put down my dog, Lucas, when vets in New York are not allowing pet owners to come inside and hold our animals as they die. You just hand over your dog to the nurse in the vestibule between the sidewalk and the vet office and say goodbye there: So long, my tail-wagging pal! Here's a stranger who's going to kill you. Sorry. Please don't hate me. We had a good run these past thirteen years, didn't we? Woof.

In a sense, I am giving myself permission to grieve by writing these stories while still recovering from a virus whose destruction feels ongoing and endless. To translate the pain of not being able to see or hug my older children, who are back in the States but still refugees from my infected home. To mark the loss of friends and their parents. To capture the feelings of not being able to breathe; of too many Zoom funerals to count; of everyone dying alone, without their loved ones by their sides; of all of us losing the connective social threads holding life's batting in place.

Meanwhile, I have to keep up with all of my Alzheimer's writing and responsibilities for my Silicon Valley job as well: Zoom meetings, op-eds, app-writing, social media posts, all from my bedroom, coughing up a lung. My recovery is slow. It will be months before I can breathe properly or walk up stairs without feeling faint, but I put on a nice shirt over my pajama bottoms, sit at a desk, and feign wellness whenever I meet with colleagues online. I even purchase a ring light to soften the dark shadows on my wan face. I want them to know they can count on me, with or without oxygen.

On the morning of May 6, 2020, I wake up, have my coffee, open my computer, and continue to ghostwrite a new op-ed for Elli, on the nature of communal grief and its effects on the brain. We've partnered with several insurance companies, who want to provide our app as a perk to their long-term care customers, and my job is to get my boss's name out there as an expert in the field. I've also just helped her put the finishing touches on another op-ed, but it's still in its final round of revisions. When her private Slack message arrives at 12:15 P.M., as I'm toasting a frozen bagel for lunch, I assume it's about that.

"Are you around?" she writes over Slack. Weird. Normally she texts my phone when she wants to chat.

"Yup!" I type back. Where else would I be?

"Did you get the notice for the all hands?"

No, I have not seen the email she sent less than an hour earlier. I've been writing her new op-ed and editing an old one. Plus normally emails from the West Coast don't start arriving in my inbox until just after noon my time.

I dial in to the Zoom meeting and see only a blank white screen. I've missed it entirely. Double weird. Normally our all hands Zoom meetings last between forty-five minutes and an hour. At night. Suddenly, a new Slack channel appears: #goodbye.

"Wait, is the company folding?" I type to Elli.

It takes an unusually long time for the word layoffs to appear. She'd hoped to explain all of this during the public Zoom, then over a private discussion later. A representative from HR will have to join us on a Zoom link later. Meaning, I am about to get fired . . . over Zoom?

I click on the recording of the all hands meeting I missed. Instead of twenty-five tiny Zoom boxes, it contains one large rectangle of our CEO, wearing a black shirt and sitting under the familiar white eaves of her beige home office. Or maybe that's her bedroom, who knows? Though we've all become intimate with the color, shape, and decoration of one another's homes, they hardly paint a full picture of who we are, how we grieve, or what keeps us up at night when those walls reflect neither light nor color.

In the video, she mentions the ravages of Covid-19 on our business and the rationale behind the significant reduction in force of our ranks: RIF for short, I'll later learn, after the acronym gets batted around so many times in a subsequent meeting, I have to secretly google it mid-Zoom. The last half of her announcement is taken up by a heartfelt, moving, tearful apology, replete with an acknowledgment of the pain she knows this will inflict on our lives and on those of our families, particularly now.

At the appointed hour for my own video conference layoff, I click on the Zoom link. A Doom link, I think, as my image appears vertically between Elli's and Vien's, our head of HR. In *Brady Bunch* terms, I'd be Alice, my boss would be Carol, and our head of HR would be Mike.

"I'm so sorry," says Elli. Her eyes water anew. She has made this same call multiple times over the course of this day.

"I'm so sorry, too," I said, choking back my own tears. "But this is an unprecedented time, and I get it. Are you okay? I'm worried about you."

Hyperempathy, my shrink once labeled this propensity to avoid my own pain by over-identifying with the pain of others: A trait that is simultaneously self-protective and self-destructive.

"I should write about this for *The Atlantic*, getting fired over Zoom," I say. When people talk about the hazards of being a writer, this is what they mean. I'm literally saying these words out loud to my boss and to the head of HR, already composing the odd little story I could stuff into a bottle and float out into the grief ocean as my shame-reducing offering to everyone else getting fired over Zoom about getting fired over Zoom while getting fired over Zoom. I even consider it a small victory to imagine processing the suffering while living through it. The time gap between those two used to be longer. Decades longer, in some cases.

Luckily, I have not taken a single day of vacation since starting this job two years ago. After being penalized in my performance review at the PR firm for taking off two weeks to work on *Younger* in L.A. (*Leslie also said she had to pick up your slack when you were off gallivanting in Hol-*

lywood . . .), I've been afraid of taking one day off from this job, even while working on *Emily in Paris*. I simply scheduled my Zoom calls during lunch and took the evening hours after work to complete the rest of the day's Alzheimer's research and writing.

This, I know, is crazy. In fact, from all of my Alzheimer's research, I've learned that giving up life and sleep and socializing and a proper break from work is pretty much the worst thing you can do for both your brain and your body. But now, at least, I've bought myself an extra month of vacation pay to figure out what's next.

I will need it.

After crying what I believe to be all the tears, I'm interrupted by worse news. A classmate from college, the mother of five who range in age from grade school to young teen, has succumbed to the trauma of this period and killed herself. "We may never fully understand the whys of this," her husband writes, "but we do understand that the human heart, with the right mix of circumstances, may in a moment choose the unthinkable."

Will walks in on me weeping in the living room as I'm reading the announcement of my classmate's death, two hours after my fifth job loss in seven years—the first for spending too much time at Sloan Kettering; the second for not dumbing it down and making it shorter; the third for not fucking my boss; the fourth for not being a "good fit"; and now the fifth due to Covid-19. It seems wrong for me to worry about how I will pay for food and my half of the rent when my classmate's husband's and children's burdens are so much greater. And yet I was just fired over Zoom during an economic extinction event. It hurts. I'm worried about my future, my children's future, Earth's future. Will knows me well enough at this point to read all of this on my face. "I have an idea," he says, "but it's really more of an order. We're going on a bike ride."

A quick note about Will and love, because he will hate this paragraph when he stumbles upon it. Which is one of the things I love about him: his abhorrence of the Instagramization of happy coupledom; his fierce protection of the sacred and private. But it must be said, as I finally retire WhatifLovewerereal?49 as my computer password, that not only is love with Will real, it is because of him—because of us—that I finally understand love as a verb, not a noun. "Here," he'll say, "I thought you might need this," handing me a cozy wool-covered hot-water bottle, which he's already filled with boiling water, when it's cold outside, and I'm working. Or I'll awake to the aroma of coffee and spot the latte he's frothed and hand-pulled and quietly slipped onto the bedside table, so as not to wake me. Or he'll send me a link to a photography class he thinks my son might like. Or he'll find me weeping in the living room and know exactly what I need before my grieving brain even has time to think it.

"Yes," I say, grateful. "A bike ride. That would be nice."

We ride out to Red Hook in time to stare out at the sun setting behind the Statue of Liberty.

"Still standing," I say.

"For now," says Will. "I'll be right back." He returns five minutes later with a key lime pie. "Thought you might like this," he says, securing the pie box to his bicycle's basket with a couple of masks.

The Cost of Oxygen

MAY–JULY 2020

At the end of May, still struggling to breathe, I visit a pulmonologist and get a chest X-ray and a new prescription for a steroid inhaler. I also start tackling the unexpected final section of this book.

Writing, post-Covid, has been a challenge. Many days, I give up after a couple of paragraphs. On the days I do push through, I often lose the end of a sentence, word, or thought before it makes it onto the page. Simple words and concepts feel beyond my grasp to name. I have to thesaurus-hop my way to them. Take that last sentence: I couldn't come up with the word *grasp*. I remembered only that it meant "hold on to."

At the same time, over in Minneapolis, George Floyd shouts, "I can't breathe!" as Derek Chauvin kneels on his neck and slowly suffocates him. Suddenly, after three months of sheltering in place, Americans exit quarantine en masse and take to the streets in protest. As do my kids and I. It feels both disorienting and exhilarating to be standing so close to so many other bodies, although I'm glad to see, as we shout "I can't breathe!" that every single one of us is wearing a mask.

Over the next month, dressed in either black or dark clothes, we march. From City Hall to Washington Square Park. From Union Square to Times Square. From the Barclays Center over the Manhattan Bridge. From McCarren to Domino. From Bed Stuy to Bushwick.

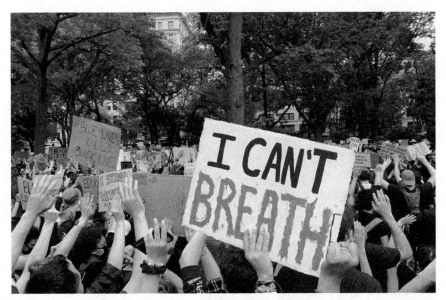

Washington Square Park, June 2, 2020, © Deborah Copaken

More than 10,000 Americans will be taken into police custody this June, for performing their constitutionally guaranteed right to peaceful protest. My older son will be maced. Unidentified goon squads will push protestors into unmarked cars. I would be lying if I said all of this police brutality and shattered norms don't scare me—at my age, in this body—but I've covered enough stories of antidemocratic forces in the world by now to understand we have been reduced to a binary choice: Either we put our bodies on the line and risk physical harm and arrest, or we remain complicit with state-sanctioned terrorism against our Black neighbors.

"Never again!" we Jews are brought up saying. They practically feed it to us with our baby gruel. Well, never is now. And so we march.

My older son has become radicalized. He's taken it upon himself to be one of the growing group of demonstrators who buys and hands out free bottles of water and hand sanitizer during the marches. My daughter and younger son usually march with me, but we stop periodically to let the little one, who's not yet five feet tall, hop up on barriers and benches to take photos like it's his job. Which it kind of is.

At least one of us has a job, I think. At the same time, I know if I had my full-time job right now, I would not have this time to demonstrate

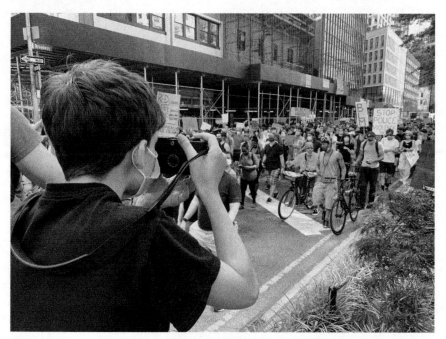

Columbus Circle, June 7, 2020, © Deborah Copaken

with my kids, so that's one good thing to come out of getting sacked in a pandemic. The other good thing is that, having been paid a chunk of the cash for this book, once I'd handed it in in March, I've taken this time with a little bit of financial runway to put together a pitch to turn it into a TV show.

Darren can keep Emily, I'll think. I can no longer empathize with or write dialogue for a white woman selling luxury whiteness to other white people. At some point, I'd told him early on as we were working on the pilot, Emily would have to have her come-to-Jesus moment, when she realizes she is selling air to those who can already breathe. When she actually sees Paris for Paris: a multicultural melting pot where real people, who have critical life lessons to teach her, reside.

On the sixth day of Black Lives Matter demonstrations, June 2, 2020, my two younger kids and I are marching up Fifth Avenue through the Washington Square Arch, tired and thirsty, when my daughter, spotting a man in a mask handing out water off in the distance, suddenly squeals and sprints ahead to reach him. My younger son and I rush to catch up with her before the bottles of water are all gone. "Can I have one, too?" I ask the man in the mask, before realizing I gave birth to him.

"Purell, Mother?" my firstborn says, laughing. Now all three of my kids are laughing at me, for having failed to recognize my own child behind his mask, and I'm laughing at me, too. There is, in fact, such unbridled joy in this moment of serendipity that my older son says, "Uh-oh, watch out. Mom's gonna cry now," at the precise moment my tears spill out over my eyes and onto my mask.

I carried this recently maced, newly radicalized baby home from the hospital exactly a quarter century ago—his twenty-fifth birthday co-incided with the first night of demonstrations—and then I took him to Peshawar when he was six, and drove him to college on the day my marriage ended. And then he flew off to Samos. And his little sister joined the Peace Corps. And then Covid-19 stole these auspicious starts to both of their lives.

But now, miraculously, here we are: my little family, minus their father and the womb in which they grew, but intact, whole. Soon more people are clamoring for free water and squirts of Purell, so my daughter and younger son say goodbye to their older brother, and we march on.

One block north, another squeal erupts from my daughter as she spots her old friend Hannah, who lived in The Commune in Harlem. I half expect to see Ralph Edwards shouting, "Deb Copaken, this is your life!" I have hugged no one but Will and my kids in three long months, but when I see Hannah, I can't help myself. "Hannah!" I scream, and we're hugging and crying and holding each other's faces for several long minutes. The last time I saw her was five years earlier, when she came over for Thanksgiving dinner to our new home in Inwood after she'd had to move back in with her mother. Then she left for college, as did my daughter, and life moved on. Now here she is, in a crop top and green pants, looking snazzy, cool, adult. "I'm so sorry for how everything ended," I say. "I'm sorry I couldn't hold on to you or that home."

Before moving out of The Commune, I'd pulled Hannah aside several weeks earlier and said I could no longer house her. She would have to move back in with her mother. I was upset over a typical teenage breach of trust: a small gathering with alcohol she'd thrown in our absence, after I'd asked her not to do that while I was away with the kids visiting my mom. I blamed my decision on this breach and on the fact that we were all going to have to vacate the home soon anyway. Both true. But I was also struggling, at the time, to keep it together psychologically and to pay for food, and I'd been ashamed to admit that her extra mouth had become a burden I could no longer carry. I'm about to explain all of this to her when Hannah cuts me off.

"Deb! Are you kidding? Stop," she says. "I was literally just writing you a letter to say how grateful I am for all of the times you took me in. No apologies. Ever."

We hug one last time on the corner of Fifth Avenue and East 10th Street. I tell her to come visit us in Brooklyn. She promises she will and asks a stranger to snap a commune reunion photo of the four of us, after which we continue marching north, shouting, "No justice, no peace!" and "I can't breathe!"

"Actually," I tell my kids, a few blocks later, "I really can't breathe."

Back home, I take a quick puff of my steroid inhaler and feel an immediate sense of relief. I breathe in and out. In and out. Fully, deeply, finally. I know it won't last for more than an hour, this unlabored exchange of oxygen for carbon dioxide, so I remind myself to remember this moment and relish an automatic reflex I used to take for granted. I look up the cost of the Qvar inhaler without insurance, wondering how I will breathe when my coverage runs out at the end of September. $543.98 for one inhaler. Jesus. On top of the $603 a month for Aimovig. I guess I can live, albeit poorly and without being able to earn a living, with daily migraines, but I cannot live without air. I wonder how long I can make one inhaler last if I ration it. I do the math in my head. The Qvar has 120 puffs. I take four puffs a day: That's a thirty-day supply, if I keep going at that rate. If I cut back my puffs to two a day, I can make one inhaler last for two months, bringing my monthly cost of breathing down to $271.99. Doable, if I cut back on food, too.

Among first world citizens, only Americans are doing this kind of math.

Fireworks Redux

JULY 4, 2020

My youngest has informed me he will not be celebrating the Fourth of July this year because the signers of the Declaration of Independence owned slaves; and Blacks in this country are still not free; and women are still paid less than men; and Indigenous people were murdered so that we could take over their land; and there's a fascist in the White House holding unmasked rallies and keeping immigrant children in Covid-infected cages; so what, exactly, is there to celebrate?

"Hope?" I say.

He has none, he says.

My job is to try to convince this rapidly sprouting fourteen-year-old American boy otherwise, even as I struggle to hold on to it myself. "Be that as it may," I say, "maybe we could just sit outside and watch the fireworks?" I tell him I read that they're supposed to explode above the Brooklyn Bridge, which means we can probably see them from our balcony, which has just enough room for three camping chairs.

"Okay, fine," he says, rolling his teen eyes, and he joins me outside where I have been staring out at the East River, watching the sun set. The Statue of Liberty, from our vantage point, has been reduced to the size of a pixel. Will joins us as her microscopic light turns on. The sky is now dark, fireworks-ready. So we wait. And we wait. And we steal glimpses at our watches and phones and wait some more. "It's 9:35," says my son, "shouldn't they already have started?"

"Yes," I say. Bootleg fireworks are going off all around our Brooklyn neighborhood, as they've been every night, all night, since the beginning of June, but because of the position of our balcony, we can only hear them, not see them. Occasionally, we see their reflections in the windows of the buildings around us.

Will goes inside to check on the TV version of the celebration and comes back to inform us that the Macy's fireworks are being launched over Coney Island, not the Brooklyn Bridge. The organizers changed it at the last minute, fearing Covid-spreading crowds. It's now 9:40 P.M.

"Bummer," I say. My son has been away at camp for the past six summers, so he hasn't seen any Fourth of July fireworks since he was seven years old, just before his dad left. That summer, 2013, my friend Tanya had lent me her house near the ocean for the long weekend, both to escape my crumbling marriage and to squeeze in some time when my son was asleep to write the novel I would soon toss in the trash before starting my job at *Health Today*. We'd carried a picnic blanket and some food to the edge of the water to join the festivities. I snapped one of my favorite photos of him that dusk, as he twirled a Hula-Hoop around his waist in front of the setting sun, just before the start of the fireworks.

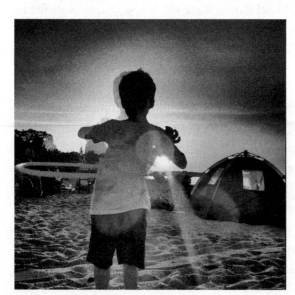

July 4, 2013, Sag Harbor, NY,
© Deborah Copaken

Does some sentimental if irrational part of me want to recapture that sun-kissed moment, after everything I've put him through since? Yes. That weekend was hardly the first time I'd been alone with one of my kids, but it was the first time I'd been alone with one of them realizing that state would be permanent. Can I really do this? I'd wondered. Can the two of us make it on our own after his brother and sister leave for college? The answer was twirling right in front of me, backlit orange: Happy Independence Day.

"Come on," I say to my son, practically grabbing him. I have no desire to watch the fireworks in two dimensions. Our life has been mediated through a screen for too long. "Let's go to the roof, before it's too late. Maybe we can see some of the unofficial fireworks from up there. You wanna come, Will?"

"Nah, I'll watch it down here." Will is highly attuned to the needs of others. He can tell, without my having to say anything—without my even understanding this yet myself—that I need this moment alone with my child. My son had been an honors student until Covid-19 hit, but distance learning combined with his own bout with the virus, isolation from his friends, and this new round of financial insecurity from my job loss destroyed both his concentration and his drive. "I just . . . can't," he'd said, when all of his eighth grade final projects were due. "I can't."

"Then don't," I said. No one will care if he messes up the last quarter of middle school during a pandemic. Least of all his teachers, who've had their own struggles trying to coax thirty adolescents in tiny boxes to learn. I'm normally the one saying, "You can't go out until you finish your homework." But life, right now, is not normal. And it won't be for a while.

My son follows me upstairs to the forbidden ladder, which goes from the corner of our kitchen/living/dining room area up through a small hatch leading up to the roof. We've been banned by our landlord from going up there. The roof has no fence, for one, and he would be liable if we fell off; plus it's not properly covered for walking on it with shoes. After we moved in, I'd strung three sets of Tibetan prayer flags I'd bought in Kathmandu along the entire length of the ladder's steps, as teen deterrent. The only times I've ever climbed it was to pop my head through, Whac-A-Mole style, to see the double rainbow I'd spotted obliquely through my bedroom window—"Hi, Dad!" I'd said, greeting my father without irony—and to open the hatch to release smoke whenever we sear something on the poorly vented stove top that sets off the fire alarm.

"Wait, are we allowed?" says my son. He's a rule-follower. So am I, but I am trying to be less of one. Ripping up marriage contracts that don't work. Allowing my son to neglect his homework during a pandemic. Taking corporations to task for illegal, immoral, or exploitative business practices. Speaking publicly about my private parts, both physical and emotional.

"You just can't *do* that," a good friend scolded me, after overhearing me telling one of our mutual friends, who'd asked about my summer, the story of the two surgeries that had defined it: the trachelectomy in June; the bleed-out in July. "No one wants to hear about your bleeding vagina at a party. It's gross." She was trying to save me, she said, from myself.

This woman and I have been friends for over twenty years. Her generosity is unparalleled, her kindness a balm. I love and trust her. In fact, the only time we'd ever previously disagreed was just after my marriage broke up, when she urged me to dye the gray streak in my hair brown, start wearing a little makeup, and maybe think about getting sexier shoes before heading out into the dating world. No, I'd said, putting my Doc-Martened foot down. I understood and appreciated her concerns. And I loved her for voicing them and worrying about me. But anyone with whom I'd actually want to share the rest of my life would have to accept me as is. Graying. Lug-heeled. Unadorned.

What if I'd been in a car accident? I asked her. Would I have been allowed to talk about that at a party?

That's different, she said.

So it's not about blood in general. Just giant blood clots shooting out of my vagina?

The clots, specifically, yes, she said, laughing. No one wants to hear about those.

I get that, I said, but what if I were a man, and I'd had surgery to remove cancer in my prostate, but then three weeks later, due to some postoperative complication, I was rushed back to the hospital with *internal* bleeding? Would that be an inappropriate topic of conversation if someone had asked me, "How was your summer?"

I wasn't listening to her, my friend said, growing frustrated. She was telling me this for my own good. People—not just her—were talking.

But I nearly died, I said. From complications from an operation so common in America that a uterus is excised here, on average, once every minute. Shouldn't I not only be allowed to talk about this stuff but rather be compelled to do so?

No, she said. It's not appropriate.

By whose measure? That is always the question we must be asking ourselves. By whose measure is talking about our bleeding ladyparts not appropriate, when they are as much a part of our bodies as eyes, lips, hands, and hair? By whose measure are the normal processes of our childbearing bodies weaponized into insult, as when Trump derided a female journalist for having "blood coming out of her wherever" or when my daughter and I were not allowed near my orthodox father-in-law's grave to bury him, for fear that the existence of women's menstrual blood near the gravesite might contaminate it? By whose measure is describing illnesses and surgical complications of our internal reproductive organs wrong? And what do they have to gain from our silence?

I'm reminded of *The Ladies' Book of Etiquette*, Chapter 1, "Conversation":

> Avoid, at all times, mentioning subjects or incidents that can in any way disgust your hearers. Many persons will enter into the details of sicknesses which should be mentioned only when absolutely necessary, or describe the most revolting scenes before a room full of people, or even at table. Others speak of vermin, noxious plants, or instances of uncleanliness. All such conversation or allusion is excessively ill-bred. It is not only annoying, but absolutely sickening to some, and a truly lady-like person will avoid all such topics.

I love you, I said to my friend. And I hear you. And I appreciate your concern. But *The Ladies' Book of Etiquette* was written in 1860, and I respectfully disagree with every word of it. Our ignorance, avoidance, and silencing of all discussions of female-associated viscera is not polite. It's killing us.

The next morning, I sat down and pounded out the first chapter of this book.

"Tonight, yes," I say to my son. "We're allowed to break the rules and go on the roof, just this once. Take off your shoes. It'll be fine." I climb up the ladder barefoot, open the hatch, and hoist my body out onto the roof. It's slightly slanted, our roof, but not *Fiddler on the Roof* slanted. You just have to get used to the pitch and adjust your body accordingly. Suddenly, I'm surrounded by booming noise, color, and bursting lights. "Oh my god," I yell down through the hatch. "Quick! Come now! There's like an entire 360 view of the city from up here and so many fireworks going off *everywhere!*"

But my son will only come halfway up the ladder. "I'm afraid of heights," he says, looking small and scared.

"Seriously?" I say. "Since when?"

"Since forever," he says.

Maybe I shouldn't push it. Maybe we should just watch it on TV downstairs with Will.

Just then, professional fireworks erupt out of the Empire State Building's art deco spire. Yes, erupt. Like ejaculate. Impossible to see it otherwise, and I can't imagine the effect wasn't at least considered if not explicitly planned. What must it feel like, I wonder, to be a man? To see monuments to your genitalia everywhere?

"Hi, Nora," I say to the ejaculating leitmotif of *Sleepless in Seattle,* and it suddenly strikes me—how had it not before?—that a phallic symbol has replaced my surrogate mother, a circle my father, and every morning, when I sit down to write, I have to line up my chair exactly between them: Nora in front, Dad rising up to illuminate her from some unseen position on the horizon behind me. There's only one specific spot in the corner of my north-facing living room from which its far left window perfectly frames the Empire State Building to the northwest. It is there and only there where I superstitiously begin each writing day, between my ghosts.

"The only thing a uterus is good for after a certain point is causing pain and killing you," she'd said. "Why are we even talking about this? If your doctor says it needs to come out, yank it out."

I was afraid, Nora. That's why I didn't want to lose my uterus. Or get divorced. Or move to a new apartment or go on app dates or parent alone or, frankly, write the rest of this book, once I'd pounded out the first chapter. Particularly after the slut-shaming, rape-blaming reaction to my last memoir, the one that made us friends. It felt safer doing nothing. To stand, like my son, halfway up the ladder between two dimensions and three. To follow my friend's advice, play my proper lady part, and stay silent. To accept the suffering, because it felt familiar, rather than finding a pathway out. To wallow, like the dad Tom Hanks plays in *Sleepless in Seattle*, in solo-parenting inertia. I half expect to see a red heart glowing in the windows of the Empire State Building, like during the final scene in that film. Didn't it also end with fireworks? It did, didn't it?

There is nothing new under the sun, indeed. Or moon, as it were, tonight. Even *Sleepless in Seattle* was an homage to an *Affair to Remember*. Which itself was a remake of *Love Affair*. "I'm gonna get out of bed every morning," says Sam, played by Tom Hanks, during a particularly hopeless moment, "breathe in and out all day long. Then after a while, I won't have to remind myself to get out of bed every morning and breathe in and out. And then after a while, I won't have to think about how I had it great and perfect for a while."

Resignation, in the face of adversity, is just easier. Nora, who never resigned herself to anything—not even her own death—knew this. Non-resignation was her secret sauce, what she taught by example, in every word written, in every frame shot, in every dinner party thrown. Yes, life can be shitty. And hard. And the obstacles can feel insurmountable, especially in a woman's body. But you still get to be the hero of your own story. You are still allowed a cupful of grace. That's why she and my dad got along so well that night at my book party, laughing off in the corner. Not because they were both dying. But because they were both *living*.

Of course, all of us face down terminal illness every day. That's what it means to live in a dying body: to accept that all of this—I stare up at the sky, down at my son, my feet, the roof, our home[*]—is on loan. We are but brain scaffolding, for passing on genes. If you're lucky, you get to lease your body for about eighty years or so. Dad got sixty-seven. Nora got seventy-one. If I live as long as my dad, that gives me another thirteen years. If I live as long as Nora, I get seventeen.

"Come on," I tell my son. There's no time to waste! "The Empire State Building is exploding! Right now. Just push through the fear. I'm here. I've got you. You have to see this!"

He makes his way to the top of the ladder and pokes only his head

---

[*] In two months, we will receive written notice from our landlord's lawyer, saying our two-year lease will not be renewed.

through the hatch while the rest of his body stays below. "Cool," he says, without climbing farther.

"Dude, you're not even looking at it," I say. The hatch door is blocking his view. I hold out my hand. "You can do this. You're going to want to see this. I promise. Give me your hand!"

"No!"

Finally, after several more back-and-forths, he holds out his shaking hand, and I yank him through the hatch. "Oh my god," he says, witnessing the full 360-degree effect of standing five stories tall, surrounded by light and sound and an ejaculating skyscraper. "I'm scared of the tilt," he says, gripping my arm.

"We're all afraid of the tilt," I say. But without it there would be no seasons, no balance, no chance of a life-sustaining future. "Come. Let's sit." I walk him over to the middle of the parapet dividing our roof from our neighbor's, halfway between the unfenced ledges on either side, and he finally calms down and starts to take it all in. The colors. The sky. The full moon. The rocket's red glare and bombs bursting in air and the unfettered freedom of rising above the rooms in which we've been imprisoned. For the next twenty minutes, we sit in near silence as the world explodes around us into color, light, and sound. Boom! Red! Boom! Blue! Boom! White sparkly trails! Boom! Boom! Boom!

"Don't give up on this country," I say. "It still has a chance."

"But what if Trump gets reelected?" He's been reading up on fascism and voter suppression, posting memes about their dangers alongside pleas for Breonna Taylor's killers to be arrested and for police budgets to be redirected to schools, healthcare, and social programs.

"We'll move to France," I say, missing Paris, wondering if we'll even be allowed over the border. "Or . . . somewhere."

"But I want to stay here," he says. "This is my home."

"I know, sweetie. Same. But let's wait until after the election to start panicking, okay?"

Two days before I'll head to the polls to vote, Ken Kurson will be arrested and charged by federal prosecutors for cyberstalking, based on the research I provided the FBI after my #MeToo essay in *The Atlantic* unleashed "The Others." I will listen in on the public call between the judge and Kurson—in-person court appearances during Covid will not be possible—and feel both a profound sense of relief and so many PVCs I'll faint when I stand up too quickly afterward.

That same day—that same hour, in fact, of Kurson's hearing, on October 23, 2020—I will close a deal to executive produce and write a TV show based on this book, a coincidence of timing not lost on me. We women have to work twice as hard to get half as far, and the moats are filled with Kursons and Weinsteins and Lauers and Cosbys and Kellys and Batalis and Nassers and Aileses and Trumps and Moonveses and Browns and Roses and C.K.s and Ratners, plus untold others. But eventually, if we live long enough and fight hard enough, some of us will get to the other side with our bodies still intact.

On November 3, 2020, Trump will be voted out of office. My first thoughts, upon hearing the election finally called for Biden on the morning of November 7, will be those of unbridled relief and elation. I will scream. I will cry. I will combust into human confetti. My second thoughts will leave me drenched in the cold sweat of panic: *Shit*, I'll think, *now he'll pardon Ken "I come from a grudge-holding desert people" Kurson.*

"'Ken Kurson' Trump pardon," I'll keep googling, day after day, hoping to find nothing. On December 23, 2020, Trump will pardon Paul Manafort, Roger Stone, and Charles Kushner, Jared's father. I'm sunk. If Jared can get his daddy off the hook, he's definitely working behind the scenes to save his best buddy Ken from going to jail, too. Every day, I'll keep scanning the headlines for more pardons, waiting for the Kurson shoe to drop. Maybe the president will be too busy spreading lies about voter fraud and inciting violent insurrection to even think about pardoning Kurson or anyone.

For the next thirteen days, I'll keep hearing more pardons are forthcoming, but none will come forth. I'll go to bed late on the night of January 19, 2021, breathing a sigh of relief. The White House pussy grabber will be out of office the next day by noon. Justice prevails! Pussies triumph! God bless America.

"Bad news," Will will say, waking me up at 4 A.M. on the morning of Biden's inauguration. "He pardoned Kurson."

"Fuck."

"What do I do?" I'll ask Special Agent Eckstut, the FBI agent who showed up at my apartment in Inwood wearing sensible flats. Two other federal agents are listening in on the line, Zack Goodman and Andrew Taff. "I gave you guys the information that led to his arrest!" I'll say. "Remember his email? 'I come from a grudge-holding desert people'? You arrested him for his acts of revenge. *This is who he is.*"

"If there's an imminent threat to your safety," Emily will say, "call 911. If it's less imminent, let us know, and we'll certainly look into it."

"That's it? Call 911? I have no other recourse to guarantee my safety?"

"I mean, as a last resort, there's always witness protection," one of the male agents listening in on the line will offer. I have no idea which one. They're just disembodied voices on the line.

Yeah, no, I'll think. I am not going to go into hiding and leave everything and everyone I know and love behind because the man who carefully targeted, groomed, and sexually harassed me, as well as inflicted emotional and reputational pain on many others, has been pardoned by the fucking president of the United States.

Reader, I am afraid.

The bootleg fireworks are going nuts now all around us, becoming more intense and numerous.

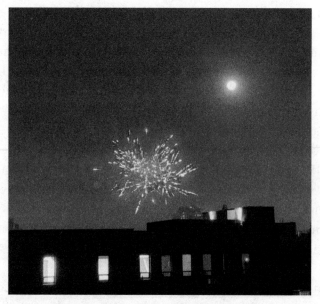

Brooklyn, July 4, 2020, © Deborah Copaken

"Oh my god! Is that a heart?" says my son.

Indeed, it is. An Ephronesque red heart exploding next to the full moon. A "Buck Moon," they call it, because it coincides with the time of year when young male deer grow their antlers. A deer bar mitzvah, I think, since the main purpose of antlers is to attract females. And the main purpose of attracting females is to continue propagating the species. And the main purpose of propagating the species is god knows what, but I'm sitting here atop the slanted world with the final fruit of my excised womb watching hearts explode beneath the full Buck Moon, so hey. Thanks, genes!

My son's baby fat, I notice, has melted down overnight into angles and planes after his own bar mitzvah last year, at that nightclub in Bushwick with the dildo chandeliers my freshly widowed aunt loved so much, she giggled and posed for pictures with them. The House of Yes, it was called. I chose it because Dani, one of their employees, had sent me an invitation on LinkedIn, and when I googled her place of work and read its core beliefs—art heals, weird is wonderful—I thought yes. Just yes. Plus, I mean, the name alone: The House of Yes? Sign me up.

"Do you do bar mitzvahs?" I wrote.

They'd never done one before, said Dani, but why not? Would I like to come by and check out the space? *What a perfect "Yes, and . . ."* I thought. Of course the House of Yes would follow improv protocol. They also rented me the space for a steal, since we'd be the bar mitzvah guinea pigs, plus hardly anyone booked Saturday afternoons, so it was found revenue. I paid the bill out of the advance for these words.

It was only after I'd sent out the invitations that a friend who'd received one told me what goes on there at night.

"Wait, *it's a sex club*?!" said my son.

"Only at night!" I said. "Your bar mitzvah's at four." Besides, what better place to mark one's passage into manhood?

Another heart explodes on the horizon. And another. And another. In my brain, watching these hearts explode, neurotransmitters light up at the same time to form this thought: Had you died three years ago, during that other Fourth of July weekend, when the stitches at the top of your vaginal canal came undone, you would have missed this perfect moment. You would have missed meeting Will; your daughter's graduation; Aunt Marilyn laughing at the dildo chandeliers; your mother's hand in yours as you spun around and around in a giant circle of love during the hora. You would have missed the look of pure shock on your sister Jen's face, after she realized dozens of her closest friends and family had gathered for her surprise fiftieth birthday; and you would have missed those four perfect minutes a couple of days later, when you and Will were driving north along the Pacific Coast Highway, Kacey Musgraves's "Oh, What a World" came on the radio, and you burst into tears.

"That was my favorite moment of my life," you'll later tell Will, "the way the ocean suddenly appeared over the horizon as the song came on, and then I looked at you," and he'll pause for a moment, cock his head, and say, "I think mine was at a Grateful Dead show." So you would have missed chortling at this response, too. You would have missed climbing that hill outside Kathmandu and swimming naked in that lake in Maine and bearing witness to 1,098 sunsets in between, some of which you know were breathtaking, in the pre-Covid sense of the word, because you keep evidence of them in your phone.

"You ready to head back down?" I ask my son. It's getting late.

"Five more minutes?"

"Sure."

After a minute or so of silence he speaks. "Why is there a moon?"

I have no idea. Why is there anything? "For the tides," I say.

"No," he says. "I mean, how did it form?"

Chaos, buddy. "Oh, um . . ." I mumble what little I can remember about impact theory from my dad's astronomy lessons in my childhood bedroom, when he pretended to be the sun, and I, the earth, twirled around him, a blur of nightgown and dizzy glee. "I think, like, Earth bumped into another planet, and then the moon formed from all the pieces of orbiting debris that remained. Or something like that." I put my arm around my son. It's rare these days that he allows this, but tonight he does.

"Every time I think about the universe, my brain hurts," he says.

"Mine, too."

"Still," he says. His eyes remain fixed on the moon. "It's cool that something that beautiful could grow out of something so violent."

"Yeah," I say, breathing in oxygen, blowing it out for the plants. "It is."

Acknowledgments

Just as no human springs forth fully formed without egg, sperm,[*] uterus, and forty weeks, no book is the spontaneous creation of one person. Since this is a book about the body, it seems only fitting to assign each collaborator a specific body part. I might regret this a few organs in, but let's try.

UTERUS: In late fall of 2014, Lisa Leshne took me out for lunch at a restaurant down the street from my office at *Cafe*. Over mussels and fries, with my boss in earshot at the next table, she made her (quiet) pitch: *Shutterbabe* was one of her favorite books; I needed to write a follow-up; and she should be the one to help me birth it. I laughed. Yeah, right. That I was already represented by another agent; that I had no time to write a dating profile, let alone a book; that the proposal itself would eventually take four years, two failed incarnations, and so many rejection letters we lost count did not faze her. Her multiple acts of grace are already mentioned herein, but I will add one more: a souvenir from the day I went in front of a judge to reclaim my birth name, and she insisted on not only joining me at the courthouse, but on taking me out afterward to celebrate.

BRAIN: In March of 2018, Mark Warren—then a stranger, now my editor— reached out after reading my *Atlantic* story about being sexually harassed by Ken Kurson. "Your piece," he wrote, "is kind of Rosetta stone to understanding not just Ken, but people like Ken. I'm really sorry that you had to go through that." After thanking him for these and other kind words, I wrote, "I feel ruined

---

[*] At least for now. If you're reading this in the future and we've figured out human cloning, god help us.

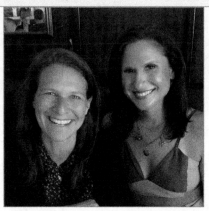

 Lisa Leshne is 🍽 eating **lunch** with **Deborah Copaken** at **The Odeon Restaurant**. ...
September 12, 2017 · New York · 👥

Post-courthouse lunch with my author and dear friend Deborah Copaken to celebrate reclaiming her name! 🖤

by it and him in ways I can't even articulate. He dangled a dream that was never mine to have. The ploy was always my pants, not my brain. And I hate him for that." To which Mark, having just been hired as an executive editor at Random House after twenty-eight years at *Esquire*, wrote back, "I would encourage you to write your way through this sentence: 'I feel ruined by it and him in ways I can't even articulate.'" *Ladyparts* is the result of this encouragement. Of forcing myself to sit down every morning for sixteen months to try to articulate what had felt so inarticulable, I'd given up trying. Mark is a gifted editor and the sweetest deus ex machina to ever drop from the sky, but more saliently, he is a feminist. I wish more men were like him.

EYES: Tad Friend has loaned me his eyes for each of my books. He is my first and most generous reader, my beloved friend of nearly four decades. When I think back on the years described in these pages, mostly I picture myself sitting at his and and his wife Amanda Hesser's kitchen table laughing, occasionally crying, but always feeling loved, heard, and well-fed while our little ones chased one another through the apartment. Diane Sokolow, running charades maestro, read the Uterus section in its early incarnation, after I'd asked her to please help me make sure I got the essence and verbal cadence of our much-missed Nora just right. Tommy Siegel, Stephen Alexander, Elizabeth Perkins, James Tucker, Zibby Owens, Joaquín Güell, Hara Woltz, Marion Mertens, Darren Star, Samantha Morrice, Eric Alterman, Monique El-Faizy, and Matt Whitaker read various early versions or chapters and provided valuable thoughts and suggestions. Ayelet Waldman, Mary Pender, Kate Adler, and Whitney Berry not only were early readers, it's thanks to them that *Ladyparts* might make it out of my computer and onto your TV. Suzi Schiffer Parrasch took on the thankless role of editing the entire manuscript in the three days leading up to its deadline. If every apostrophe is finally removed from each mention of an era, it's thanks to Suzi. (I thought it was the 60's and 70's, not the '60s and '70s. What? It still looks wrong to me.)

BREAST: It is impossible to overstate how grateful I am to be back in the bosom of Random House after a twenty-year absence. The last time I'd been to the mothership was in 2000, when I hand-delivered a printed-out version of the *Shutterbabe* manuscript—plus floppy disc—in a cardboard box held tight with rubber bands. My next visit was in the spring of 2019, after I'd written the first chunk of this book. The late Susan Kamil gleefully squeezed my hands and exclaimed, "We are so excited about *Ladyparts*! Welcome back!" She died of complications from lung cancer four months later. I hope I have honored her early enthusiasm, her love of words, and her memory. Andy Ward was equally welcoming, inviting me into his office for a long, amiable chat, as if he had all the time in the world instead of a giant publishing house to run. Cheyenne Skeete kept us in line and on schedule, dealt with all the rights, and laughed with me—not at me—as we pored over every ad hominem attack in our tear sheet photo gallery ("Yes, such 'poor judgment' to get yourself raped," she tut-tutted). Ella Laytham tirelessly designed over a dozen different covers, and Robbin Schiff—who coincidentally worked on the *Shutterbabe* cover—not only was not annoyed by my input during the design process, she actively welcomed it. The minute we all saw this one, we knew: Ella had nailed it. Thanks, too, to Marlene Glazer, for her critical legal reads and video conference calls at all hours of the day and night plus weekends as well ("What's a weekend?"); to Liz Carbonell, for her witty marginalia and for making sure every *i* was dotted, every *t* crossed, every repetition noted, and every ~~cervix~~ typo excised; to Cindy Berman, for overseeing the book's production editing under a tight deadline, when Trump's last-minute pardon of Kurson set us back yet another two weeks; to Jo Anne Metsch, for her beautiful design inside these pages, which she nailed on the first try; to Thomas Perry, for being this book's champion; and to Rachel Rokicki, Barbara Fillon, Ayelet Gruenspecht, and Penny Belnap, for making sure this tree didn't fall in a forest: The marketing and PR departments are the unsung heroes of the publishing world. I am grateful for their efforts.

HANDS: Many hands had my back during the year and a half of writing this book. Too many, in fact, to name, but here are a few. Adrienne LaFrance gave my voice a platform in *The Atlantic* and the chance to work with Paul Bisceglio and Julie Beck, Google Docs magicians. Elli Kaplan gave me the first breathing room of my adult life—a living wage, benefits, and a flexible job in Silicon Valley that started at noon in Brooklyn, which allowed me to work at home and write this between dawn and lunch. My *Emily in Paris* family not only gave me reasons to laugh every day for three months, working in that writers' room was a daily reminder, while pushing my way through some of the darker chapters herein, to extract the humor from the sludge. (It's always there, and not even well hidden.) As for my friends, you know who you are. You're either in this book, on my phone, going on a socially distanced walk, or smiling in a sad little Zoom rectangle on my computer. Speaking of Zoom rectangles, a special shout out to my ladywriter friends spread out across the U.S. and in Paris, and to our two honorary writerdudes in their wood-beamed rectangle in Liguria for providing an imposed daily seven-minute workout and a sense of community during our strange communal moment of disconnection and isolation.

HIPPOCAMPUS: Every week, for those couple of years when I had good insurance, I spent an hour in the office of Dr. Steven Tublin. I told stories and decimated his tissue box; he listened for patterns and talked me off the ledge. I'm sorry I ran out of both money and the good insurance to keep up with this weekly practice. (Let's fix this, America. Mental health is not a separate category from general health. It's not only a critical part of the body's immune system, the less financially secure you are, the more you need it.)

HEART: My children have given me more than I could ever give them: not just love, but life, texture, joy, awe, and all the other corny nouns in between. This cri de coeur—which literally translates as "cry from the heart"—is for them. I don't want my daughter to have to face the decades of sexism and inequality my mother and I faced, and I don't want my sons to grow up in a world that would ever treat their sister as less worthy of income, scientific study, or respect; or her body as a commodity, object, baby factory, or bargaining chip in an employment negotiation. I also don't want my kids to have to choose between their professional passions and health insurance. If this book can shine one tiny light on our unwinnable, shameful game of healthcare Frogger, *dayenu*. To my sisters, Jen, Julie, and Laura Copaken: You got me through those penniless three months in the summer of 2014, and I will never forget it; I look forward to paying you back in limitless Kohr's as soon as we're all vaccinated. Aunt Marilyn? You've kept me sane and made me laugh: the best medicine I know. And Mom? I hope it's clear from these words herein that I not only love you, but I see you, I appreciate you, and I know that, however hard my generation of women had it, yours had it worse. To my new family, the Betts, Perkins, and Danas: Thank you for saving me a spot around your hearth. Its warmth has been a soothing balm. And Will. My god, Will. You are the still point of my turning world.

Notes

PREFACE

xiv *flip Mulvey's male gaze*: Laura Mulvey, "Visual Pleasure and Narrative Cinema," *Screen*, 1975, asu.edu/courses/fms504/total-readings/mulvey-visualplea
sure.pdf.

xvn **the decision was not mine**: Deborah Copaken, "My So-Called 'Post-Feminist' Life in Arts and Letters," *The Nation*, April 9, 2013, thenation.com/article/archive/my-so-called-post-feminist-life-arts-and-letters/.

TWO: LUNCH WITH NORA, FREDS

20 **minus a clitoris**: Julia Unteregger, "Yes, This Is a Sexist Term and Here Is Why . . . ," TEDx Vienna, April 6, 2019, tedxvienna.at/blog/yes-this-is-a-sexist
-term-and-here-is-why/.

21 **average of sixty-five minutes**: Laura Kiesel, "Women and pain: Disparities in experience and treatment," *Harvard Health Publishing*, Harvard Medical School, October 9, 2017, health.harvard.edu/blog/women-and-pain-disparities
-in-experience-and-treatment-2017100912562.

21 **only half as likely**: "Researcher says women less likely to get painkillers," *UPI* archives, March 11, 1989, upi.com/Archives/1989/03/11/Researcher-says
-women-less-likely-to-get-painkillers/2047605595600/.

21 **7 on a scale of 10**: Diane E. Hoffmann, Anita J. Tarzian, "The Girl Who Cried Pain: A Bias Against Women in the Treatment of Pain," *The Journal of Law, Medicine & Ethics*, 2001, ssrn.com/abstract=383803.

21 **"almost as bad as a heart attack"**: Olivia Goldhill, "Period pain can be 'al-

most as bad as a heart attack.' Why aren't we researching how to treat it?,"
Quartz, February 15, 2016, qz.com/611774/period-pain-can-be-as-bad-as-a
-heart-attack-so-why-arent-we-researching-how-to-treat-it/.

21 **trial of sildenafil citrate:** R. Dmitrovic, A. R. Kunselman, R. S. Legro, "Sildenafil citrate in the treatment of pain in primary dysmenorrhea: a randomized
controlled trial," *Human Reproduction*, Volume 28, Issue 11, November 2013,
academic.oup.com/humrep/article/28/11/2958/628626.

21 **when I first read that in a book:** Caroline Criado Perez, *Invisible Women:
Exposing Data Bias in a World Designed for Men* (New York: Abrams, 2019).

21 **"did not see dysmenorrhea":** Ibid.

22 **"men don't care about":** Radhika Sanghani, "Period pain can feel 'as bad as a
heart attack'—so why is it being ignored?," *The Telegraph*, September 6, 2017,
telegraph.co.uk/women/life/period-pain-can-feel-bad-heart-attack-ignored/.

23 **Nora's "A Few Words About Breasts":** Nora Ephron, "A Few Words About
Breasts," *Esquire*, May 1, 1972, classic.esquire.com/article/1972/5/1/a-few-words
-about-breasts.

FIVE: EMPATHY

43 **needs become misaligned:** Daniel Schöttle, Peer Briken, et al., "Sexuality in
autism: hypersexual and paraphilic behavior in women and men with high-
functioning autism spectrum disorder," *Dialogues in Clinical Neuroscience*, Volume 19, Issue 4, December 2017, pp. 381–393, ncbi.nlm.nih.gov/pmc/articles
/PMC5789215/.

43 **"too tired for an encounter":** Ashley Stanford, *Asperger Syndrome and Long-
Term Relationships* (London: Jessica Kingsley Publishers, 2014).

SIX: ESCAPE

46 **A few weeks after 9/11:** Deborah Copaken, "I am very sad because my heart is
bleeding," *O, The Oprah Magazine*, March 15, 2002, deborahcopaken.com/#
/essaysjournalism/.

SEVEN: LUNCH WITH NORA, E.A.T.

54 **Malcolm Gladwell wrote a profile:** Malcolm Gladwell, "The Formula,"
The New Yorker, October 9, 2006, newyorker.com/magazine/2006/10/16/the
-formula.

54 **Dad later wrote on:** Richard Copaken, "Plumbing the Depths," *Happy Dick is
Sick*, August 17, 2008, happydickissick.com/2008/08/17/plumbing-the-depths/.

55 **Couldn't he divine that:** Deborah Copaken, "La Vie en Rose, the Takeout Version," *The New York Times*, April 15, 2007, nytimes.com/2007/04/15/fashion
/15love.html.

EIGHT: WHERE'S THE HUSBAND?

66 **an accurate 3D model:** Minna Salami, "This is a 3D model of a clitoris—and
the start of a sexual revolution," *The Guardian*, September 15, 2016, theguard

ian.com/commentisfree/2016/sep/15/3d-model-clitoris-sexual-revolution-sex
-education-womens-sexuality.

73   **NHS would allow me:** "Overview—Hysterectomy," NHS, nhs.uk/conditions
       /hysterectomy/.

73   **get up to four:** Gillian Harvey, "My Operation in France: Hysterectomy," *The
       Connexion*, February 21, 2018, connexionfrance.com/Practical/Health/My
       -operation-in-France-Hysterectomy; "Hysterectomy—Topic Overview," Alberta
       Health Services, myhealth.alberta.ca/Health/pages/conditions.aspx?Hwid=hw
       212587.

76   **refers to this as Cassandra syndrome:** Kenneth Roberson, PhD, "Adult As-
       perger's and the Cassandra Phenomena," kennethrobersonphd.com/adult
       -aspergers-and-the-cassandra-phenomena/.

NINE: LANDSLIDE

81   **"more hospitable to cancer":** Markham Heid, "How stress affects cancer
       risk," The University of Texas MD Anderson Cancer Center, December 2014,
       mdanderson.org/publications/focused-on-health/how-stress-affects-cancer-risk
       .h21-1589046.html.

82   **speed the development of cancer:** Valentina-Fineta Chiriac, Adriana Baban,
       Dan L. Dumitrascu, "Psychological stress and breast cancer incidence: a sys-
       tematic review," *Clujul Medical*, January 15, 2018, ncbi.nlm.nih.gov/pmc
       /articles/PMC5808262/.

83   **false framing of the opt-out narrative:** Joan C. Williams, Jessica Manvell,
       Stephanie Bornstein, "'Opt Out' or Pushed Out?: How the Press Covers Work/
       Family Conflict, The Untold Story of Why Women Leave the Workforce,"
       The Center for WorkLife Law, UC Hastings College of the Law, 2006, psy
       chologytoday.com/files/attachments/47131/optoutorpushedoutreportfinal.pdf.

84   **crucial first three months:** Robert Winston, Rebecca Chicot, "The impor-
       tance of early bonding on the long-term mental health and resilience of chil-
       dren," *London Journal of Primary Care*, February 24, 2016, ncbi.nlm.nih.gov
       /pmc/articles/PMC5330336/.

89   **considered to be failing:** Kate Taylor, "Harlem Schools Are Left to Fail as
       Those Not Far Away Thrive," *The New York Times*, January 24, 2017, nytimes
       .com/2017/01/24/nyregion/harlem-schools-are-left-to-fail-as-those-not-far-away
       -thrive.html.

91   **"My children have only one life":** Richard Severo, "Kenneth Clark, Who
       Fought Segregation, Dies," *The New York Times*, May 2, 2005, nytimes.com
       /2005/05/02/nyregion/kenneth-clark-who-fought-segregation-dies.html.

92   **entrenched caste system:** Isabel Wilkerson, *Caste: The Origins of our Discon-
       tents* (New York: Random House, 2020).

92   **"Conversations about racism":** UNICEF, "Talking to your kids about racism:
       How to start the important conversation and keep it going," June 9, 2020,
       unicef.org/parenting/talking-to-your-kids-about-racism.

92   **CEO-to-worker compensation ratio:** Dominic Rushe, "US bosses now earn

312 times the average worker's wage, figures show," *The Guardian*, August 16, 2018, theguardian.com/business/2018/aug/16/ceo-versus-worker-wage-american-companies-pay-gap-study-2018.

92 **largest rise in income inequality:** "Income Inequality," Inequality.org, inequality.org/facts/income-inequality/.

93 **average of $21.3 million a year:** Lawrence Mishel, Jori Kandra, "CEO compensation surged 14% in 2019 to $21.3 million," Economic Policy Institute, August 18, 2020, epi.org/publication/ceo-compensation-surged-14-in-2019-to-21-3-million-ceos-now-earn-320-times-as-much-as-a-typical-worker/.

93 **a whopping $280,621,552 a year:** "Highest Paid CEOs," AFL-CIO, 2019, aflcio.org/paywatch/highest-paid-ceos.

102 **men like to hire other men:** Dina Gerdeman, "Why Employers Favor Men," Harvard Business School *Working Knowledge*, September 11, 2017, hbswk.hbs.edu/item/why-employers-favor-men.

102 **biased against older women:** David Neumark, Ian Burn, Patrick Button, "Is it Harder for Older Workers to Find Jobs? New and Improved Evidence from a Field Experiment," National Bureau of Economic Research, October 2015, revised November 2017, nber.org/system/files/working_papers/w21669/w21669.pdf.

TEN: CHIAROSCURO

106 **I blame the industrial revolution:** Jan Riordan, RN, MN; Betty Ann Countryman, RN, MN, "Part I: Infant Feeding Patterns Past and Present," *JOGN Nursing*, Volume 9, Issue 4, July–August 1980, p. 207, sciencedirect.com/science/article/abs/pii/S0090031115303276?via%3Dihub.

115 **"relief theory":** Alex Borgella, "Science deconstructs humor: What makes some things funny?" *The Conversation*, November 1, 2016, theconversation.com/science-deconstructs-humor-what-makes-some-things-funny-64414.

115 **Humor, according to Schopenhauer:** Danny Lewis, "Finally There's a Scientific Theory for Why Some Words are Funny: The science behind Dr. Seuss," *Smithsonian Magazine*, December 7, 2015, smithsonianmag.com/smart-news/finally-theres-scientific-theory-why-some-words-are-funny-180957462/.

ELEVEN: YES, AND . . .

122 **an essay I'd written in *The Nation*:** Copaken, "My So-Called 'Post-Feminist' Life."

122 **The lede, after readers revolted:** Douglas Martin, "Yvonne Brill, a Pioneering Rocket Scientist, Dies at 88," *The New York Times*, March 30, 2013, nytimes.com/2013/03/31/science/space/yvonne-brill-rocket-scientist-dies-at-88.html.

123 **"refers to me as a stay-at-home mom":** Janet Reitman, "Bang-Bang girl," *Salon*, January 30, 2001, salon.com/2001/01/29/shutterbabe/; Rebecca Johnson, "Shutterbabe: A photojournalist chronicles love and death around the globe," *Talk*, January 2001.

123n **first used in 1982:** Miriam Peskowitz, *The Truth Behind the Mommy Wars: Who Decides What Makes a Good Mother?* (Seal Press, 2005), pp. 24–25.

123 **"Women's Prize for Fiction nominee"**: Nick Clark, "Women's Prize for Fiction nominee Deborah Copaken Kogan lifts the lid on sexism in publishing and the arts," *The Independent*, April 12, 2013, independent.co.uk/arts -entertainment/books/news/women-s-prize-fiction-nominee-deborah-copaken -kogan-lifts-lid-sexism-publishing-and-arts-8570468.html.

123 **calling me "Heroine of the Day"**: Melissa Silverstein, "Heroine of the Day: Deborah Copaken Kogan," *Women and Hollywood*, April 11, 2013, women andhollywood.com/heroine-of-the-day-deborah-copaken-kogan/.

123 **became its own meme:** "This is what sexism does best: it makes you feel crazy for desiring parity and hopeless about ever achieving it," 9Quotes, 9quotes .com/quote/deborah-copaken-kogan-395066.

124 **permanently banned from the site:** Andrew Leonard, "Wikipedia cleans up its mess," *Salon*, May 21, 2013, salon.com/2013/05/21/wikipedia_cleans_up _its_mess/.

128 **They've done studies:** Etta Kralovic, John Buell, *The End of Homework: How Homework Disrupts Families, Overburdens Children, and Limits Learning* (Boston: Beacon Press, 2000).

128 **U.S. government does not recognize the reality of our childcare costs:** Andrew Keshner, "Child-care costs in America have soared to nearly $10K per year," *MarketWatch*, March 8, 2019, marketwatch.com/story/child-care-costs -just-hit-a-new-high-2018-10-22.

128 **no state in the entire country:** Lynette M. Fraga, "Parents and the High Cost of Child Care," Child Care Aware of America, 2017 annual report, childcare aware.org/wp-content/uploads/2017/12/2017_CCA_High_Cost_Report _FINAL.pdf.

128 **37 percent of their household income:** Keshner, "Child-care costs in America."

129 **2019 Federal Reserve study:** "Report on the Economic Well-Being of U.S. Households in 2018," Board of Governors of the Federal Reserve System, May 2019, federalreserve.gov/publications/files/2018-report-economic-well-being-us -households-201905.pdf.

130 **can't afford insulin:** Sarah Jones, "Another Person Has Died After Rationing Insulin," *New York*, July 15, 2019, nymag.com/intelligencer/2019/07/another -person-has-died-from-rationing-insulin.html.

131 **"Medicine is for people, not for profits":** George W. Merck, *Time*, August 18, 1952, content.time.com/time/covers/0,16641,19520818,00.html.

131 **worth $22.6 million:** Kenneth C. Frazier, Executive Compensation, Salary .com, 2019, www1.salary.com/Kenneth-C-Frazier-Salary-Bonus-Stock-Options -for-MERCK-and-CO.html.

131 **$54.8 million in his own stock:** Jerry Useem, "The Stock-Buyback Swindle," *The Atlantic*, August 2019, theatlantic.com/magazine/archive/2019/08/the-stock -buyback-swindle/592774/.

131 **pharmaceutical industry a Ponzi scheme:** William Lazonick, Matt Hopkins, Ken Jacobson, Mustafa Erdem Sakinç, Öner Tulum, "US Pharma's Financialized Business Model," Institute for New Economic Thinking, Working Papers,

July 13, 2017, ineteconomics.org/uploads/papers/WP_60-Lazonick-et-al-US
-Pharma-Business-Model.pdf.

131 **$10 billion on research and development:** Useem, "The Stock-Buyback
Swindle."

131 **lauded in the press:** Riley Griffin, Anders Melin, "Merck Prepares for CEO's
Departure With Internal Successor Hunt," June 19, 2019, bloomberg.com
/news/articles/2019-06-19/merck-prepares-for-ceo-s-departure-with-internal
-successor-hunt.

132 **nearly $4.6 billion into lobbying:** "Industries," Center for Responsive Politics,
opensecrets.org/federal-lobbying/industries?cycle=a.

132 **hundreds of millions of dollars:** "Industry Profile: Pharmaceuticals/Health
Products," Center for Responsive Politics, opensecrets.org/federal-lobbying
/industries/summary?cycle=2019&id=h04.

132 **partly funded by pharma-dollars:** Rick Claypool, "Pharma's Orders: U.S. Rep-
resentatives Who Sided With Big Pharma in Medicare Lobbying Fight Received
82% More Industry Campaign Contributions," Public Citizen, July 11, 2016,
citizen.org/wp-content/uploads/pharmas-orders-medicare-part-b-campaign
-finance-report-july-2016.pdf.

132 **"Nobody dies because":** Kathryn Watson, "GOP congressman: 'Nobody dies
because they don't have access to health care,'" CBS News, May 6, 2017,
cbsnews.com/news/gop-congressman-nobody-dies-because-they-dont-have
-access-to-health-care/.

132 **death rates since the Supreme Court's decision:** Sara Rosenbaum, Timo-
thy M. Westmoreland, "The Supreme Court's Surprising Decision On The
Medicaid Expansion: How Will The Federal Government And States Proceed?," *Health Affairs*, August 2012, healthaffairs.org/doi/full/10.1377/hlthaff
.2012.0766.

132 **A single death is a tragedy:** attributed to Joseph Stalin, *The Washington Post*,
January 20, 1947, oxfordreference.com/view/10.1093/acref/9780191826719.001
.0001/q-oro-ed4-00010383.

133 **"the UK spends dramatically LESS":** Rob Delaney, Twitter, July 17, 2019,
twitter.com/robdelaney/status/1151567475814948866.

133 **behind the following countries:** Nisha Kurani, Daniel McDermott, Nico-
las Shanosky, "How does the quality of the U.S. healthcare system compare
to other countries?" (chart: "The U.S. ranks last in a measure of health care
access and quality, indicating higher rates of amenable mortality than peer
countries"), Peterson-KFF, Health System Tracker, August 20, 2020, health
systemtracker.org/chart-collection/quality-u-s-healthcare-system-compare
-countries/#item-healthcare-quality-and-access-haq-index-rating-2016.

133 **more on healthcare per capita:** Gerard F. Anderson, Peter Hussey, Varduhi
Petrosyan, "It's Still The Prices, Stupid: Why The US Spends So Much On
Health Care, And A Tribute To Uwe Reinhardt," *Health Affairs*, January 2019,
healthaffairs.org/doi/10.1377/hlthaff.2018.05144.

133 **higher GDP than the eight countries:** "Richest Countries In The World

2020," World Population Review, worldpopulationreview.com/country-rank ings/richest-countries-in-the-world.

133 **all but dismantled:** Nicholas Kristof, "At a Clinic Threatened by Trump's Rules, She Asks, 'Why Attack Women?'," *The New York Times,* July 27, 2019, nytimes.com/2019/07/27/opinion/sunday/women-health-trump.html.

136 **started keeping a journal:** Ruth Franklin, *Shirley Jackson: A Rather Haunted Life* (New York: Liveright, 2016).

TWELVE: HEALTH TODAY

140 **overtreatment of DCIS:** Peggy Orenstein, "Our Feel-Good War on Breast Cancer," *The New York Times Magazine,* April 25, 2013, nytimes.com/2013/04 /28/magazine/our-feel-good-war-on-breast-cancer.html.

144 **"Everything is tracked, recorded and analyzed":** Matthew Desmond, "In order to understand the brutality of American capitalism, you have to start on the plantation," *The New York Times Magazine,* August 14, 2019, nytimes.com /interactive/2019/08/14/magazine/slavery-capitalism.html.

144 **"Low-road capitalism":** Erik Olin Wright, Joel Rogers, *American Society: How It Really Works* (New York: W. W. Norton, 2011).

144 **list of seventy-one nations:** "Compare your Country," OECD, Employment Protection Legislation, compareyourcountry.org/employment-protection-legis lation.

149 **women who cry at work:** Niels van de Ven, Maartje H. J. Meijs, Ad Vinger-hoets, "What emotional tears convey: Tearful individuals are seen as warmer, but also as less competent," *British Journal of Social Psychology,* Volume 56, Issue 1, March 16, 2017, pp. 146–160, bpspsychub.onlinelibrary.wiley.com /doi/pdf/10.1111/bjso.12162.

THIRTEEN: IN FLAGRANTE DELICTO

152 **before Tinder fully entered:** Jennifer Booton, "Dating app Tinder set to ex-plode to $1 billion," *MarketWatch,* September 5, 2014, marketwatch.com /story/tinder-valuation-to-explode-to-1-billion-2014-09-04.

155 **subsequent release of oxytocin:** Valerie C. Robinson, "Support for the hy-pothesis that sexual breast stimulation is an ancestral practice and a key to understanding women's health," *Medical Hypotheses,* Volume 85, Issue 6, De-cember 2015, pp. 976–985, pubmed.ncbi.nlm.nih.gov/26386486/.

155 **can actually be detrimental:** Ibid.

FOURTEEN: YOU WON THE LOTTERY!

164n **one old study from 1994:** P. Cassoni, A. Sapino, F. Negro, G. Bussolati, "Oxytocin inhibits proliferation of human breast cancer cell lines," *Virchows Archiv,* Volume 425, Issue 5, December 1994, pp. 467–472, pubmed.ncbi.nlm .nih.gov/7850070/.

164n **reduction of the *non-lactating* breast:** Huiping Liu, Christian W. Gruber, Paul F. Alewood, et al., "The oxytocin receptor signalling system and breast cancer: a critical review," *Oncogene*, Volume 39, Issue 37, August 11, 2020, nature.com/articles/s41388-020-01415-8.

CHAPTER FIFTEEN: INWOOD

172 **PVCs—premature ventricular contractions:** "Premature ventricular contractions (PVCs)," Mayo Clinic, mayoclinic.org/diseases-conditions/premature -ventricular-contractions/symptoms-causes/syc-20376757.

174 **"last affordable neighborhood":** Matthew Haag, "It's Manhattan's Last Affordable Neighborhood. But for How Long?," *The New York Times*, September 27, 2019, nytimes.com/2019/09/27/nyregion/inwood-manhattan-affordable -housing.html.

178 **"powerfully intersects with sexism":** Jessica Bennett, "I Am (an Older) Woman. Hear Me Roar," *The New York Times*, January 8, 2019, nytimes.com /2019/01/08/style/women-age-glenn-close.html.

185 **Irene Zisblatt, née Zegelstein:** Irene Zisblatt, *The Fifth Diamond* (UK: Ithaca Press, 2008).

SIXTEEN: MONEY

198 **rise by more than 25 percent:** Rupert Neate, "Billionaires' wealth rises to $10.2 trillion amid Covid crisis," *The Guardian*, October 6, 2020, theguardian .com/business/2020/oct/07/covid-19-crisis-boosts-the-fortunes-of-worlds -billionaires.

198 **"impossible to spend":** Ibid.

198 **he brags about these wages:** Jeff Bezos, "2019 Letter to Shareholders," About Amazon, April 16, 2020, aboutamazon.com/news/company-news/2019-letter -to-shareholders.

199 **faces a loss of 41 percent:** United States Government Accountability Office, "Retirement Security: Women Still Face Challenges," Highlights of GAO-12-699, a report to the Chairman, Special Committee on Aging, U.S. Senate, July 2012, aging.senate.gov/imo/media/doc/hr250gao.pdf.

201 **bought the film rights:** Deborah Copaken, "The Last Time She Saw Paris: In her twenties, she was an intrepid war photographer. Now Deborah Copaken Kogan's memoir, *Shutterbabe*, is being made into a movie by *Sex and the City*'s Darren Star. So she went to France to walk him through her snappy past . . . ," *O, The Oprah Magazine*, August 2002.

202 **"below 200 percent of poverty":** "An Overview of America's Working Poor," PolicyLink, policylink.org/data-in-action/overview-america-working-poor.

SEVENTEEN: AT THE STILL POINT OF THE TURNING WORLD

209 **"At the still point":** T.S. Eliot, "Burnt Norton," *Collected Poems, 1909-1962* (New York: Harcourt, 1991).

209 **"psychological and physical disintegration":** Debra Umberson, Jennifer Karas Montez, "Social Relationships and Health: A Flashpoint for Health Policy," *Journal of Health and Social Behavior*, August 4, 2011, ncbi.nlm.nih .gov/pmc/articles/PMC3150158/.

210 **"emotionally sustaining qualities"**: Ibid.

211 **dating app called Hinge**: Kristin Tice Studeman, "Hinge, a Dating App, Introduces Friends of Friends," *The New York Times*, March 28, 2014, nytimes.com /2014/03/30/fashion/hinge-a-dating-app-introduces-friends-of-friends.html.

213 **"giant ten-foot vagina"**: Alison Herman, "Kara Walker Knew People Would Take Dumb Selfies With 'A Subtlety,' and That Shouldn't Surprise Us," *Flavorwire*, October 14, 2014, flavorwire.com/482585/kara-walker-knew-people -would-take-dumb-selfies-with-a-subtlety-and-that-shouldnt-surprise-us.

EIGHTEEN: BAD JUDGMENT

216 *Forbes* **asks to reprint**: Deborah Copaken, "Harvard Grad, 48, Loses Job And Insurance, Gets Rejected By Container Store," *Forbes*, November 4, 2014, forbes.com/sites/nextavenue/2014/11/04/harvard-grad-48-loses-job-and -insurance-gets-rejected-by-container-store/?sh=10ffe0c4132a.

216 **TV comes calling**: Nicole Duignan, "Good enough for an Emmy, but not The Container Store," *Yahoo! Finance*, November 7, 2014, finance.yahoo.com/news /bestselling-author—rejected—by-the-container-store-201526323.html.

216 **MIT's living wage calculator**: "Living Wage Calculation for New York-Newark-Jersey City, NY," Massachusetts Institute of Technology, livingwage .mit.edu/metros/35620.

218 **"It's easy to imagine"**: KJ Dell'Antonia, "Writer, Rejected for a Retail Job, Is Embraced and Vilified on Facebook," *The New York Times*, November 3, 2014, parenting.blogs.nytimes.com/2014/11/03/writer-rejected-for-a-retail-job-is -embraced-and-vilified-on-facebook/.

219 **"'Maybe no one liked her'"**: "An ex-photojournalist who brags about screwing half the foreign press corps is no feminist hero—she's just an opportunist," Janet Reitman, "Bang-bang girl," *Salon*, January 30, 2001, salon.com/2001/01 /29/shutterbabe/.

219 **countless other examples**: Rebecca Johnson, "Shutterbabe: A photojournalist chronicles love and death around the globe," *Talk*, January 2001; "Could there possibly be something about [Copaken] that invites these abuses?" Deborah Solomon, "Shooting star," *Women's Review of Books*, April 2001.

221 **"Sexism wears a lab coat"**: Kate Manne, *Down Girl: The Logic of Misogyny* (Oxford University Press, 2017).

221 **"do you identify with her"**: Dell'Antonia, "Writer, Rejected."

222 **hurting us, our kids**: Ayelet Waldman, "Truly, Madly, Guiltily," *The New York Times*, March 27, 2005, nytimes.com/2005/03/27/fashion/truly-madly-guiltily .html.

223 **Seventy-one out of ninety-four**: Kieran Snyder, "The abrasiveness trap: High-achieving men and women are described differently in reviews," *Fortune*, August 26, 2014, fortune.com/2014/08/26/performance-review-gender-bias/.

223 **five times as many**: Emily Khazan, Jesse Brooks Borden, Steve Johnson, Laura Greenshaw, "Examining Gender Bias in Student Evaluations of Teaching for Graduate Teaching Assistants," *North American Colleges and Teachers of Agriculture Journal*, Volume 64, November 2019–October 2020, researchgate.net

/publication/345178456_Examining_Gender_Bias_in_Student_Evaluations
_of_Teaching_for_Graduate_Teaching_Assistants.

NINETEEN: UNREQUITED

228 **Unrequited, one might:** Lisa A. Phillips, *Unrequited: Women and Romantic Obsession* (New York: HarperCollins, 2015).

228 **"She was needy":** Deborah Copaken, "Book review: 'Unrequited: Women and Romantic Obsession,' by Lisa A. Phillips," *The Washington Post*, February 6, 2015, washingtonpost.com/opinions/book-review-unrequited-women -and-romantic-obsession-by-lisa-a-phillips/2015/02/05/2294c112-8091-11e4 -81fd-8c4814dfa9d7_story.html.

TWENTY: THE CHURCH FOR WAYWARD HEARTS

240 **"You up for being":** Deborah Copaken, "After the Divorce: Returning to Paris, the Place We Fell In Love," *Glamour*, November 30, 2015, glamour .com/story/divorce-trip.

242 **launch of Rebecca Solnit's:** Rebecca Solnit, *Men Explain Things to Me* (Chicago: Haymarket Books, 2014).

TWENTY-ONE: LUNCH WITH KEN

243 **"The assumption is that":** Clyde W. Summers, "Employment At Will in the United States: The Divine Right of Employers," University of Pennsylvania *Journal of Business Law*, Volume 3, Issue 1, 2000, pp. 65–86, law.upenn.edu/jour nals/jbl/articles/volume3/issue1/Summers3U.Pa.J.Lab.&Emp.L.65(2000).pdf.

244 **"the monarchy still survives":** Ibid.

252 **full Amanda Palmer:** Amanda Palmer, "The art of asking," TED talk, February 2013, ted.com/talks/amanda_palmer_the_art_of_asking.

TWENTY-TWO: KIND OF A TINDER DATE AND KIND OF NOT

258 **publicly slut-shamed again:** Deborah Copaken, "How to Write an Anti-Feminist Profile in Six Easy Steps," *Medium*, February 23, 2016, medium.com/athena -talks/how-to-write-an-anti-feminist-profile-in-six-easy-steps-14ca9b885f39.

259 **"viewed as internalized oppression":** Elizabeth A. Armstrong, Laura T. Hamilton, Elizabeth M. Armstrong, J. Lotus Seeley, "'Good Girls': Gender, Social Class, and Slut Discourse on Campus," *Social Psychology Quarterly*, Volume 77, Issue 2, 2014, pp. 100–122, asanet.org/sites/default/files/savvy/journals/SPQ /Jun14SPQFeature.pdf?hc_location=ufi.

259 **"High-status women":** Ibid.

265 **Two in five:** "The 'Loneliness Epidemic'," Health Resources & Services Administration, last reviewed January 2019, hrsa.gov/enews/past-issues/2019/january-17 /loneliness-epidemic.

265 **as lethal as smoking:** Ibid.

265 **Alzheimer's disease:** Sarvada Chandra Tiwari, "Loneliness: A disease?," *Indian Journal of Psychiatry*, Volume 55, Issue 4, October–December 2013, pp. 320–322, ncbi.nlm.nih.gov/pmc/articles/PMC3890922/.

TWENTY-THREE: DURKHEIM

268 **"expressly mislead" creditors:** Michelle Singletary, "Consumer agency's $25 million settlement with Freedom Debt Relief shows the risks of such programs," *The Washington Post*, July 12, 2019, washingtonpost.com/business/get-there/consumer-agency-reaches-25-million-settlement-with-freedom-debt-relief/2019/07/11/cce920a4-a3f0-11e9-b8c8-75dae2607e60_story.html.

270 **my first column:** Deborah Copaken, "The Best Part of Middle Age: Letting Go of Shame," *Observer*, July 16, 2015, observer.com/2015/07/the-best-part-of-middle-age-letting-go-of-shame/.

270 **vagaries of dating:** Deborah Copaken, "Uncharted Territory: A Mother of Three Navigates the World of the Newly Single," *Observer*, September 18, 2015, observer.com/2015/09/uncharted-territory-a-mother-of-three-navigates-the-world-of-the-newly-single/.

TWENTY-FOUR: PUBLIC RELATIONS

281 **several years earlier:** Deborah Copaken, "La Vie En Rose, the Takeout Version," *The New York Times*, April 15, 2007, nytimes.com/2007/04/15/fashion/15love.html.

281 **"When Cupid Is":** Deborah Copaken, "When Cupid Is a Prying Journalist," *The New York Times*, November 26, 2015, nytimes.com/2015/11/29/style/modern-love-when-cupid-is-a-prying-journalist.html.

282 **illness whose primary risk factor:** Anne G. Wheaton, PhD; Yong Liu, MD; Janet B. Croft, PhD; et al., "Chronic Obstructive Pulmonary Disease and Smoking Status—United States, 2017," *Morbidity and Mortality Weekly Report*, June 21, 2019, cdc.gov/mmwr/volumes/68/wr/mm6824a1.htm.

TWENTY-FIVE: PRIVATE RELATIONS

285 **"desk-clerk law":** Elizabeth F. Emens, "Changing Name Changing: Framing Rules and the Future of Marital Names," *University of Chicago Law Review*, Volume 74, Issue 3, Summer 2007, papers.ssrn.com/sol3/papers.cfm?abstract_id=940449.

287 **"All the Young Dudes":** Deborah Copaken, "All the Young Dudes," *Observer*, June 2, 2016, observer.com/2016/06/all-the-young-dudes/.

TWENTY-SIX: ON-RAMP

292 **74 percent of those:** Sylvia Ann Hewlett, Carolyn Buck Luce, "Off-Ramps and On-Ramps: Keeping Talented Women on the Road to Success," *Harvard Business Review*, March 2005, hbr.org/2005/03/off-ramps-and-on-ramps-keeping-talented-women-on-the-road-to-success.

292 **"Off-ramps are around":** Ibid.

TWENTY-SEVEN: YOUNGER

297 **Ann Bauer, in an essay:** Ann Bauer, "'Sponsored' by my husband: Why it's a problem that writers never talk about where their money comes from," *Salon*,

January 25, 2015, salon.com/control/2015/01/25/sponsored_by_my_husband
_why_its_a_problem_that_writers_never_talk_about_where_their_money
_comes_from/.

TWENTY-EIGHT: ENFP

301 **"an elaborate Chinese fortune cookie"**: Robert Hogan, *Personality and the Fate of Organizations* (New York: Psychology Press, 2015).

301 **"no scientific basis whatsoever"**: Annie Murphy Paul, *The Cult of Personality Testing: How Personality Tests Are Leading Us to Miseducate Our Children, Mismanage Our Companies, and Misunderstand Ourselves* (New York: Free Press, 2005).

304 **sue Facebook for age discrimination**: Wendy Lee, "Former Facebook employee sues, says he faced age discrimination," *San Francisco Chronicle*, September 23, 2017, sfchronicle.com/business/article/Former-Facebook-employee-sues-claims-he-faced-12222267.php.

304 **"Young people are just smarter"**: Steven Kotler, "Is Silicon Valley Ageist Or Just Smart?," *Forbes*, February 14, 2015, forbes.com/sites/stevenkotler/2015/02/14/is-silicon-valley-ageist-or-just-smart/.

305 **published an op-ed**: Meg Halverson, "360 Reviews Often Lead to Cruel, Not Constructive, Criticism," *The New York Times*, February 26, 2016, nytimes.com/2016/02/28/jobs/360-reviews-often-lead-to-cruel-not-constructive-criticism.html.

305 **"at best, a waste"**: Marcus Buckingham, "The Fatal Flaw with 360 Surveys," *Harvard Business Review*, October 17, 2011, hbr.org/2011/10/the-fatal-flaw-with-360-survey.

THIRTY: BLOODY MOTHER'S DAY

315 **listed at $28.5 million**: "30 E 85th St #PH30A, New York, NY 10028," Zillow, zillow.com/homedetails/30-E-85th-St-PH30A-New-York-NY-10028/2082639466_zpid/.

316 **80 percent of all cervical cancers**: "Should I get the HPV vaccine?," Planned Parenthood, plannedparenthood.org/learn/stds-hiv-safer-sex/hpv/should-i-get-hpv-vaccine.

THIRTY-ONE: HOSPITALS ARE NOT MY THING

323 **"deaths of despair"**: Anne Case, Sir Angus Deaton, "Mortality and morbidity in the 21st century," *Brookings Papers on Economic Activity*, Spring 2017, ncbi.nlm.nih.gov/pmc/articles/PMC5640267/.

323 **"a marked increase"**: Anne Case, Sir Angus Deaton, "Rising morbidity and mortality in midlife among white non-Hispanic Americans in the 21st century," *PNAS*, Volume 112, Issue 49, December 8, 2015, pnas.org/content/112/49/15078.

329 **wasn't even a clinical diagnosis**: Jean Endicott, "History, evolution, and diagnosis of premenstrual dysphoric disorder," *The Journal of Clinical Psychiatry*, 2000, pubmed.ncbi.nlm.nih.gov/11041378/.

THIRTY-TWO: MY DAY IN COURT (MY AFTERNOON IN HOSPITAL)

333 **pro se divorce:** Deborah Copaken, "The DIY Divorce: How I got divorced without hiring a lawyer," *The Atlantic*, February 12, 2019, theatlantic.com /family/archive/2019/02/how-i-got-divorced-without-hiring-lawyer/582508/.

334 **"potted plant" parent:** Leanne Lester, Jacinth Watson, Stacey Waters, Donna Cross, "The Association of Fly-in Fly-out Employment, Family Connectedness, Parental Presence and Adolescent Wellbeing," *Journal of Child and Family Studies*, Volume 25, 2016, link.springer.com/article/10.1007/s10826-016-0512 -8; Suniya S. Luthar, Shawn J. Latendresse, "Comparable 'risks' at the socioeco- nomic status extremes: Preadolescents' perceptions of parenting," *Development and Psychopathology*, Volume 17, Issue 1, Winter 2005, pp. 207–230, ncbi .nlm.nih.gov/pmc/articles/PMC4373649/; Lisa Damour, "What Do Teenagers Want? Potted Plant Parents," *The New York Times*, December 14, 2016, nytimes .com/2016/12/14/well/family/what-do-teenagers-want-potted-plant-parents .html.

334 **still earn 80.5 cents:** National Committee on Pay Equity fact sheet, pay-equity .org/info-time.html.

THIRTY-THREE: EMPTY BRAIN

348 **the resulting stories:** Deborah Copaken, "How One Woman Found Healing in the Himalayas," Oprah.com, November 29, 2017, oprah.com/inspiration /deborah-copaken-how-one-woman-found-healing-in-the-himalayas; Deborah Copaken, "I fled to Nepal to heal after a near-death experience, and found it to be surprisingly spiritual," *Business Insider*, March 13, 2018, insider.com /spiritual-healing-trip-to-kathmandu-nepal-2018-3.

354 **any number beyond two:** Peter Schumer, "When did humans first learn to count?," *The Conversation*, June 5, 2018, theconversation.com/when-did -humans-first-learn-to-count-97511.

356 **Weinstein's multiple assaults:** Jodi Kantor and Megan Twohey, "Harvey Wein- stein Paid Off Sexual Harassment Accusers for Decades," *The New York Times*, October 5, 2017, nytimes.com/2017/10/05/us/harvey-weinstein-harassment -allegations.html.

358 **"Vaginal cuff dehiscence":** Myung Ji Kim, Seongmin Kim, Hyo Sook Bae, et al., "Evaluation of risk factors of vaginal cuff dehiscence after hysterectomy," *Obstetrics & Gynecology Science*, Volume 57, Issue 2, March 2014, pp. 136– 143, ncbi.nlm.nih.gov/pmc/articles/PMC3965697/.

358 **"Despite being rare":** Yacine Ben Safta, Montassar Ghalleb, Aymen Baccari, et al., "Vaginal cuff dehiscence and evisceration 11 years after a radical hyster- ectomy: A case report," *International Journal of Surgery Case Reports*, October 28, 2017, ncbi.nlm.nih.gov/pmc/articles/PMC5686219/pdf/main.pdf.

358 **"between 0% and 7.5%":** Kim, et al., "Evaluation of risk factors."

359 **600,000 hysterectomies:** "Hysterectomy," National Women's Health Net- work, nwhn.org/hysterectomy/.

359 **incidence of erectile dysfunction:** "Sexual dysfunction after prostate surgery

is more common than previously reported, says Hutchinson Center study," Fred Hutch, January 18, 2000, fredhutch.org/en/news/releases/2000/01/JAMA prostatectomy.html.

359 **"would be quite costly"**: Beth Cronin, Vivian W. Sung, Kristen A. Matteson, "Vaginal cuff dehiscence: risk factors and management," *American Journal of Obstetrics & Gynecology*, April 2012, ajog.org/article/S0002-9378(11)01077-5 /pdf.

360 **"Narrative medicine"**: Rita Charon, MD, PhD, "Narrative Medicine: A Model for Empathy, Reflection, Profession, and Trust," *Journal of the American Medical Association*, October 17, 2001, jamanetwork.com/journals/jama /fullarticle/194300.

361 **effects of Tibetan singing bowl**: Tamara L. Goldsby, Michael E. Goldsby, et al., "Effects of Singing Bowl Sound Meditation on Mood, Tension, and Well-being: An Observational Study," *Journal of Evidence-Based Complementary & Alternative Medicine*, August 15, 2016, ncbi.nlm.nih.gov/pmc/articles /PMC5871151/pdf/10.1177_2156587216668109.pdf.

361 **"Rituals trigger"**: Ted Kaptchuk, "Placebo studies and ritual theory: a comparative analysis of Navajo, acupuncture and biomedical healing," *Philosophical transactions of the Royal Society of London*, June 27, 2011, ncbi.nlm.nih .gov/pmc/articles/PMC3130398/.

THIRTY-FOUR: #METOO

370 **hits the publish button**: Deborah Copaken, "How to Lose Your Job From Sexual Harassment in 33 Easy Steps," *The Atlantic*, March 9, 2018, theatlantic.com /entertainment/archive/2018/03/how-to-lose-your-job-from-sexual-harassment -in-33-easy-steps/555197/.

372 **funded in part by Yuri Milner**: Jesse Drucker, "Kremlin Cash Behind Billionaire's Twitter and Facebook Investments," *The New York Times*, November 5, 2017, nytimes.com/2017/11/05/world/yuri-milner-facebook-twitter-russia.html.

372 **necessarily ethical**: Jon Swaine, "Company part-owned by Jared Kushner got $90m from unknown offshore investors since 2017," *The Guardian*, June 10, 2019, theguardian.com/us-news/2019/jun/10/jared-kushner-real-estate-cadre -goldman-sachs.

373 **Keith Kelly's byline**: Keith J. Kelly, "Ex-Observer editor joked about my breasts: writer," *New York Post*, March 12, 2018, nypost.com/2018/03/12/ex -observer-editor-joked-about-my-breasts-writer/.

373 **disembodied man**: Keith J. Kelly, "Observer fashion editor denies knowing about freelancer's sex harassment claims," *New York Post*, March 13, 2018, nypost.com/2018/03/13/observer-editor-denies-knowing-about-freelancers-sex -harassment-claims/.

377 **"Concerning Ms. Copaken's"**: Jesse Drucker, "The Trump Administration Considers an Old Friend: Ken Kurson," *The New York Times*, May 11, 2018, nytimes.com/2018/05/11/business/media/ken-kurson-trump-administration .html.

379 **Jesse's second story:** Jesse Drucker, Emily Steel, Danny Hakim, "A Kushner Ally Was Up for a Federal Post. Then the F.B.I. Began Digging," *The New York Times*, July 26, 2018, nytimes.com/2018/07/26/business/ken-kurson-jared-kushner.html.

THIRTY-FIVE: COGNITIVE HEALTH

383 **FINGER study in Finland:** Tiia Ngandu, Jenni Lehtisalo, Alina Solomon, et al., "A 2 year multidomain intervention of diet, exercise, cognitive training, and vascular risk monitoring versus control to prevent cognitive decline in at-risk elderly people (FINGER): a randomised controlled trial," *The Lancet*, March 11, 2005, thelancet.com/journals/lancet/article/PIIS0140-6736(15)60461-5/fulltext.

385 **Divorcing without a lawyer:** Copaken, "The DIY Divorce."

386 **it costs $1.30:** "Surprising divorce costs from around the world revealed," *Love Money*, January 14, 2019, lovemoney.com/gallerylist/80925/surprising-divorce-costs-from-around-the-world-revealed.

386 **publish it on *Medium*:** Deborah Copaken, "Exploring the Link Between Menopause and Alzheimer's," *Medium*, May 30, 2019, medium.com/neurotrack/menopause-and-alzheimers-1c455f29fe16.

388 **"Have you looked at your brain scan?":** Maria Shriver, "Neuroscientist studies possible link between Alzheimer's and menopause," *Today*, November 1, 2019, today.com/video/neuroscientist-studies-possible-link-between-alzheimer-s-and-menopause-72570437699.

388 **study had so many flaws:** James H. Clark, "A critique of Women's Health Initiative Studies (2002-2006)," *NURSA (Nuclear Receptor Signaling)*, October 30, 2006, ncbi.nlm.nih.gov/pmc/articles/PMC1630688/pdf/nrs04023000.pdf.

388 **women like me without uteri:** Garnet L. Anderson, Rowan T. Chlebowski, Aaron K. Aragaki, et al., "Conjugated equine oestrogen and breast cancer incidence and mortality in postmenopausal women with hysterectomy: extended follow-up of the Women's Health Initiative randomised placebo-controlled trial," *The Lancet*, March 7, 2012, thelancet.com/journals/lanonc/article/PIIS1470-2045(12)70075-X/fulltext.

388 **only 20 percent of ob-gyn:** Jennifer Wolff, "What Doctors Don't Know About Menopause," *AARP*, August/September 2018, aarp.org/health/conditions-treatments/info-2018/menopause-symptoms-doctors-relief-treatment.html.

389 **reaching out to me over Twitter:** Rachel S. Rubin, MD, @rachelsrubin1, May 3, 2019, twitter.com/rachelsrubin1/status/1124324324251459585?s=20.

THIRTY-SIX: FUCK YOUR DUMB FIRE

392 **Many ladies, moving:** Florence Hartley, *The Ladies' Book of Etiquette, and Manual of Politeness: A Complete Hand Book for the Use of the Lady in Polite Society* (Boston: G.W. Cottrell, 1860), Chapter XVI, gutenberg.org/files/35123/35123-h/35123-h.htm#CHPTR_XVI.

393 **a letter written to:** Deborah Copaken, "The Letter I Wrote My Rapist," September 18, 2018, deborahcopaken.com/blog/2018/9/23/the-letter-i-wrote-to-my-rapist.

396 **rapist apology story:** Deborah Copaken, "My Rapist Apologized," *The Atlantic*, September 21, 2018, theatlantic.com/ideas/archive/2018/09/copaken-kavanaugh/571042/.

398 **Katherine Schwarzenegger reaches out:** Katherine Schwarzenegger Pratt, *The Gift of Forgiveness: Inspiring Stories from Those Who Have Overcome the Unforgivable* (New York: Pamela Dorman Books, 2020).

THIRTY-SEVEN: MAKE A WISH

404 **"Cancel everything!":** Yascha Mounk, "Cancel Everything," *The Atlantic*, March 10, 2020, theatlantic.com/ideas/archive/2020/03/coronavirus-cancel-everything/607675/.

405 **major risk factors:** Rina Marie Doctor, "Women Love High Heels But It Causes Morton's Neuroma And That's Not Wow: What To Know," *Tech Times*, June 22, 2015, techtimes.com/articles/62389/20150622/women-love-high-heels-but-it-causes-mortons-neuroma-and-thats-not-wow-what-to-know.htm.

410 **"Star studied French":** Alexis Soloski, "Darren Star Finds Sex in Another City With 'Emily in Paris': What do women want? Star, who created 'Sex and the City' and 'Younger,' seems to know," *The New York Times*, October 2, 2020, nytimes.com/2020/10/02/arts/television/darren-star-emily-in-paris.html.

410 **Actress Mira Sorvino:** Molly Redden, "Peter Jackson: I blacklisted Ashley Judd and Mira Sorvino under pressure from Weinstein," *The Guardian*, December 16, 2017, theguardian.com/film/2017/dec/15/peter-jackson-harvey-weinstein-ashley-judd-mira-sorvino.

411 **lost their twenty-three-year-old daughter:** Deborah Copaken, "Finding a Way Through an Unspeakable Loss," *The Atlantic*, December 28, 2018, theatlantic.com/family/archive/2018/12/finding-way-through-unspeakable-loss/579130/.

413 **roughly 10,000:** Derek Watkins, Josh Holder, James Glanz, et al., "How the Virus Won," *The New York Times*, June 24, 2020, nytimes.com/interactive/2020/us/coronavirus-spread.html.

413n **women were prescribed the wrong antibiotic:** Anne Mobley Butler, "Most Women Receive Inappropriate Treatment for Urinary Tract Infections," *Infection Control & Hospital Epidemiology*, February 24, 2021, https://www.shea-online.org/index.php/journal-news/press-room/press-release-archives/899-most-women-receive-inappropriate-treatment-for-urinary-tract-infections.

415 **estrogen loss and Alzheimer's:** Deborah Copaken, "What Menopause Does to Women's Brains," *The Atlantic*, November 8, 2019, theatlantic.com/health/archive/2019/11/menopause-alzheimers/601642/.

415 **Even migraines:** "Headaches and hormones: What's the connection?," Mayo Clinic, December 10, 2020, mayoclinic.org/diseases-conditions/chronic-daily-headaches/in-depth/headaches/art-20046729.

415 **"health-care gaslit":** Ashley Fetters, "The Doctor Doesn't Listen to Her. But the

Media Is Starting To," *The Atlantic*, August 10, 2018, theatlantic.com/family /archive/2018/08/womens-health-care-gaslighting/567149/.

415–416 **calcitonin gene-related peptide (CGRP):** "Are the new migraine medications working?" Harvard Health Letter, October 2019, health.harvard.edu /diseases-and-conditions/are-the-new-migraine-medications-working.

416 **three times more prevalent:** "Migraine is an extraordinarily prevalent neurological disease, affecting 39 million men, women and children in the U.S. and 1 billion worldwide," Migraine Research Foundation, migraineresearchfoun dation.org/about-migraine/migraine-facts/.

416 **Recent research suggests:** Nu Cindy Chai, B. Lee Peterlin, Anne H. Calhoun, "Migraine and estrogen," *Current Opinion in Neurology*, July 17, 2014, ncbi.nlm.nih.gov/pmc/articles/PMC4102139/.

416 **33 percent more often:** Neil Sherman, "Women See Doctors More than Men," *HealthDay*, July 27, 2001, consumer.healthday.com/public-health-information -30/centers-for-disease-control-news-120/women-see-doctors-more-than-men -400589.html.

416 **76 percent of all doctors:** Jeffrey A. Singer, "Women Should Not Have to Visit a Doctor for Birth Control," *Time*, January 14, 2016, time.com/4180612/birth -control-prescriptions/.

416 **more than 100 countries:** "Global Oral Contraceptive Availability," The Oral Contraceptives (OCs) Over-the-Counter (OTC) Working Group, ocsotc.org /world-map.

416 **fourteen times more likely:** Raisa O Platte, Krystal Reynolds, "Why are urinary tract infections (UTIs) more common in women than in men?" Medscape, October 8, 2019, medscape.com/answers/452604-54622/why-are-urinary-tract -infections-utis-more-common-in-women-than-in-men.

417 **story about coming down:** Deborah Copaken, "My Whole Household Has COVID-19," *The Atlantic*, March 27, 2020, theatlantic.com/family/archive /2020/03/my-whole-household-has-covid-19/608902/.

417 **shared custody under quarantine:** Deborah Copaken, "How Are Parents Supposed to Deal With Joint Custody Right Now?," *The Atlantic*, April 8, 2020, theatlantic.com/family/archive/2020/04/navigating-joint-custody-under -coronavirus-quarantine/609676/.

417 **put down my dog:** Deborah Copaken, "On Top of Everything Else, My Dog Died," *The Atlantic*, April 22, 2020, theatlantic.com/family/archive/2020/04 /when-your-dog-dies-during-pandemic/610339/.

419 **"getting fired over Zoom":** Deborah Copaken, "I Got Fired Over Zoom," May 12, 2020, theatlantic.com/business/archive/2020/05/fired-zoom-layoffs -coronavirus/611509/.

THIRTY-EIGHT: THE COST OF OXYGEN

423 **More than 10,000:** Michael Sainato, "'They set us up': US police arrested over 10,000 protesters, many non-violent," *The Guardian*, June 8, 2020, theguard ian.com/us-news/2020/jun/08/george-floyd-killing-police-arrest-non-violent -protesters.

THIRTY-NINE: FIREWORKS REDUX

431 **when Trump derided:** Philip Rucker, "Trump says Fox's Megyn Kelly had 'blood coming out of her wherever'," *The Washington Post*, August 8, 2015, washingtonpost.com/news/post-politics/wp/2015/08/07/trump-says-foxs -megyn-kelly-had-blood-coming-out-of-her-wherever/.

431 **"Avoid, at all times":** Hartley, *The Ladies' Book of Etiquette*, Chapter I, guten berg.org/files/35123/35123-h/35123-h.htm#CHPTR_I.

434 **arrested and charged:** Nicole Hong, Jesse Drucker, "Trump Family Ally Is Arrested on Cyberstalking Charge," *The New York Times*, October 23, 2020, nytimes.com/2020/10/23/nyregion/ken-kurson-arrest-cyberstalking.html.

ABOUT THE AUTHOR

DEBORAH COPAKEN is *The New York Times* bestselling author of several books, including *Shutterbabe, The Red Book,* and *Between Here and April.* A contributing writer at *The Atlantic,* she was also a TV writer on *Emily in Paris,* a performer (The Moth, etc.), and an Emmy Award–winning news producer and photojournalist. Her photographs have appeared in *Time, Newsweek,* and *The New York Times.* Her writing has appeared in *The New Yorker, The New York Times, The Guardian, The Financial Times, Observer, The Wall Street Journal, The Nation, Slate, O, the Oprah Magazine,* and *Paris Match,* among other publications. Her column "When Cupid Is a Prying Journalist" was adapted for the *Modern Love* streaming series. She lives in Brooklyn with her family.

deborahcopaken.com
Twitter: @dcopaken